OKU

Orthopaedic Knowledge Update:

Musculoskeletal Infection

AAOS

AMERICAN ACADEMY OF
ORTHOPAEDIC SURGEONS

OKU

Orthopaedic
Knowledge
Update:

Musculoskeletal Infection

EDITORS
George Cierny III, MD
Alex C. McLaren, MD
Montri D. Wongworawat, MD

Developed by the
Musculoskeletal Infection Society

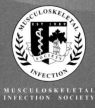

MUSCULOSKELETAL
INFECTION SOCIETY

AAOS
AMERICAN ACADEMY OF
ORTHOPAEDIC SURGEONS

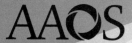

AMERICAN ACADEMY OF ORTHOPAEDIC SURGEONS

The material presented in **Orthopaedic Knowledge Update: Musculoskeletal Infection** has been made available by the American Academy of Orthopaedic Surgeons for educational purposes only. This material is not intended to present the only, or necessarily best, methods or procedures for the medical situations discussed, but rather is intended to represent an approach, view, statement, or opinion of the author(s) or producer(s), which may be helpful to others who face similar situations.

Some drugs or medical devices demonstrated in Academy courses or described in Academy print or electronic publications have not been cleared by the Food and Drug Administration (FDA) or have been cleared for specific uses only. The FDA has stated that it is the responsibility of the physician to determine the FDA clearance status of each drug or device he or she wishes to use in clinical practice.

Furthermore, any statements about commercial products are solely the opinion(s) of the author(s) and do not represent an Academy endorsement or evaluation of these products. These statements may not be used in advertising or for any commercial purpose.

Published 2009 by the
American Academy of Orthopaedic Surgeons
6300 North River Road
Rosemont, IL 60018

Copyright 2009
by the American Academy of Orthopaedic Surgeons

ISBN 978-0-89203-573-1
Printed in the USA

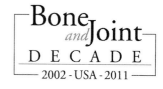

Acknowledgments

Orthopaedic Knowledge Update: Musculoskeletal Infection Editorial Board

George Cierny III, MD
REOrthopaedics, Inc.
San Diego, California

John L. Esterhai Jr, MD
Professor of Orthopaedic Surgery
University of Pennsylvania School of Medicine
Chief of Orthopaedics
Philadelphia Veterans Administration Medical Center
Philadelphia, Pennsylvania

Alex C. McLaren, MD
Assistant Professor of Clinical Orthopaedic Surgery
University of Arizona College of Medicine
Program Director, Banner Good Samaritan Orthopaedic Residency
Phoenix, Arizona

Robin Patel, MD
Professor of Medicine
Professor of Microbiology
Division of Clinical Microbiology
Mayo Clinic
Rochester, Minnesota

Michael J. Patzakis, MD
Professor and Chair
Vincent and Julia Meyer Chair
Department of Orthopaedic Surgery
Keck School of Medicine
University of Southern California
Los Angeles, California

Montri Daniel Wongworawat, MD
Associate Professor
Department of Orthopaedic Surgery
Loma Linda University
Loma Linda, California

Musculoskeletal Infection Society Executive Board, 2008-2009

John L. Esterhai Jr, MD
President

Charalampos G. Zalavras, MD, PhD
Vice President

Elli Berbari, MD
Secretary-Treasurer

Arvind Nana, MD
Member at Large

Douglas R. Osmon, MD
First Past President

George Cierny III, MD
Second Past President

Contributors

Abass Alavi, MD
Professor of Radiology
Director of Research Education
Hospital of the University of Pennsylvania
Philadelphia, Pennsylvania

Jason H. Calhoun, MD, FACS
Frank J. Kloenne Chair in Orthopaedic Surgery
Professor and Chair, Department of
  Orthopaedics
The Ohio State University Medical Center
Columbus, Ohio

J. Robert Cantey, MD
Professor
Division of Infectious Diseases
Medical University of South Carolina
Charleston, South Carolina

George Cierny III, MD
REOrthopaedics, Inc.
San Diego, California

John W. Costerton, PhD, FRCS
Director, Center for Biofilms
School of Dentistry
University of Southern California
Los Angeles, California

Carl A. Deirmengian, MD
Clinical Assistant Professor of Orthopaedic
  Surgery
University of Pennsylvania School of Medicine
Philadelphia, Pennsylvania

Jose L. Del Pozo, MD, PhD
Division of Infectious Disease
Department of Medicine
Mayo Clinic College of Medicine
Rochester, Minnesota

Doreen DiPasquale, MD
REOrthopaedics, Inc.
San Diego, California

Frank J. Eismont, MD
Professor and Chair
Department of Orthopaedics
University of Miami Miller School of Medicine
Miami, Florida

John L. Esterhai Jr, MD
Professor of Orthopaedic Surgery
University of Pennsylvania School of Medicine
Chief of Orthopaedics
Philadelphia Veterans Administration Medical
  Center
Philadelphia, Pennsylvania

J. Timothy Feltis, MD, FRCPC
Chief of Laboratory Medicine
The Credit Valley Hospital
Mississauga, Ontario, Canada

Felipe N. Gutierrez, MD, MPH
Director, Antimicrobial Management Team
Division of Infectious Diseases
Banner Good Samaritan Medical Center
Phoenix, Arizona

Arlen D. Hanssen, MD
Professor of Orthopaedic Surgery
Mayo Clinic
Rochester, Minnesota

Jack L. LeFrock, MD
Private Practice
Sarasota, Florida

Benjamin A. Lipsky, MD, FIDSA, FACP
Professor of Medicine
University of Washington
Director of Primary Care
VA Puget Sound Health Care System
Seattle, Washington

M.M. Manring, PhD
Research Assistant Professor
Department of Orthopaedic Surgery
University of Missouri, Columbia
Columbia, Missouri

Camelia E. Marculescu, MD, MSCR
Assistant Professor of Medicine
Division of Infectious Diseases
Medical University of South Carolina
Charleston, South Carolina

Mary Martin, PharmD
Infectious Disease Clinical Manager
Associate Director, Antimicrobial Management
  Team
Banner Good Samaritan Medical Center
Phoenix, Arizona

Alex C. McLaren, MD
Assistant Professor of Clinical Orthopaedic
  Surgery
University of Arizona College of Medicine
Program Director, Banner Good Samaritan
  Orthopaedic Residency
Phoenix, Arizona

Ryan McLemore, PhD
Orthopaedic Research Associate
Banner Orthopaedic Residency
Banner Good Samaritan Hospital
Phoenix, Arizona

William B. Morrison, MD
Associate Professor of Radiology
Director, Musculoskeletal Imaging
Department of Radiology
Thomas Jefferson Hospital
Philadelphia, Pennsylvania

Douglas R. Osmon, MD, MPH
Associate Professor of Medicine
Division of Infectious Diseases
Department of Internal Medicine
Mayo Clinic College of Medicine
Rochester, Minnesota

Javad Parvizi, MD, FRCS
Vice Chair for Research
Professor of Orthopaedic Surgery
Rothman Institute at Thomas Jefferson
  University Hospital
Philadelphia, Pennsylvania

Robin Patel, MD
Professor of Medicine
Professor of Microbiology
Division of Clinical Microbiology
Mayo Clinic
Rochester, Minnesota

Michael J. Patzakis, MD
Professor and Chair
Vincent and Julia Meyer Chair
Department of Orthopaedic Surgery
Keck School of Medicine
University of Southern California
Los Angeles, California

Nalini Rao, MD, FACP, FSHEA
Clinical Professor of Medicine and Orthopaedics
Department of Medicine
University of Pittsburgh Medical Center
Pittsburgh, Pennsylvania

Michael A. Saubolle, PhD, ABMM, FAAM,
  FIDSA
Medical Director
Laboratory Sciences of Arizona/Banner Health
Associate Clinical Professor of Medicine
University of Arizona
Phoenix, Arizona

Stephen B. Schnall, MD
Professor of Clinical Orthopaedics and Surgery
Chief of Hand Surgery
Department of Orthopaedics
Keck School of Medicine
University of Southern California
Los Angeles, California

Kevin Tetsworth, MD, FRACS
Director of Orthopaedics
Department of Orthopaedics
Royal Brisbane and Women's Hospital
Brisbane, Queensland, Australia

Seth K. Williams, MD
Assistant Professor of Clinical Orthopaedics
Department of Orthopaedics
University of Miami Miller School of Medicine
Miami, Florida

Montri Daniel Wongworawat, MD
Associate Professor
Department of Orthopaedic Surgery
Loma Linda University
Loma Linda, California

Edwin Yu, MD
Clinical Assistant Professor of Medicine
Division of Infectious Disease
University of Arizona College of Medicine
Banner Good Samaritan Medical Center
Phoenix, Arizona

Charalampos G. Zalavras, MD, PhD
Associate Professor
Department of Orthopaedic Surgery
University of Southern California
Los Angeles County–University of Southern
  California Medical Center
Los Angeles, California

Preface

The Musculoskeletal Infection Society (MSIS) is proud to present *Orthopaedic Knowledge Update: Musculoskeletal Infection*. Founded in 1989, the MSIS is a multidisciplinary educational and scientific forum dedicated to advancing knowledge in the field of study of infection and treatment. The MSIS mission is education of its clinician and research members, the medical community and the general public; and the promotion and maintenance of professional standards in efforts to provide the best professional care to patients with musculoskeletal infection.

The update begins with a discussion of current knowledge about the biology of microbes, biofilms, and the host-microbe interactions that link pathophysiology with diagnosis and treatment. Similarly, the patterns of musculoskeletal infectious diseases are referenced to microbial behavior and the formation of antimicrobial resistance. The relationships between specific microbes, clinical syndromes, and important risk factors related to therapeutic success are profiled.

The next two sections include diagnostic and general treatment concepts when managing musculoskeletal infections. Planning takes into account the patient-specific local and systemic immune status of the host and the individual socioeconomic, cultural, and functional parameters that determine the treatment. When eradication is the goal, surgical débridement requires complete resection of the nidus of infection. Antimicrobial management is an obligate, adjuvant treatment delivered locally, systemically, or both to assist the host in eliminating any residual microbial phenotypes. The dynamics of antimicrobial delivery (local and systemic) and the coordination of medical and surgical care are outlined.

Commonly encountered musculoskeletal infections are reviewed in the final section by the involved tissue or structure (bone, joint, implant), the anatomic site (hand, foot, spine), or the specific clinical scenario (postoperative or nosocomial infection, atypical microbes, diabetes). Each chapter applies nuances of the concepts developed in the earlier sections. Authors analyze classic, key, and current publications for up-to-date treatment.

The editors thank the 16 members, the 17 guest authors, and the publications staff of the American Academy of Orthopaedic Surgeons for their dedication, knowledge, and time in completing this work. The MSIS's commitment to the philosophy of collaborative surgical and medical care is reflected by the coauthorship of many of the chapters in this book. The MSIS hopes soon to publish *OKU: Musculoskeletal Infections 2*, with new discussions of these and additional topics on infection, including pediatric infections, diagnostic pathways, soft-tissue infections, and host immunity.

George Cierny III, MD

Alex C. McLaren, MD

Montri D. Wongworawat, MD

Editors

Table of Contents

Section 1

General Considerations

SECTION EDITORS:

JOHN L. ESTERHAI JR, MD
ALEX C. MCLAREN, MD

Chapter 1

The Epidemiology of Musculoskeletal Infections

John L. Esterhai Jr, MD   Nalini Rao, MD, FACP, FSHEA

Introduction

The epidemiology of musculoskeletal infections is the study of the causes, distribution, and control of disease, including the characteristics of the organisms; affected populations; mechanisms of transmission; occurrence; clinical manifestations; and the treatment of bone, joint, implant, and soft-tissue infections. Epidemiologists attempt to quantify the frequency of disease by calculating its incidence (the number of new occurrences in a population during a defined period, expressed as an annual rate or percentage; the calculation is performed by dividing the number of newly diagnosed cases by the number of persons observed during the period). One purpose of analytic epidemiology is to identify the risk factors associated with a specific infection.

Public health officials use statistics on the incidence of different diseases to allocate scarce resources. To prevent and control infection, interventions are developed to identify reservoirs of infectious agents and their mechanisms of transmission. Over time, changes in the incidence of an infection can reveal emerging patterns of infection and determine the effectiveness of prevention and control measures. The ultimate goal of public health officials is to control and prevent infection by interrupting or preventing its transmission, preventing the colonization of infectious organisms, and preventing a developing infection from causing illness. Physicians play an important role by educating patients, ensuring appropriate prophylaxis and treatment, and recognizing and reporting issues related to public health.

This discussion of the epidemiology of musculoskeletal infections includes nosocomial infections; guidelines for modifying trends in nosocomial infection; reservoirs in adult and pediatric long-term care facilities; the increasing vulnerability of the population resulting from aging, transplant medicine, and human immunodeficiency virus (HIV); the accelerating development of hospital-acquired and community-acquired methicillin-resistant *Staphylococcus aureus* (MRSA), vancomycin-intermediate sensitive *S aureus* (VISA), vancomycin-resistant enterococci (VRE), and multidrug-resistant organisms; infections associated with military operations in Iraq and Afghanistan; and occupationally acquired HIV among health care workers. The general epidemiologic principles are directly applicable to the care of patients with a musculoskeletal disorder, including musculoskeletal infections.

Nosocomial Infections

The most common complication affecting hospitalized patients is nosocomial infection. Nosocomial is defined as "denoting a new disorder, not the patient's original condition, associated with being treated in a health care environment." Two million patients (5% to 10% of all patients admitted to an acute care hospital in the United States) each year develop at least one nosocomial infection, and as many as 90,000 deaths result.[1] Surgical site infection (SSI) is the third most common type of nosocomial infection. Approximately 17% of all hospital-acquired infections are SSIs, and more than 29% of these infections are caused by MRSA.[2]

In the 1960s, the US Centers for Disease Control and Prevention (CDC) recommended that hospitals begin the surveillance of infections acquired by hospitalized patients. The Joint Commission in 1964 made surveillance a responsibility of the medical staff and in 1976 made surveillance of hospital-acquired infections mandatory for Joint Commission hospital accreditation. The Institute of Medicine's 1999 report *To Err Is Human: Building a Safer Health System* listed health care–associated infection as a preventable adverse patient event.

Reported rates of SSI in part are determined by the definition of infection and the intensity and duration of observation. The National Nosocomial Infections Surveillance (NNIS) system of the CDC, a voluntary, confidential, hospital-based reporting system, is the only national source of systematically gathered data on infection. The NNIS system classifies an SSI as follows: (1) a superficial incisional infection involving only the skin or subcutaneous tissue; (2) a deep incisional infection involving the deeper soft tissues; or (3) an organ-space infection involving any part of the anatomy other than an incised body wall layer. The NNIS system includes all SSIs that occur within the first 30 days after surgery or within 1 year of surgery if an implant was placed and the infection is related to the surgery.

The duration of observation is an especially important factor because of the decreased average length of hospitalization after many orthopaedic procedures. Decreases in hospital length of stay compromise the completeness of SSI data that require inpatient surveillance. There is no consensus as to the best methods of postdischarge surveillance; data based on surgeon records or patient memory have been shown to lack both specificity and sensitivity. The US Department of Veterans Affairs has an excellent systemwide electronic medical record-keeping system that enables health care workers to thoroughly capture the NNIS data.[3]

The Surgical Care Improvement Program
In 2002, the US Centers for Medicare and Medicaid Services (CMS) and the CDC implemented the National Surgical Infection Prevention project, with the goal of decreasing SSI morbidity and mortality among hospitalized Medicare patients by promoting the appropriate selection and timing of prophylactic antibiotics. In 2003, this program was expanded into the Surgical Care Improvement Project (SCIP), which was implemented in 2005. The American Academy of Orthopaedic Surgeons is a member of the expert panel that advises the SCIP steering committee. The goal of SCIP is to achieve a 25% reduction by 2010 in preventable surgical morbidity and mortality from SSIs, cardiovascular complications, and venous thromboembolisms.[4,5] To receive full Medicare payment, hospitals must comply with ostensibly voluntary reporting of SCIP process measures, including antibiotic prophylaxis. Furthermore, value-based payment adjustments mandated by the Deficit Reduction Act of 2005, which took effect October 1, 2008, forbid the CMS from reimbursing hospitals for the treatment of a multitude of specific complications during the same hospitalization, including an SSI after an elective total knee replacement.

Reservoirs in Nosocomial Infections
Health care workers, patients, medical equipment and supplies, and the surrounding physical environment constitute the reservoir for nosocomial infections. Patients and health care workers can carry *Streptococcus pyogenes, S aureus,* or VRE for months. Patients in long-term care facilities are an important reservoir of hospital-acquired infection caused by these organisms. Chronically ill patients who have received multiple courses of antibiotic agents frequently are colonized with resistant bacteria, and they can reintroduce resistant bacteria to an acute care institution with each admission. The emergence of resistant organisms in adult long-term care facilities is associated with several factors: the presence of patients who are immunocompromised or malnourished, have a percutaneous feeding tube or a dialysis catheter, or have a decubitus ulcer;

the transfer of patients from an acute care facility who are colonized with multidrug-resistant bacteria; the excessive use of broad-spectrum antibiotic agents; and repeated cycles of hospitalization and long-term institutional care. Patients in pediatric extended care facilities are even more susceptible to transmission from carriers because of close physical contact in playrooms and classrooms and the need for intensive caregiver interaction, as occurs when an infant is cuddled or consoled.[6]

Transmission of Nosocomial Infections
Nosocomial infection with MRSA can occur through transmission from another patient or from a transiently or persistently colonized health care worker. Inadequate hand hygiene or sharing of equipment such as stethoscopes and blood pressure cuffs may be responsible for the colonization. A seriously ill patient in an intensive care unit (ICU) may be at risk through contact with multiple consultants, each of whom is accompanied by additional physicians. A reservoir of infection in a specific hospital location can lead to an outbreak of infection from a common source. For example, water-borne microbes in scrub sinks can be transmitted to multiple patients in the procedure suite. Cross contamination is closely related to the concept of colonization pressure, which is defined as the proportion of patients colonized with the causative bacteria in an individual hospital or unit.[7,8]

Vulnerable Populations
The emergence of new infectious pathogens has paralleled technical advances in medical care and an increase in the population of immunocompromised patients, especially those with HIV infection. These patients have increased susceptibility to a variety of bacterial, fungal, and viral organisms that rarely cause illness in patients who are immunocompetent.

The relationship between infection and social change or technological advancement has been documented since the Middle Ages, when overpopulation, urbanization, and advances in agriculture contributed to the emergence and transmission of *Pasteurella pestis.* The resulting bubonic plague destroyed one quarter of the population of Europe between 1334 and 1351. Recent trends in infectious disease, such as the emergence of antimicrobial resistance, also are strongly influenced by social change and technology. The emergence of resistance is related to selective pressure from the increasing use of antimicrobial agents in animals and humans as well as factors that are increasing the transmission of drug-resistant organisms. Strains of *Mycobacterium tuberculosis* and enterococci essentially have become untreatable using existing antibiotic agents.

Certain patient characteristics are associated with an increased risk of infection: extreme old or young age, diabetes, systemic steroid use, obesity, malnutrition, tobacco use, and immunosuppression necessitated by organ transplantation.[9,10] The use of disease-modifying antirheumatic drugs such as methotrexate, hydrochloroquine, azathioprine, and, especially, the new biologics infliximab, etanercept, adalimumab, and anakinra also are associated with an increased risk of infection. Surgical techniques including effective hemostasis, prevention of hypothermia and hyperglycemia, adequate débridement with removal of all devitalized tissue, judicious use of surgical drains, and postoperative oxygenation have an impact on decreasing infection risk.

Multidrug-Resistant Organisms

Multidrug-resistant microorganisms are resistant to one or more classes of antimicrobial agents.[11] Although some multidrug-resistant organisms are named for a specific antimicrobial agent (for example, MRSA, VRE), frequently the organism is resistant to most available agents. Certain gram-negative bacilli, including those producing extended-spectrum β-lactamases, are resistant to multiple classes of antimicrobial agents (for example, *Escherichia coli*, *Klebsiella pneumoniae*, and *Acinetobacter baumannii*). Most of these bacilli are opportunistic pathogens that colonize the skin and mucous membranes without producing infection. When there is a breakdown in the host immunologic or physical defenses, however, the colonizing bacteria can cause infection and even death.

Three methicillin-resistant isolates were reported in 1961, only 6 months after methicillin was commercially introduced.[12] Methicillin resistance is defined as a minimum inhibitory concentration for oxacillin that is at least 4 µg/mL. It is encoded on the *mec* gene, which produces penicillin-binding protein PBP2a. By 1968, methicillin resistance had been reported in Switzerland, France, Denmark, Australia, India, and the United States. By the early 1990s, MRSA accounted for 20% to 25% of the *S aureus* isolates found in hospitalized patients in the United States. In 1999, MRSA accounted for more than 50% of *Staphylococcus* isolates from patients in ICUs, and that proportion increased to 60% by 2003.[13] The number of deaths attributed to MRSA in 2005 surpassed the combined number of deaths that occurred from acquired immunodeficiency syndrome (AIDS) and during Hurricane Katrina. In 2007, the CDC estimated that MRSA causes 94,000 severe infections annually, and 19,000 patients die from the infection. In major urban centers, MRSA now accounts for more than 80% of upper extremity staphylococcal infections of the skin or soft tissue.[14]

Vancomycin, a glycopeptide antibiotic agent, is the most widely used agent for treating serious infection caused by gram-positive bacteria.[15] The first staphylococci with reduced susceptibility to vancomycin were found in Japan in 1997. The minimum inhibitory concentration of these so-called VISA isolates ranges from 4 to 8 µg/mL. However, MRSA strains that are heteroresistant to vancomycin are more common; these hVISA strains contain subpopulations with reduced susceptibility to vancomycin. The first hVISA strain

was isolated in 2002 in Michigan, and five isolates have been recovered to date. Enterococci possess several systems capable of transmitting the genetic material responsible for resistance: transposons transpose DNA sequences to plasmids intracellularly, and plasmids transmit DNA to other bacteria. High-grade vancomycin resistance from VanA protein encoded on the *VanA* gene (VanA-mediated vancomycin resistance) can be transferred from VRE to MRSA.

The emergence of new strains of MRSA in patients with no known health care–associated risk factors was first reported in 1993 in Australia. The MRSA strains isolated from patients with a community-acquired infection usually are distinct from the strains endemic in health care settings; genotypic analysis with pulsed-field gel electrophoresis, detection of the Panton-Valentine leukocidin gene, staphylococcal cassette chromosome *mec* typing, multilocus sequence typing, and staphylococcal protein A typing are used for this determination.[16] The two pulsed-field types responsible for most community-acquired infections are USA 300 and USA 400; USA 100 and USA 200 are the genetic types from health care settings. Community-acquired infections are sensitive to most antibiotic agents other than β-lactams and macrolides, perhaps as a result of the overuse of the first-generation cephalosporins and penicillinase-resistant penicillin.[17] These infections carry gene complexes for the Panton-Valentine leukocidin cytotoxin, which causes severe abscesses and necrotizing pneumonias in otherwise healthy individuals; they also carry staphylococcal chromosomal cassette *mec* type IVa for methicillin resistance.[18] This genetic cassette is smaller than types I, II, and III, which typically are found in health care–associated MRSA. Type IVa is thought to be more transferable between *S aureus* strains. There is increasing concern that community clones combining virulence, transmissibility, and resistance will become established in hospitals.[19,20]

The prevalence of VRE increased from less than 1% of all *Enterococcus* isolates in any patient to approximately 15% by 1997 and then rose to 25% in 1999 and 30% in 2003.[21]

The CDC recommends that health care providers follow 12 steps for preventing the spread of resistant infections among hospitalized adults[22] (**Table 1**). The Society for Healthcare Epidemiology of America, the Association of Professionals in Infection Control and Epidemiology, and the Healthcare Infection Control Practices Advisory Committee promote the use of active surveillance cultures to screen patients for colonization upon hospital admission. These organizations also promote hand hygiene, the use of gowns and gloves, the judicious use of antibiotic agents (antibiotic stewardship), health care worker education, environmental cleaning, an automatic alert system for readmission of a colonized patient, and tracking and monitoring of infection control initiatives. Unfortunately, as of 2008, screening cultures taken from the anterior nares alone were able to identify only 80% of carriers.[7,8,23]

1: General Considerations

Table 1

The CDC's 12 Steps for Preventing Antimicrobial Resistance Among Hospitalized Adults

Prevent infection.

1. Vaccinate.
   - Give influenza or pneumococcal vaccine to at-risk patients before discharge.
   - Get influenza vaccine annually.
2. Limit the use of catheters.
   - Use catheters only when essential.
   - Use the correct catheter.
   - Use proper insertion and catheter care protocols.
   - Remove catheters when they are no longer essential.

Diagnose and treat infection effectively.

3. Target the pathogen.
   - Culture the patient.
   - Target empiric therapy to likely pathogens and the local antibiogram.
   - Target definitive therapy to known pathogens and antimicrobial susceptibility test results.
4. Access the experts.
   Consult an infectious diseases expert for patients with serious infections.

Use antimicrobial agents wisely.

5. Practice antimicrobial control.
   Engage in local antimicrobial control efforts.
6. Use local data.
   - Know your antibiogram.
   - Know your patient population.
7. Treat infection, not contamination.
   - Use proper antisepsis for blood and other cultures.
   - Culture the blood, not the skin or catheter hub.
   - Use proper methods to obtain and process all cultures.
8. Treat infection, not colonization.
   - Treat pneumonia, not the tracheal aspirate.
   - Treat bacteremia, not the catheter tip or hub.
   - Treat urinary tract infection, not the indwelling catheter.
9. Know when to say "no" to vancomycin.
   - Treat infection, not contaminants or colonization.
   - Understand that fever in a patient with an intravenous catheter is not a routine indication for vancomycin.
10. Stop antimicrobial treatment
    - when infection is cured.
    - when cultures are negative and infection is unlikely.
    - when infection is not diagnosed.

Prevent transmission.

11. Isolate the pathogen.
    - Use standard infection control precautions.
    - Contain infectious body fluids. (Follow airborne, droplet, and contact precautions.)
    - When in doubt, consult infection control experts.
12. Break the chain of contagion.
    - Stay home when you are sick.
    - Keep your hands clean.
    - Set an example.

(Adapted from Centers for Disease Control and Prevention: Campaign to Prevent Antimicrobial Resistance in Healthcare Settings: 12 steps to prevent antimicrobial resistance among hospitalized adults. http:www.cdc.gov/drugresistance/healthcare/ha/12steps_HA.htm. Published November 2003. Accessed March 4, 2009.)

Nosocomial infections cause significant morbidity and mortality in hospitalized children as well as adults. The treatment of infections caused by gram-positive bacteria is becoming increasingly more difficult because of antimicrobial resistance. Fifteen species of coagulase-negative staphylococci colonize the skin. The majority of *Staphylococcus epidermidis* and 60% of *S aureus* recovered from hospitalized pediatric patients are methicillin resistant; MRSA is associated with a higher mortality rate than methicillin-susceptible *S aureus*. VISA has been rarely described in children. Because some children with resistant staphylococcal infections require prolonged and repeat hospitalization, the CDC guidelines for discontinuing contact precautions in this population are strict: assume that carriers of multidrug-resistant organisms are permanently colonized; reculture 6 to 12 months after the child last required antibiotic agents, an indwelling device, or hospitalization; and discontinue contact precautions only after three or more negative surveillance cultures are obtained over a 1- to 2-week period and the patient has no signs of infection, such as profuse respiratory secretions or a draining wound.[11]

Military Operations

A significant number of soldiers are surviving severe blast injuries incurred during military operations in Iraq or Afghanistan, often because they were protected by body armor and a helmet. Some patients with massive wounds have infections caused by new types of antimicrobial-resistant bacteria. Frequently, the wounds are colonized with soil- and water-based bacteria indigenous to the region, particularly gram-negative, multidrug-resistant *Acinetobacter baumannii-calcoaceticus*. The rate of infection is correlated with the number of host-nation patients in the combat support hospital ICU or ward as well as the length of the patient's ICU stay.[24]

Although there is no standard definition of multidrug resistance, the definition from the Walter Reed Army Medical Center Department of Pathology specifies that gram-negative bacteria that are resistant to at least three of five classes of antibiotics (aminoglycosides, carbapenems, cephalosporins, penicillins, and quinolones) are considered multidrug resistant.[25] From 2000 to 2006, there was a decrease in the percentage of *Acinetobacter* isolates that were susceptible to six classes of antibiotics.[25]

Occupationally Acquired HIV Infection

In 1991, the CDC developed a standardized protocol to investigate the incidence of HIV infection in individuals employed in health care or laboratory settings who had no identifiable risk factors. Of the 57 health care workers documented to have occupationally acquired HIV infection by December 2001, 86% had been exposed to blood, and 88% had a percutaneous injury. "Documented occupationally acquired infection" occurred if the health care worker had evidence of seroconversion in temporal association with an occupational exposure and no other known exposure to HIV. Seroconversion was determined using either a serum specimen that was negative for HIV antibodies as long as 1 year before or 1 month after exposure and a subsequent serum sample that was positive for HIV antibodies within 1 year of exposure; or infection with an HIV strain that was determined by DNA sequencing to be related to the occupational source. Of the 51 percutaneous exposures, 41% occurred after a procedure; 35% during a procedure; and 20% during disposal of a sharp object.[26]

During the same period, 138 additional health care workers had a "possible occupationally acquired infection." These workers had no identified behavior or transfusion risk factors and a positive history of exposure; however, the time and source of the HIV infection could not be documented, and therefore seroconversion to HIV as a result of occupational exposure could not be documented.[26] Highly active combination antiretroviral therapy regimens have dramatically improved the survival and health of patients infected with HIV.

Prevention strategies for health care workers should emphasize the elimination of exposure to blood. It is especially important for health care workers to be educated about postexposure prophylaxis options and procedures. The most recent CDC guidelines on health care worker exposure to HIV and other blood-borne viral pathogens, risk factors, and postexposure protocols were published in 2005.[27]

Epidemiology of Specific Musculoskeletal Infections

Septic Arthritis

Septic arthritis is caused by a bacterial invasion of the synovial space. The host responds with an acute inflammatory reaction and phagocytosis by the polymorphonuclear leucocytes. Toxins and enzymes released by the bacteria and stimulated T cells lead to destruction of articular cartilage and loss of function.[28]

The yearly incidence of native septic arthritis in the general population ranges from 2 to 10 per 100,000; in patients with rheumatoid arthritis, the range is 30 to 70 per 100,000. Despite adequate treatment, as many as 50% of patients have an irreversible loss of function. The risk factors for septic arthritis include joint disease, chronic systemic disease, immunocompromise, trauma, intravenous drug abuse, and endocarditis[29,30] (**Table 2**).

Bacterial septic arthritis usually is hematogenously acquired. Other routes of infection include direct inoculation through trauma, injection, aspiration, or a surgical procedure; and contiguous spread. The infection can be caused by a diverse range of microorganisms. Bacterial arthritis can have an acute onset, and it has the potential to rapidly destroy the joint. The knee is involved in more than 50% of patients. Mycobacterial or fungal arthritis usually is a chronic, slowly progressing monoarticular arthritis. Viral arthritis often involves multiple joints and

Table 2

Common Risk Factors for Bacterial Septic Arthritis

Systemic
AIDS
Alcoholism
Anti–tumor necrosis factor-α suppression therapy
Chronic renal failure
Diabetes mellitus
Endocarditis
Glucocorticosteroid therapy
Hemodialysis
Hemophilia
Hypogammaglobulinemia
Immunosuppressive drug therapy
Intravenous drug abuse
Liver disease
Malignancy
Organ transplantation
Psoriasis
Rheumatoid arthritis

Local
Direct joint trauma
Joint-specific rheumatoid arthritis
Knee or hip prosthesis
Open fracture reduction
Recent joint surgery

Age-Related
Age older than 80 years
Age 6 months to 2 years

Socioeconomic
Low socioeconomic status (risk factor for tuberculosis)
Occupational exposure to animals (risk factor for brucellosis)

(Adapted with permission from Garcia-De La Torre I: Advances in the management of septic arthritis. *Rheum Dis Clin N Am* 2003;29:61-75.)

may occur as infection with intra-articular viral particles or a reactive immune response with arthralgia. Table 3 outlines the microbiology of bacterial septic arthritis as related to age, and Table 4 describes septic arthritis as a complication of specific clinical settings.[29,31]

Osteomyelitis

Osteomyelitis is an infection of bone and the medullary cavity. There are 50,000 hospital admissions for osteomyelitis annually in the United States; in 80% of patients, the disease is caused by *S aureus*. The prevalence of MRSA ranges from 33% to 55% among adult patients hospitalized for osteomyelitis. MRSA osteomyelitis can be difficult to control, and its incidence is on the rise worldwide.

The severity of the disease is staged based on its pathogenesis, the extent of bone involvement, and host factors. The source of osteomyelitis can be hematogenous seeding, direct inoculation, or contiguous spread of nearby infection. Hematogenous osteomyelitis primarily is a disease of children; 85% of patients are younger than 17 years. As many as 47% to 50% of adult patients have posttraumatic osteomyelitis. The major risk factors include penetrating trauma, intravenous drug abuse, diabetes mellitus, immunocompromise, perioperative infection, contiguous soft-tissue infection, vascular insufficiency, and open fracture.[32,33] Tables 5 and 6 outline the pathogenesis and microbiology of osteomyelitis in specific clinical settings.

Prosthetic Joint Infection

Prosthetic joint infection involves an interaction among the implant, host, and microorganism. In the hip or shoulder, the incidence of implant-related infections is less than 1%, and in the knee it is less than 2%. Approximately 60% of prosthetic joint infections occur through direct contamination during the surgical procedure. Infection also can spread from a contiguous focus. Bacteremia is a risk factor for hematogenous

Table 3

Microbiology of Bacterial Septic Arthritis as Related to Patient Age

Organism	Child (Age 6 Months to 5 Years)	Young Adult Engaging in High-Risk Sexual Behavior	Adult	Elderly Adult
S aureus	10% to 20%	15% to 20%	60% to 70%	45% to 65%
Streptococcus species	5% to 10%	1% to 5%	15% to 20%	10% to 15%
Gram-negative bacterium	1% to 5%	Rare	10% to 15%	15% to 35%
Haemophilus influenzae	Rare*	Rare*	Rare*	Rare*
Neisseria gonorrhoeae	1% to 5%	60% to 80%	1% to 5%	Rare

*with widespread immunization
(Adapted with permission from Liu NY, Giansiracusa DF: Septic arthritis, in Gorbach SL, Bartlett JG, Blacklow NR (eds): *Infectious Diseases*, ed 2. Philadelphia, PA, WB Saunders, 1998, p 1345.)

Table 4

The Microbiology of Septic Arthritis as Related to Patient Physiologic Status

Condition Affecting Physiologic Status	Associated Risk Factors for Septic Arthritis	Common Pathogens (Incidence)	Treatment Considerations
Rheumatoid arthritis	Disabling arthritis Skin lesions Infected rheumatoid nodule Tumor necrosis factor-α suppression therapy Malnutrition Cytotoxic drugs Corticosteroids (systemic and local to joint)	*S aureus* (40% to 60%) *S pyogenes* (10% to 20%) *Salmonella* species (rare) *Moraxella catarrhalis* (rare) *Listeria,* with tumor necrosis factor-α suppression therapy (rare)	Patient education Early diagnosis Surgical débridement Antibiotics Special caution required with tumor necrosis factor-α suppression therapy
Age older than 80 years	Diabetes mellitus Urinary tract infection Biliary tract infection Diverticulitis	*S aureus* (30% to 40%) Gram-negative bacilli (10% to 20%)	Poor outcome if treatment started later than 7 days after symptom onset
Bacterial endocarditis	Septic immobilization Reactive immune arthritis Intravenous drug abuse	*S aureus* (10% to 30%) *S pyogenes* (40% to 60%) *Pseudomonas aeruginosa* (5% to 10%)	Adverse effects of long-duration antibiotic treatment (4 to 6 weeks)
Prosthetic joint infection	Dental procedures Systemic lupus erythematosus Immunosuppression Diabetes mellitus Hemophilia Urinary tract infection Skin infection Prior joint infection (≤ 2 years after surgery)	Staphylococci (40% to 60%) Streptococci (10% to 30%) Gram-negative bacilli (10% to 15%)	Antibiotic prophylaxis indicated
Immunosuppression, AIDS, stem cell transplantation	Immunosuppression Decreased humoral and cell-mediated immunity	*Stenotrophomonas* (rare) *Salmonella* (rare) *Rhizobium* (rare) Fungi (rare) Atypical mycobacteria (rare)	Responsible organisms are unusual and otherwise nonpathogenic.
Whipple disease		*Tropheryma whippelii* (rare)	
Hypogammaglobulinemia	Decreased humoral immunity	*Ureaplasma* species (rare)	
Hemoglobinopathy	Microinfarcts in intestinal wall	Salmonella (rare) *S aureus* (rare)	Osteomyelitis is more common than septic arthritis.
Human or animal bite wound	Inoculation of indigenous mouth flora	*Pasteurella multocida* (rare) *Eikenella corrodens* (rare) *Streptobacillus moniliformis* (rare)	Septic arthritis occurs near injury site. Knuckle osteomyelitis occurs with clenched fist injury.
Intravenous drug abuse	Endocarditis Diskitis	*S aureus* (60% to 80%) *P aeruginosa* (rare) *Serratia* (rare) *Candida* species (rare)	Occurs in sacroiliac, sterno-costal, and sternoclavicular joints.
Plant thorn	Puncture wound Foreign body	*Pantoea agglomerans* (rare) *Sporothrix schenckii* (rare) Atypical mycobacteria (rare) *Nocardia* (rare) *Clostridium sordellii* (rare) *Actinomyces israelii* (rare)	Foreign body is detected using radiographs of joint.
Tick (in Lyme-disease endemic area)	Tick bite	*Borrelia burgdorferi*	
Exposure to contaminated seawater	Skin breaks	*Mycobacterium marinum*	Septic arthritis in small joints of hand
Positive tuberculin skin test	Malnutrition HIV Immunosuppression	*M tuberculosis*	Septic arthritis in axial skeleton and large joint

prosthetic joint infection. *S aureus* bacteremia is associated with a 34% risk of implant-associated infection. Host factors that predispose a patient to prosthetic joint infection are older age, poor nutritional status, inflammatory joint disease, diabetes mellitus, obesity, prior native joint infection, remote infection, and advanced HIV disease. Patients with rheumatoid arthritis have a 2.6 times greater risk of prosthetic joint infection than those with osteoarthritis. The infection rate associated with revision surgery is 4.2%, compared with 0.54% after primary arthroplasty.[34-36]

The most commonly cultured microorganisms are coagulase-negative staphylococci (30% to 43%) and *S aureus* (12% to 23%). Mixed flora (10% to 12%), streptococci (9% to 10%), gram-negative bacilli (3% to 6%), enterococci (3% to 7%), and anaerobes (2% to 4%) also are found. No microorganism is detected in approximately 11% of infections.[35]

A microorganism's ability to form a biofilm is a virulence factor in prosthetic joint infections. This is particularly true for coagulase-negative staphylococci and *Propionibacterium acnes*. The organisms in the biofilm can be in a stationary phase of growth, and they are relatively unlikely to be cultured in the artificial medium used in the microbiology laboratory. The traditional intraoperative swab culture has been replaced by multiple biopsy specimens and specimens from sonicated implants, both of which are incubated for prolonged periods. Although polymerase chain reaction has the potential to improve microbe identification in culture-negative implant infections, the techniques have limitations and are not commercially available for routine use.[34]

Table 5

Microorganisms in Acute Hematogenous Osteomyelitis

Population	Microorganisms
Infants	*S aureus* Group B *Streptococcus* E coli
Children (1 to 4 years)	*S aureus* *S pyogenes*
Healthy adults (21 to 79 years)	*S aureus*
Elderly adults (80 years or older)	Gram-negative rods
Patients with intravascular device	*Candida* species
Patients who abuse intravenous drugs	*S aureus* *P aeruginosa*

Table 6

Clinical Risk Factors for Nonhematogenous Osteomyelitis

Risk Factor	Organisms	Anatomic Sites
Intravenous drug abuse	*S aureus* *P aeruginosa*	Axial skeleton Sternoclavicular joint
Hemoglobinopathy	*Salmonella*	Long bones
Tooth abscess	Anaerobes	Mandible
Diabetic foot abscess	Polymicrobial	Small bones of feet
Human bite	*E corrodens* *S aureus*	Hands
Animal bite	*P multocida*	Hands, feet, face
Puncture wound of foot	*P aeruginosa*	Calcaneus
Median sternotomy	*S aureus* *S epidermidis*	Sternum
Meat handling	*Brucella*	Flat bones
Fish handling	*M marinum*	Small bones of hand
Hemodialysis	*S aureus* *S epidermidis*	Axial skeleton
Positive tuberculin skin test	*M tuberculosis*	Thoracic spine
Exposure to tuberculosis, residence in tuberculosis-endemic area	*M tuberculosis*	
Prosthetic device	*S aureus* *S epidermidis*	Extremities and joints

Spine Infections

Osteomyelitis occurs in the axial skeleton in 2% to 7% of patients. The predisposing factors include advanced age, diabetes mellitus, malnutrition, substance abuse, malignancy, long-term steroid use, renal failure, septicemia, and HIV-AIDS. The commonly responsible organisms include *S aureus* and streptococci. In patients who are intravenous drug abusers, gram-negative bacilli such as *P aeruginosa* and *Serratia marcescens* frequently are isolated. *M tuberculosis* and fungi usually are found in patients who are immunocompromised. Organisms of low virulence, such as *Streptococcus viridans* and coagulase-negative staphylococci, can cause an indolent infection. *Salmonella osteomyelitis* may be responsible for infection in a patient with sickle cell disease. The infecting organism cannot be identified in approximately one third of patients.[37-39]

Diabetic Foot Infections

Infected foot ulcers account for 25% of hospital admissions of patients with diabetes, and 85% of lower limb amputations in these patients are preceded by an infected foot ulcer. The epidemiology, pathogenesis, and treatment of diabetic foot ulceration have not been fully investigated, despite the impact of the condition on patients and society.[40]

The spectrum of foot infections in a patient with diabetes includes paronychia, cellulitis, myositis, abscess, necrotizing fasciitis, septic arthritis, and osteomyelitis. The most common manifestation is an infected ulcer. Neuropathy is the most important predisposing factor for ulcer formation.d society.[41]

Gram-positive cocci, including *S aureus* and β-hemolytic streptococci, especially group B streptococci, are the predominant organisms in mild and moderate infections. Chronic wounds develop more complex microbial flora including Enterobacteriaceae, *Pseudomonas,* and enterococci. The significance of *Pseudomonas* and enterococci in this setting is not entirely clear. Severe, limb-threatening infections with impending gangrene usually are caused by mixed aerobic, gram-positive cocci; Enterobacteriaceae; nonfermenting gram-negative bacilli; or obligate anaerobes.[42,43]

Diabetic foot infection caused by MRSA is a growing problem worldwide. In two separate studies from diabetic foot clinics in the United Kingdom, the prevalence of MRSA infections increased twofold over a 3-year period.[43]

Summary

Epidemiology is the study of the causes, distribution, and control of disease, with identification of the factors affecting the health and illness of populations. Epidemiology provides the foundation for public health intervention, and epidemiologic data provide information to educate patients and ensure appropriate prophylaxis and treatment. Orthopaedic surgeons have the responsibility to recognize and report public health problems.

Nosocomial infections are a significant public health issue. SSIs following orthopaedic surgical procedures contribute to the incidence of nosocomial infections. SCIP, which is sponsored by the CMS, the CDC, and other public health organizations, is aimed at reducing the number of SSIs through public reporting and CMS payment penalties.

Socioeconomic factors and technical advances in medicine have increased the number of immunocompromised patients and led to an increase in the general population's risk of infection-related diseases. Individual patient factors such as extreme old or young age, diabetes, systemic steroid use, obesity, malnutrition, tobacco use, immunosuppression for organ transplantation, disease-modifying antirheumatic drugs, and surgical details (bleeding, hypothermia, hyperglycemia, adequacy of débridement, and postoperative oxygenation) can increase an individual patient's risk of infection.

Resistance to antimicrobial agents has been detailed epidemiologically. Musculoskeletal infections are a major treatment challenge, especially with the emergence of multidrug-resistant bacteria such as MRSA and VRE, resistant gram-negative bacilli such as extended-spectrum β-lactamase *Klebsiella* species, *E coli*, and multidrug-resistant *A baumannii*. The CDC recommends strict hand hygiene, patient isolation and cohorting precautions, contact precautions with the use of appropriate barriers, and antibiotic stewardship.

Annotated References

1. Burke JP: Infection control: A problem for patient safety. *N Engl J Med* 2003;348:651-656.

   Nosocomial infections are a persistent problem. The CDC and other organizations are pursuing approaches including epidemiologic analysis, active surveillance, safer devices, and quality improvement projects, with limited success.

2. Anderson DJ, Sexton DJ, Kanafani ZA, Auten G, Kaye KS: Severe surgical site infection in community hospitals: Epidemiology, key procedures, and the changing prevalence of methicillin-resistant Staphylococcus aureus. *Infect Control Hosp Epidemiol* 2007;28:1047-1053.

   The prevalence of MRSA infections almost doubled from 2000 to 2005 in 26 community hospitals. MRSA became the most frequently cultured pathogen in SSI.

3. Patel M, Weinheimer JD, Waites KB, Baddley JW: Active surveillance to determine the impact of methicillin resistant Staphylococcus aureus colonization on patients in the intensive care unit of a Veterans Administration Medical Center. *Infect Control Hosp Epidemiol* 2008;29:503-509.

Sixteen percent of patients admitted to an ICU were colonized with methicillin-susceptible *S aureus,* and 7% were colonized with MRSA. MRSA colonization was an independent predictor of death or MRSA infection onset after hospital discharge. The risk factors for MRSA colonization included dialysis and recent antibiotic use. Active risk surveillance for MRSA may identify patients at risk for these complications.

4. US Department of Health and Human Services: Hospital Compare. http://www.hospitalcompare.hhs.gov. Updated February 11, 2009. Accessed March 4, 2009.

   Hospital reporting of SCIP measures is disclosed to the public on this Web site.

5. Centers for Medicare and Medicaid Services: QualityNet. http://qualitynet.org. Accessed January 30, 2009.

   The CMS developed a comprehensive online resource for quality improvement information related to Medicare's national quality improvement priority topics. SCIP process and outcome measures related to infection can be found on this site.

6. Harris JA: Infection control in pediatric extended care facilities. *Infect Control Hosp Epidemiol* 2006;27: 598-603.

   Pediatric extended care facilities provide for both the physical and psychosocial needs of patients younger than 21 years who have self-care deficits. Infection control policies appropriate for adult long-term care facilities are not applicable in this environment.

7. Rohr U, Wilhelm M, Muhr G, Gatermann S: Qualitative and (semi)quantitative characterization of nasal and skin methicillin-resistant Staphylococcus aureus carriage of hospitalized patients. *Int J Hyg Environ Health* 2004;207:51-55.

   The study objective was to investigate MRSA carrier patterns and the intensity of colonization at different sites. A combination of nose, forehead, and groin colonization provided the highest yield. Further study must show the significance of degree of colonization for transmission.

8. Milstone AM, Perl TM: MRSA: Screening and laboratory identification. *Pediatr Infect Dis J* 2008;27: 927-928.

   MRSA screening with enhanced laboratory techniques does not in itself prevent transmission. Vigilant hand hygiene is the first line of defense. Selected patient populations may benefit from screening decolonization.

9. McGarry SA, Engemann JJ, Schmader K, Sexton DJ, Kaye KS: Surgical site infections due to Staphylococcus aureus among elderly patients: Mortality, duration of hospitalization and cost. *Infect Control Hosp Epidemiol* 2004;25:461-467.

   Among surgical patients older than 70 years, *S aureus* SSIs were independently associated with increased mortality, length of hospital admission, and cost. Postoperative length of stay increased from 9 to 13 days.

10. Fishman JA: Infection in solid organ transplant recipients. *N Engl J Med* 2007;357:2601-2614.

Although increasingly potent immunosuppressive agents have decreased the incidence of transplant organ rejection, they have increased patients' susceptibility to opportunistic infections. Exposures that are benign to a normal host can lead to a major infection after transplantation. The net state of immunosuppression refers to all factors that contribute to the patient's risk of infection, including the dosages, duration, and sequence of immunosuppressive medications.

11. Siegel JD, Rhinehart E, Jackson M, Chiarello L, Healthcare Infection Control Practices Advisory Committee: *Management of Multidrug-Resistant Organisms in Healthcare Settings, 2006.* Atlanta, GA: Centers for Disease Control and Prevention, 2006. http://www.cdc. gov/ncidod/dhqp/pdf/ar/mdroguideline2006.pdf. Accessed January 26, 2009.

    The prevention and control of multidrug-resistant organisms are a national priority. CDC has outlined recommendations to guide the implementation of strategies and practices to prevent transmission of MRSA, VRE, and other multidrug-resistant organisms. Resources must be available for infection control, expert consultation, laboratory support, adherence monitoring, and data analysis.

12. Grundmann H, Aires-de-Sousa M, Boyce J, Tiemersma E: Emergence and resurgence of methicillin-resistant Staphylococcus aureus as a public health threat. *Lancet* 2006;368:874-885.

    This is a thorough discussion of genetics and the worldwide burden of MRSA. Hospital-acquired MRSA infection increases morbidity, mortality, and cost of care (including containment of outbreaks and antibiotic prescriptions). Although molecular epidemiologic data suggest that the evolution of MRSA is predominantly clonal, horizontal transfer of bacterial DNA from other species can occur.

13. Engemann JJ, Carmeli Y, Cosgrove SE, et al: Adverse clinical and economic outcomes attributable to methicillin resistance among patients with Staphylococcus aureus surgical site infection. *Clin Infect Dis* 2003;36: 592-598.

    Compared with patients with a methicillin-susceptible *S aureus* SSI, patients with an MRSA infection had a higher 90-day mortality rate, a longer hospital stay, and increased hospital charges (control group, $29,455; methicillin-susceptible *S aureus* group, $52,791; MRSA group, $92,363).

14. Klein E, Smith DL, Laxminarayan R: Hospitalizations and deaths caused by methicillin-resistant Staphylococcus aureus, United States, 1999-2005. *Emerg Infect Dis* 2007;13:1840-1846.

    National hospitalization and resistance data were used to determine that the estimated number of *S aureus*–related hospitalizations increased 62% from 1999 to 2005 and that the estimated number of MRSA-related hospitalizations more than doubled.

15. Moellering RC Jr : Vancomycin: A 50-year reassessment. *Clin Infect Dis* 2006;42:S3-S4.

The compound now known as vancomycin was isolated in 1952 from *Streptomyces orientalis* in a soil sample in Borneo. The name vancomycin was derived from "vanquish."

16. Klevens RM, Morrison MA, Nadle J, et al: Invasive methicillin resistant Staphylococcus aureus infections in the United States. *JAMA* 2007;298:1763-1771.

    Invasive MRSA infection affects some population groups more than others. In 2005, the standardized incidence rate of invasive MRSA was 31.8 per 100,000 population. The incidence per 100,000 was highest among those who were older than 65 years (127.7), black (66.5), or male (37.5). The standardized mortality rate was 6.3 per 100,000. Molecular testing identified strains historically thought to be community acquired in hospital-onset MRSA infections.

17. Diep BA, Chambers HF, Graber CJ, et al: Emergence of multi-drug resistant, community-associated, methicillin-resistant Staphylococcus aureus clone USA300 in men who have sex with men. *Ann Intern Med* 2008;148: 249-257.

    The authors describe an increased risk of community-acquired MRSA among men who have sex with men, independent of HIV infection.

18. Daum RS: Clinical practice: Skin and soft tissue infections caused by methicillin-resistant *Staphylococcus aureus*. *N Engl J Med* 2007;357:380-390.

    Persons at risk for community-acquired MRSA include those having contact at home or in a day care center with a patient with proven MRSA infection, children, men who have sex with men, soldiers, prisoners, contact sport athletes, Native Americans, Pacific Islanders, persons with previous community-acquired MRSA, and intravenous drug abusers. The recommendations to limit the spread of community-acquired MRSA include covering draining wounds with clean bandages, washing hands after contact with an infected wound or dressing, regularly bathing with soap, laundering clothes and linens that have come into contact with drainage, avoiding sharing of personal items such as razors or towels, and cleaning sports equipment with an Environmental Protection Agency–approved detergent or disinfectant.

19. Gould IM: Community-acquired MRSA: Can we control it? *Lancet* 2006;368:824-826.

    This is a discussion of the ability to control community-acquired MRSA and the potential impact of an influenza pandemic complicated by community-acquired MRSA infections.

20. Paintsil E: Pediatric community acquired methicillin-resistant Staphylococcus aureus infection and colonization: Trends and management. *Curr Opin Pediatr* 2007; 19:75-82.

    The author reviews the spreading epidemic of MRSA and urges effective active surveillance programs and infection control.

21. Levine DP: Vancomycin: A history. *Clin Infect Dis* 2006;42:S5-S12.

Vancomycin-resistant enterococci were reported in Europe in 1986 and the United States in 1987. Vancomycin-resistant *S aureus* appeared in the United States in 2002.

22. Centers for Disease Control and Prevention: Campaign to Prevent Antimicrobial Resistance in Healthcare Settings: 12 steps to prevent antimicrobial resistance among hospitalized adults. http:www.cdc.gov/drug resistance/healthcare/ha/12steps_HA.htm. Published November 2003. Accessed March 4, 2009.

23. Carroll KC: Rapid diagnostics for methicillin resistant Staphylococcus aureus: Current status. *Mol Diagn Ther* 2008;12:15-24.

    The availability of rapid molecular diagnostics has strengthened infection control programs by providing results in hours rather than days. Probe-based and amplification rapid diagnostic methods are available for surveillance using nasal swab and blood specimens.

24. Griffith ME, Gonzalez RS, Holcomb JB, Hospenthal DR, Wortmann GW, Murray CK: Factors associated with recovery of Acinetobacter baumannii in a combat support hospital. *Infect Control Hosp Epidemiol* 2008;29:664-666.

    The US military has reported an increase in the rate of *A baumannii* infections in combat support hospitals in Iraq and Afghanistan. The rate of infection was found to be correlated with the number of host-nation patients in the ICU or ward and with ICU length of stay.

25. Zapor MJ, Erwin D, Erowele G, Wortman G: Emergence of multidrug resistance in bacteria and impact on antibiotic expenditure at a major army medical center caring for soldiers wounded in Iraq and Afghanistan. *Infect Control Hosp Epidemiol* 2008;29:661-663.

    Clinical isolation of multidrug-resistant microorganisms, particularly gram-negative bacteria, have become more frequent at Walter Reed Army Medical Center since the US invasions of Iraq and Afghanistan. Antibiotic prescribing has mirrored this pattern.

26. Do AN, Ciesielski CA, Metler RP, Hammett TA, Li J, Fleming PL: Occupationally acquired human immunodeficiency virus (HIV) infection: National case surveillance data during 20 years of the HIV epidemic in the United States. *Infect Control Hosp Epidemiol* 2003;23: 86-96.

    National surveillance systems based on voluntary case reporting were used to determine the incidence of HIV infection among heath care workers.

27. Solomon SL: Updated US public health guidelines for the management of occupational exposures to HIV and recommendations for postexposure prophylaxis. *MMWR* 2005;54:RR-9. http://www.cdc.gov/mmwr/ PDF/rr/rr5409.pdf. Accessed February 9, 2009.

    The CDC provides guidelines on health care worker exposure to HIV and other blood-borne viral pathogens, risk factors, and postexposure protocols.

28. Rao N: Septic arthritis. *Curr Treat Options Infect Dis* 2002;4:279-287.

Antibiotic therapy and surgical management are reviewed, with discussion of septic arthritis in special clinical settings. Acute septic arthritis is a medical and surgical emergency that can lead to rapid joint destruction, resulting in irreversible loss of joint function. *Staphylococcus* and *Streptococcus* species are the predominant organisms. Successful treatment depends on early diagnosis, systemic antimicrobial therapy, and urgent decompression of the infected joint.

29. Smith JW, Chalupa P, Shabaz Hasan M: Infectious arthritis: Clinical features, laboratory findings and treatment. *Clin Microbiol Infect* 2006;12:309-314.

Native joint infections can be monoarticular or polyarticular; the latter usually occurs during bacteremia. Bacterial infections lead to suppurative joints. Viral infections involve multiple joints producing inflammation. Chronic granulomatous monoarthritis is caused by infection with mycobacteria and fungi and must be differentiated from other chronic infectious arthritis. Sterile arthritis may occur as postinfectious or reactive arthritis.

30. Garcia-De La Torre I: Advances in the management of septic arthritis. *Rheum Dis Clin North Am* 2003;29:61-75.

Septic arthritis is reviewed with a focus on the risk factors and pathogenesis of nongonococcal bacterial arthritis, with differential diagnosis and treatment.

31. Ross JJ: Septic arthritis. *Infect Dis Clin North Am* 2005;19:799-817.

The epidemiology, pathogenesis, risk factors, clinical presentation, bacteriology, treatment, and outcomes of septic arthritis are outlined.

32. Calhoun JH, Manring MM: Adult osteomyelitis. *Infect Dis Clin North Am* 2005;19:765-786.

The major classification systems for adult osteomyelitis are reviewed, with a brief discussion of hematogenous, contiguous, and chronic osteomyelitis. The role of imaging techniques and the approaches to treatment of different types of adult osteomyelitis are discussed, with cases involving special populations.

33. Calhoun JH, Rao N, Manring MM: Osteomyelitis. Epocrates Online. https://online.epocrates.com/u/2911354/Osteomyelitis. Updated August 5, 2008. Accessed March 4, 2009.

This review of osteomyelitis outlines the epidemiology, risk factors, clinical features, diagnosis, and treatment (including empiric and culture-directed antibiotic regimens for adults and children).

34. Zimmerli W: Infection and musculoskeletal conditions: Prosthetic-joint-associated infections. *Best Pract Res Clin Rheumatol* 2006;20:1045-1063.

This review of prosthetic joint–associated infections focuses on predisposing factors, the role of biofilm in pathogenesis, microbiology, and diagnostic pitfalls. Antimicrobial therapy must be combined with algorithm-based surgical treatment.

35. Zimmerli W, Trampuz A, Ochsner PE: Prosthetic-joint infections. *N Engl J Med* 2004;351:1645-1654.

The pathogenesis, clinical classification, diagnosis, and treatment of prosthetic joint infections are outlined, including medical and surgical treatments.

36. Lidgren L, Knutson K, Stefansdottir A: Infection and arthritis: Infection of prosthetic joints. *Best Pract Res Clin Rheumatol* 2003;17:209-218.

The significance of prosthetic joint infection and the diagnostic puzzle are highlighted, with microbiology and treatment modalities.

37. Govender S: Spinal infections. *J Bone Joint Surg Br* 2005;87:1454-1458.

The epidemiology, mode of infection, clinical features, diagnosis, and management of spinal infections are outlined.

38. Jevtic V: Vertebral infection. *Eur Radiol* 2004;14:E43-E52.

Vertebral infections represent 2% to 4% of all cases of osteomyelitis. Pyogenic and granulomatous infectious spondylitis can cause serious neurologic compromise. MRI is the method of choice for early diagnosis and follow-up.

39. Tali ET, Gultekin S: Spinal infections. *Eur Radiol* 2005;15:599-607.

This overview of spinal infections in epidural, intradural, and intramedullary compartments provides diagnostic clues pertaining to MRI and other imaging modalities.

40. Jeffcoate WJ, Harding KG: Diabetic foot ulcers. *Lancet* 2003;361:1545-1551.

The epidemiology, pathogenesis, and management of diabetic foot infections are described, as well as their effects on patients and society. This condition deserves more attention from those who provide care or fund research.

41. Boulton AJM: The diabetic foot: Grand overview, epidemiology and pathogenesis. *Diabetes Metab Res Rev* 2008;24:S3-S6.

The epidemiology and causal pathway of diabetic foot disease are reviewed, with an assessment of current understanding of the pathogenesis and management of diabetic foot infections. Recent developments are highlighted.

42. Lipsky BA, Berendt AR, Deery HG, et al: Diagnosis and treatment of diabetic foot infections. *Clin Infect Dis* 2004;39:885-910.

Practice guidelines for the diagnosis and treatment of diabetic foot infections were developed from evidence-based literature and issued on behalf of the Infectious Diseases Society of America.

43. Rao N, Lipsky BA: Optimizing antimicrobial therapy in diabetic foot infections. *Drugs* 2007;67:196-214.

The current status of the diagnosis, clinical classification, microbiology, and antimicrobial therapy of diabetic foot infections is reviewed.

Chapter 2

The Microbiology of Musculoskeletal Infections

Jose L. del Pozo, MD, PhD   Arlen D. Hanssen, MD   *Robin Patel, MD

Introduction

The specific microbial cause of a musculoskeletal infection should be determined whenever possible, to ensure a directed therapeutic approach and optimal patient outcome. The musculoskeletal infections most commonly encountered in clinical practice can be caused by a wide variety of microorganisms including bacteria, mycobacteria, fungi, viruses, and parasites. The manifestations of these infections vary with the causative microorganism.

Cellulitis

Cellulitis is an acute, spreading pyogenic inflammation of the dermis and subcutaneous tissue. There is no sharp demarcation between the affected and uninvolved skin.[1] Cellulitis is most commonly caused by β-hemolytic streptococci, especially those in group A or B. Less often, the responsible organism is a group C or G streptococcus or *Staphylococcus aureus*. The management of cellulitis caused by community-acquired methicillin-resistant *S aureus* (MRSA) is increasingly difficult.[2] In the era before routine childhood immunization with *Haemophilus influenzae* type b conjugate vaccine, infections caused by *H influenzae* were responsible for as much as 25% of facial cellulitis in children age 3 to 24 months.[3] This type of cellulitis is now rare.

Identifying a patient's cellulitis as inoculation, contiguous extension, or bacteremic can be helpful in determining the causative microorganism (Table 1). After a human or other animal bite, cellulitis can develop from the bite recipient's skin flora or the biter's oral flora, including *P multocida* or *E rhusiopathiae*. A specific causative pathogen is suggested when an infection occurs after exposure to seawater (*V vulnificus*), fresh water (*Aeromonas hydrophila*), aquacultured fish (*S in-*

iae), or aquarium water or fish (*M marinum*).[1] Subcutaneous injection of illicit drugs can lead to cellulitis caused by an unusual bacterial species such as *Clostridium tetani*, *Clostridium botulinum*, *Clostridium sordellii*, *Clostridium novyi*, or *Bacillus cereus*. Lymphedema in the ipsilateral arm after radical mastectomy can predispose the patient to streptococcal or staphylococcal cellulitis.

Table 1

Variables Related to Unusual Bacterial Causes of Cellulitis

Variable	Possible Cause of Cellulitis
Diabetic foot ulcer	Aerobic gram-negative bacilli (Enterobacteriaceae, *Pseudomonas aeruginosa*, *Acinetobacter* species) Anaerobes (*Bacteroides* species, *Peptostreptococcus* species)
Human bite wound	*Bacteroides* species *Peptostreptococcus* species *Eikenella corrodens* Viridans group streptococci *S aureus*
Dog or cat bite wound	*Pasteurella multocida* *S aureus* *Streptococcus intermedius* *Neisseria canis* *Haemophilus felix* *Capnocytophaga canimorsus* Anaerobes
Exposure to salt water	*Vibrio vulnificus*
Exposure to fresh water Therapeutic use of leeches	*Aeromonas* species
Occupational exposure to meat, fish, shellfish, or live animals (by a butcher or veterinarian, for example)	*Erysipelothrix rhusiopathiae* *Streptococcus iniae* *Mycobacterium marinum*

(Adapted with permission from Swartz MN: Cellulitis. *N Engl J Med* 2004;350: 904-912.)

*Robin Patel, MD or the department with which she is affiliated has received research or institutional support from the Orthopaedic Research and Education Foundation. Robin Patel, MD has filed a patent application for an implant sonication apparatus and technique but has foregone the right to receive royalties.

1: General Considerations

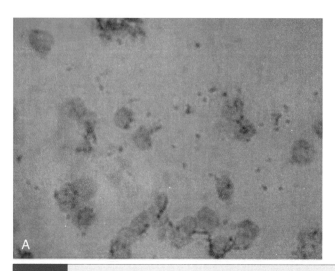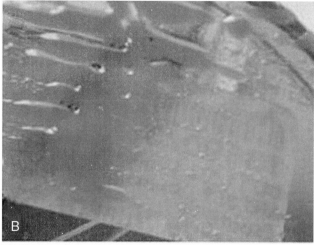

Figure 1   **A,** Gram-negative rods are often seen in smears; no specific morphologic characteristics differentiate *P aeruginosa* from enteric or other gram-negative rods in a specimen. **B,** On MacConkey agar, *P aeruginosa* does not ferment lactose and forms mucoid colonies as a result of overproduction of alginate, an exopolysaccharide.

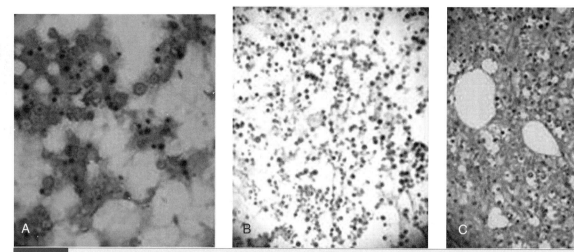

Figure 2   Subcutaneous cryptococcosis associated with blood-borne cellulitis is shown at low magnification (40×). The patient was immunocompromised. **A,** Gram staining shows encapsulated yeast cells in subcutaneous tissue. **B,** Gomori methenamine silver staining shows extracellular *C neoformans* yeast of varying size in an alveolar space. **C,** Hematoxylin and eosin staining of *C neoformans* organisms shows a clear capsule surrounding a pale blue nucleus. (Courtesy of A. Rodriguez, MD, Pamplona, Spain.)

Streptococcal or staphylococcal cellulitis also can occur in the leg of a patient whose saphenous vein has been harvested for coronary artery bypass. Crepitant cellulitis is produced by clostridia or non–spore-forming anaerobes such as *Bacteroides* species or *Peptostreptococcus* species, either alone or with facultative bacteria (particularly, *Escherichia coli*, *Klebsiella* species, or *Aeromonas* species).[1] Polymicrobial crepitant cellulitis of the left thigh can be associated with a colonic diverticular abscess.

Cellulitis only infrequently develops as a result of bacteremia. Pneumococcal cellulitis can occur on the face or limbs of a patient with diabetes mellitus, alcoholism, systemic lupus erythematosus, nephrotic syndrome, or a hematologic malignancy. Meningococcal cellulitis is rare and can affect children (typically as periorbital cellulitis) or adults (typically as cellulitis of an extremity). In a patient with cirrhosis, hemochromatosis, or thalassemia, *V vulnificus* can cause bacteremic cellulitis with prominent hemorrhagic bullae after the ingestion of raw oysters.[4] Bacteremia caused by gram-negative bacteria such as *E coli*, *Enterobacter* species, or *Proteus* species occasionally leads to soft-tissue infection, including cellulitis. *P aeruginosa* cellulitis can follow bacteremia in a patient with neutropenia (**Figure 1**). In an immunocompromised patient, less common opportunistic pathogens such as *Helicobacter cinaedi* (in a patient with human immunodeficiency virus [HIV]), *Cryptococcus neoformans*, or *Fusarium* species can cause blood-borne cellulitis[5-7] (**Figure 2**).

1: General Considerations

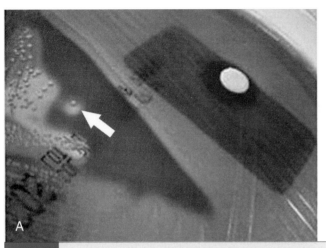
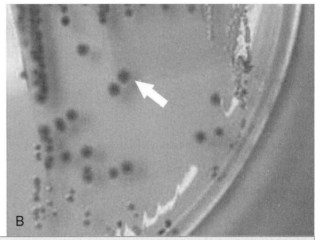

Figure 3 **A,** *Streptococcus pyogenes* (a group A streptococcus) forms β-hemolytic colonies *(arrow)* with inhibition of growth by bacitracin. **B,** Colonies on Granada agar are orange pigmented *(arrow)* and correspond to *Streptococcus agalactiae* (a group B streptococcus).

Erysipelas is a rapidly progressing infection of the dermis, with prominent lymphatic involvement and extension into the subcutaneous fat. It has an erythematous, indurated appearance with a raised border that demarcates it from adjacent normal skin.[1] The cause almost always is a group A or B *Streptococcus* (**Figure 3**). Serotype determination, exotoxin production, and clonality suggest that heterogeneous strains of group A streptococci can cause erysipelas. Other β-hemolytic streptococci, including those in group C and G, less commonly cause erysipelas but have a notable propensity to produce cellulitis in a patient with underlying venous or lymphatic compromise. Other microorganisms, including *S aureus*, *Streptococcus pneumoniae*, enterococci, and a variety of aerobic gram-negative bacilli, are rare causes of erysipelas.

Necrotizing Infections of the Skin and Fascia

Necrotizing infections of the skin and fascia, including necrotizing forms of cellulitis and fasciitis, can cause fulminant destruction of tissue, systemic signs of toxicity, and high mortality rates. However, some serious skin and subcutaneous tissue infections mimic the systemic collapse of necrotizing infections before significant areas of fascia or subcutaneous tissue become necrotic and before the development of interstitial gas or the classic mottled discoloration of the skin. These typically are monomicrobial infections, usually with a group A *Streptococcus* or MSRA. They infiltrate large areas of subcutaneous tissue in otherwise healthy patients, with deceivingly mild hypotension, tachycardia, and fever for several days, ultimately leading to rapid deterioration, cardiovascular collapse, multiorgan dysfunction, and death when homeostatic mechanisms are overwhelmed by the cytokine storm induced by bacterial exotoxins. A high index of suspicion and careful examination of the soft tissues for edema and faint hyper-

emia are essential for diagnosis and intervention before these patients develop shock.

Necrotizing Cellulitis

Several types of necrotizing cellulitis exist, including clostridial and nonclostridial anaerobic infections of the skin and subcutaneous tissue. Gas develops in the subcutaneous tissue. The fascia and deep muscle are generally spared. Nonclostridial anaerobic cellulitis typically is caused by infection with mixed anaerobic and aerobic organisms. Meleney ulcer, a progressive, synergistic gangrene that occurs after abdominal surgery, is characterized by an indolent, slowly expanding ulceration that is confined to the superficial fascia and subcutaneous tissue. It results from a synergistic interaction between *S aureus* and microaerophilic streptococci.[8] Synergistic necrotizing cellulitis is a variant of type I necrotizing fasciitis that involves the skin, fat, fascia, and muscle. It usually occurs in the leg or perineum of a patient with diabetes.

Necrotizing Fasciitis

Necrotizing fasciitis is a bacterial infection that spreads along fascial planes leading to progressive necrosis of fascia and subcutaneous fat. Type I necrotizing fasciitis is a mixed infection caused by aerobic and anaerobic bacteria. It most commonly occurs after a surgical procedure or in a patient who has diabetes, peripheral vascular disease, or both. In a 17-year study of the microbiologic and clinical characteristics of 83 patients with necrotizing fasciitis, aerobic or facultative bacteria were recovered from 10% of specimens; anaerobic bacteria, from 22%; and mixed aerobic-anaerobic flora, from 68%.[9] On average, 4.6 isolates per specimen were found; the 375 isolates included 105 aerobic or facultative bacteria and 270 anaerobic bacteria. The predominant aerobes were *S aureus*, *E coli*, and group A streptococci; the predominant anaerobes were

Peptostreptococcus species, *Prevotella* species, *Porphyromonas* species, the *Bacteroides fragilis* group, and *Clostridium* species. A correlation was found between specific clinical findings and bacteria: edema was associated with the *B fragilis* group, *Clostridium* species, *S aureus*, *Prevotella* species, and group A streptococci; gas and crepitus, with Enterobacteriaceae and *Clostridium* species; and foul odor, with *Bacteroides* species. In addition, a correlation was found between certain predisposing conditions and specific organisms: trauma, with *Clostridium* species; diabetes, with *Bacteroides* species, *S aureus,* and Enterobacteriaceae; and immunosuppression and malignancy with *Pseudomonas* species and Enterobacteriaceae. In the perineal area, penetration of the gastrointestinal or urethral mucosa by enteric organisms was found to cause Fournier gangrene (necrotizing fasciitis of the male genitalia).[10]

Type II necrotizing fasciitis is a monomicrobial infection usually caused by group A streptococci. Although group A streptococci are well known as a cause of necrotizing fasciitis, recognition and reporting of such infections have dramatically increased. Type II necrotizing fasciitis is commonly associated with early-onset shock and organ failure, called streptococcal toxic shock syndrome. Clinical reports and epidemiologic studies have repeatedly shown an association between streptococcal toxic shock syndrome and group A streptococcal strains of M protein types 1, 3, 12, and 28. Necrotizing fasciitis as a monomicrobial infection caused by MRSA also has been described.[11]

Myonecrosis

Myonecrosis is characterized by necrosis of muscle tissue without suppuration, vascular thrombosis, and histologic evidence of myositis. *Clostridium* species, typically *Clostridium perfringens*, are the usual causative organisms, but myonecrosis can occur as a component of necrotizing cellulitis caused by other organisms. A rare variant of necrotizing cellulitis of the head and neck caused by group A streptococci is associated with myonecrosis.[12] Systemic shock can develop, with acute renal failure and acute respiratory distress syndrome. Systemic shock is associated with superantigen production when *S pyogenes* is involved. Infection with *Clostridium septicum* causing gas gangrene usually arises from bacteremia secondary to a gastrointestinal tract lesion, which often represents a colonic malignancy. *Clostridium tertium* has been associated with spontaneous myonecrosis, typically caused by bacteremia in a patient who has received a long course of antimicrobial therapy. The bowel is the probable source of bacteremia; neutropenia also is a risk factor. *E coli* can cause myonecrosis associated with cellulitis, usually in a patient who is immunocompromised or has cirrhosis.[13] *Aeromonas* species can be very aggressive and should be considered in the differential diagnosis of a skin and soft-tissue infection with myonecrosis, especially in a

traumatic wound after freshwater exposure. *A hydrophila*, the most common *Aeromonas* species infecting humans, often occurs in combination with other organisms, leading to cellulitis, myonecrosis, or ecthyma gangrenosum. Although *A hydrophila* can exist in any aquatic environment, the infection typically is associated with fresh water and often with the anaerobic environment in mud at the bottom of a lake, pond, or river. *Edwardsiella tarda* was reported as the cause of myonecrosis in an immunocompetent patient after forearm laceration by a brick submerged in brackish water.[14]

Clinical entities including pyomyositis, necrotizing infection caused by *V vulnificus,* and some viral infections are sometimes confused with myonecrosis. Pyomyositis, a primary muscle abscess, can be caused by *S aureus* or occasionally another organism (Figure 4). Pyomyositis is most commonly found in patients who live in tropical areas or are HIV positive, as well as children who are infected with community-acquired MRSA. A necrotizing infection caused by *V vulnificus* can involve skin, fascia, and muscle, mostly commonly in a patient with cirrhosis, a person who consumed raw seafood, or an inhabitant of a coastal region. Viral infections, including acute influenza type A, can produce skeletal muscle injury and lead to rhabdomyolysis.

Septic Bursitis

Septic bursitis is an inflammation of the bursa from an infection caused by direct bacterial inoculation (such as from a puncture wound), contiguous spread of infection from nearby soft tissues (cellulitis), or hematogenous spread (bacterial endocarditis). In at least 80% of patients with culture-proven septic bursitis, *S aureus* is the causative organism. The next most commonly reported cause is a group A or B β-hemolytic *Streptococcus* species.[15] Infrequently reported causative organisms include coagulase-negative staphylococci, *Enterococcus* species, *E coli*, *P aeruginosa*, and anaerobes. Between 10% and 36% of patients with non–*S aureus* bursitis have a polymicrobial infection.[16] Subacute or chronic bursitis may be caused by *Brucella* species, mycobacteria such as *Mycobacterium tuberculosis* or nontuberculous mycobacteria, fungi, or algae such as *Prototheca* species.

Septic Arthritis

Infectious arthritis of one or more joints can be caused by diverse microorganisms (Table 2). Bacterial arthritis, the most common joint infection, is a medical emergency because it has the potential to cause rapid joint destruction with irreversible loss of function. In a native joint, bacterial arthritis is usually secondary to hematogenous seeding during transient or persistent bacteremia. Bacteria also can be introduced during joint surgery, joint aspiration, or local corticosteroid injec-

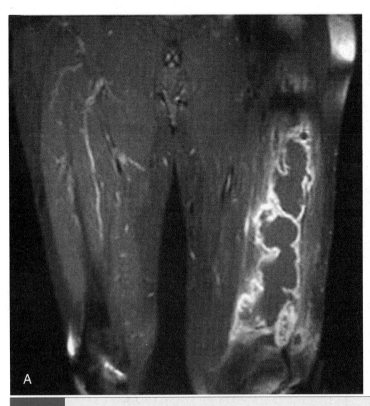
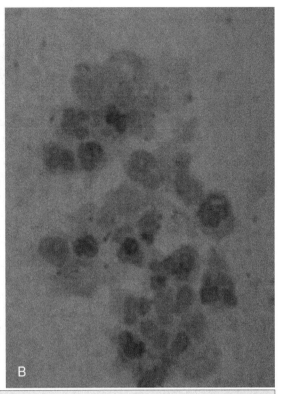

Figure 4 **A,** MRI of both upper legs shows an extensive encapsulated collection characteristic of primary muscle abscess affecting the external muscles of the left leg. **B,** Gram stain (100× magnification) of aspirated fluid shows gram-positive cocci in clusters identified as *S aureus*.

tion. A direct puncture wound does not usually serve as a portal of entry. In children, a focus of osteomyelitis in the metaphysis or epiphysis can spread to the adjacent joint.[17] Viral arthritis often involves multiple joints as a component of a systemic infection but generally does not lead to long-term morbidity. In contrast to acute bacterial or viral arthritis, a joint infection caused by mycobacteria or non–*Candida* fungi usually leads to chronic, slowly progressive monoarticular arthritis.

Nongonococcal bacterial arthritis can be the most dangerous and destructive form of acute arthritis. Although virtually any bacterium is capable of causing septic arthritis, *S aureus* and groups A, B, C, and G streptococci are more likely to cause joint infection than gram-negative bacilli, which typically produce joint infection only in a patient who has sustained trauma or has an underlying immunocompromised condition. Most patients with septic arthritis have a monomicrobial infection. Polymicrobial infection is rare and primarily occurs in patients with penetrating trauma that involves the joint space. *S aureus* is the bacterium that most commonly infects the joints of an adult, causing 80% of joint infections in patients who have concurrent rheumatoid arthritis or diabetes. *S aureus* also is the primary pathogen in hip infection and polyarticular septic arthritis.[18] Gram-negative bacilli are present more often than *S aureus* in neonates and people who are immunocompromised, older than 65

years, or users of illicit intravenous drugs. People who use illicit injected drugs may develop bacterial arthritis in an axial joint such as the sternoclavicular or sternomanubrial joint caused by *S aureus*, *P aeruginosa*, or *Candida albicans*.[19] Gram-negative bacilli are the most common pathogens in neonates and other children younger than 5 years (**Figure 5**). *S pneumoniae* causes a small but significant percentage of cases of septic arthritis in adults.[20] Anaerobes are occasionally involved in septic arthritis in a patient with diabetes. Between 10% and 20% of clinically diagnosed instances of bacterial arthritis are never confirmed by a positive synovial fluid or blood culture.[21]

In the United States, the most common form of bacterial arthritis in young, sexually active adults is disseminated gonococcal infection (**Figure 6**). Gonococcal arthritis can appear as acute monoarthritis, although migratory polyarthritis and tenosynovitis are more typical. Disseminated infection develops in 1% to 3% of patients with untreated gonorrhea.

Mycoplasma species can cause arthritis with many of the features of other forms of septic arthritis, and it has a predilection for patients who have hypogammaglobulinemia, are immunocompromised, have recently undergone urinary tract manipulation, or have recently given birth (**Figure 7**). A patient with Lyme disease may develop acute monoarthritis weeks or months after the appearance of the characteristic rash, fever, and migratory arthralgias. These patients usually live in or visited

Table 2

Microorganisms Isolated From Patients With Infectious Arthritis

Patient Characteristics	Common Microorganisms	Uncommon Microorganisms
Monoarthritis or oligoarthritis Age younger than 5 years	*S aureus* *Streptococcus* species *H influenzae* (if not vaccinated)	*Neisseria meningitidis* *Salmonella* species Gram-negative bacilli (*Kingella kingae* if age younger than 2 years)
Monoarthritis or oligoarthritis Age 5 to 60 years No immunocompromise	*S aureus* *Streptococcus* species *Neisseria gonorrhoeae*	*M tuberculosis* *Brucella* species *Borrelia burgdorferi* *P multocida* (animal bite) *Coccidioides immitis* *Blastomyces dermatitidis* Filariae
Monoarthritis or oligoarthritis Age older than 60 years Illicit intravenous drug use Comorbidity Immunocompromise	*S aureus* Gram-negative bacilli (*E coli*, *Pseudomonas* species, *Salmonella* species) *Streptococcus* species Oropharyngeal bacteria (*Fusobacterium* species, *Prevotella* species, *Pasteurella* species, *E corrodens*, *Peptostreptococcus* species, *Bacteroides* species)	*Nocardia* species *Mycobacterium* species (such as *M tuberculosis*, *M marinum*) *Mycoplasma hominis* *Ureaplasma urealyticum* *Candida* species Filamentous fungi (*Sporothrix schenckii*, *Aspergillus* species, *Pseudallescheria* species)
Prosthetic joint infection	Coagulase-negative staphylococci *Propionibacterium* species *S aureus* *Corynebacterium* species	*Candida* species *Brucella* species *Francisella tularensis* *Yersinia enterocolitica* *Campylobacter* species *Listeria monocytogenes* *P multocida* *M hominis* *S pneumoniae* *Tropheryma whippelii* *M tuberculosis* *Mycobacterium fortuitum* *Mycobacterium chelonae* *Aspergillus fumigatus*
Polyarthritis	*S aureus* Virus	*Neisseria* species *Streptobacillus moniliformis* *Treponema pallidum* *T whippelii* *Mycobacterium leprae*
Reactive arthritis	*Shigella* species *Y enterocolitica* *Chlamydia trachomatis*	*Salmonella* species *Campylobacter* species *Clostridium difficile* *Ureaplasma* species *Mycoplasma* species *Brucella* species *B burgdorferi* *N meningitidis* *Chlamydia pneumoniae* Parvovirus B19 *Giardia lamblia* *Schistosoma* species *S pyogenes*

an area with endemic Lyme disease and may or may not have discovered a tick bite. When arthritis appears, almost every patient has immunoglobulin G antibodies to *B burgdorferi*. Acute monoarthritis also can be caused by other spirochetes, including *T pallidum*.

Mycobacterial or fungal arthritis is much less common than bacterial arthritis. Although the reported incidence of tuberculous arthritis has not increased, the re-

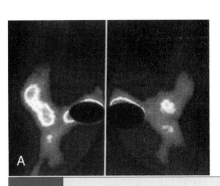
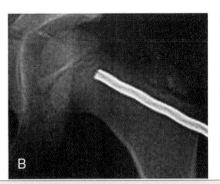
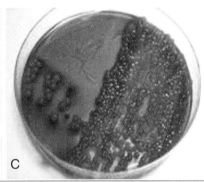

Figure 5   A, Left- and right-hip bone scans using ^{99m}Tc-phosphate show markedly increased perfusion in the left hip joint of a young child with arthritis, with extension to the femoral head. B, Tissue obtained for diagnosis through core biopsy. C, Lactose-fermenting colonies on a MacConkey agar plate were identified as *E coli*.

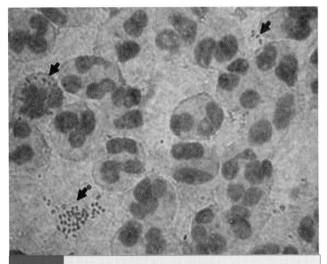

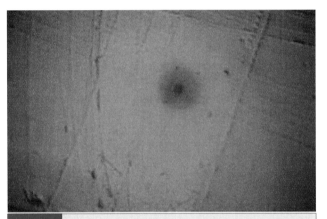

Figure 7   Colonies of *M hominis* on *Mycoplasma* glucose agar medium exhibit a characteristic fried egg appearance.

Figure 6   A synovial fluid Gram stain (×100) shows polymorphonuclear leukocytes and gram-negative diplococci *(arrows)* corresponding to *N gonorrhoeae*. Synovial fluid Gram staining is positive in fewer than 25% of patients with gonococcal arthritis. (Courtesy of M. Alonso, MD, Pamplona, Spain.)

cent increase in the incidence of pulmonary tuberculosis has revived awareness that mycobacteria can infect joints.[22] Nontuberculous mycobacterial infections can involve the synovium and should be considered in the differential diagnosis of synovitis, especially if the patient is immunocompromised or has received frequent joint injections with a corticosteroid.[22] Fungal arthritis is usually indolent, but acute monoarthritis caused by *B dermatitidis*, *C immitis*, *S schenckii*, *Scedosporium prolificans*, or *Candida* species has been reported.[23]

Septic arthritis is less common than osteomyelitis in patients with sickle cell disease. A prospective study of 14 patients with sickle cell disease and septic arthritis found that *S aureus* was the infecting organism in 11 patients, and *Salmonella* in 2 patients.[24]

Arthritis and arthralgia are well-recognized, relatively common consequences of viral infection. The viruses that most commonly cause arthritis or arthralgia include hu-

man parvovirus B19. The rubella virus, including the live attenuated virus in the rubella vaccine, is believed to grow preferentially in synovial tissues. Direction infection gives rise to symptoms. In 2004, the US Centers for Disease Control and Prevention announced that rubella (adult and congenital rubella syndrome) had been eliminated from the United States, and this clinical entity is no longer encountered in the United States. In patients who are HIV positive, arthritis sometimes occurs as painful articular syndrome, reactive arthritis, or septic arthritis. Joint symptoms and arthritis develop in 10% to 25% of patients with hepatitis B virus and 2% to 20% of patients with hepatitis C virus. Patients with cytomegalovirus or Epstein-Barr virus also can develop arthritis.[25] Acute monoarthritis is associated with mumps and many other viral infections, including infections from enteroviruses, adenovirus, coxsackievirus, echovirus, and herpes simplex virus.

Osteomyelitis

Normal bone is highly resistant to infection, which usually requires a very large inoculum, trauma, or a

1: General Considerations

foreign body. Identification of the causative microorganism is essential for diagnosis and treatment (**Table 3**). S aureus is by far the most common microorganism in any type of osteomyelitis.[26] The ability of S aureus to adhere and form biofilm is considered crucial for the early colonization of host tissues.

Acute osteomyelitis appears as a suppurative infection with acute inflammatory cells, accompanied by edema, vascular congestion, and small-vessel thrombosis. If both the medullary and periosteal blood supplies are compromised, large sequestered areas of dead bone can form. The pathologic features of chronic osteomyelitis include necrotic bone, new bone formation, and exudation of polymorphonuclear leukocytes as well as lymphocytes, histiocytes, and occasional plasma cells. Microbiologic culturing of the infected bone is required for diagnosis and appropriate treatment of chronic osteomyelitis (**Figure 8**). S aureus was isolated from 29% of specimens in one study. Also isolated, in descending order of frequency, were Enterobacteriaceae (16%); *Enterococcus* species (14.67%); anaerobic bacteria (10.67%); and, less frequently, *P aeruginosa*, coagulase-negative staphylococci, *Streptococcus* species, and the *Acinetobacter calcoaceticus-baumannii* complex. Anaerobic bone culturing yielded 16 organisms in 7 (14%) of 92 patients, primarily in association with violent trauma.[27]

Trauma and surgical procedures are the most common causes of adult osteomyelitis. In posttraumatic osteomyelitis, the infection often is polymicrobial. The pathogens may include normal skin flora or organisms from contaminated soil, water, clothing, or other environmental sources. Coagulase-negative staphylococci, S aureus, gram-negative aerobic bacilli, and anaerobic organisms were found to account for more than 75% of cultured bacteria in posttraumatic osteomyelitis.[28] Soil contamination of an open fracture can lead to an indolent infection caused by *Clostridium* species, *Bacillus* species, or *Nocardia* species (**Figure 9**). Contamination with fresh water can lead to infection with *Aeromonas* species or *Plesiomonas* species. *P aeruginosa* is the most common organism identified in osteomyelitis occurring after a puncture wound of the foot, in both adults and children.[29] Organisms such as MRSA or multidrug-resistant *P aeruginosa* can cause osteomyelitis as a complication of trauma, immunocompromise, or intravenous drug abuse.

Osteomyelitis associated with vascular insufficiency typically occurs in patients with diabetes, almost always after a soft-tissue infection of the foot spreading to bone. Although S aureus usually is responsible, other gram-positive or gram-negative aerobic or anaerobic bacteria also should be considered.

Hematogenous osteomyelitis usually occurs in prepubertal children and patients older than 65 years and is characterized by seeding of bacteria to bone that may be associated with minor blunt trauma. In children, the infection usually occurs as a single focus in the metaphyseal area of a long bone, particularly the tibia or femur.[26] The organisms most commonly encountered in neonates and infants include S aureus, coagulase-negative staphylococci, group B streptococci, and other streptococci.[30] Vaccination for H influenzae has substantially reduced the incidence of this cause of osteomyelitis in children. S aureus is the predominant cause after infancy, and gram-negative rods are found in people older than 65 years.[31]

Osteomyelitis is a common complication of sickle cell disease in children and young adults.[32] Blood cultures taken during sepsis associated with sickle cell disease most commonly yield S pneumoniae or H influenzae; however, osteomyelitis usually is caused by Salmonella species.[33]

Many other microorganisms are sometimes isolated from patients with osteomyelitis. The type of organism is related to epidemiologic factors and the presence of underlying disease. *Brucella* species, M tuberculosis, C burnetii, and endemic fungi are prevalent in some patient populations. Fungal osteomyelitis can be a complication of catheter-related fungemia, the use of drugs contaminated by *Candida* species, or prolonged neutropenia. *P aeruginosa* can be isolated from a patient who uses illicit injected drugs or has had a urinary catheter for a long period of time.[28]

Vertebral osteomyelitis typically involves two adjacent vertebral bodies in the lower thoracic or lumbar spine as well as the intervening disk space. Hematogenous spreading usually is responsible. In most studies conducted in a developed country, S aureus was found to account for more than 50% of infections.[34] The importance of MRSA as a cause of vertebral osteomyelitis has increased over time. Other important but less common pathogens include enteric gram-negative bacilli (particularly in infection after urinary tract instrumentation), *P aeruginosa*, and *Candida* species (frequently associated with intravascular catheter-related bacteremia or illicit injected drug use), group B and G streptococci (especially in patients with diabetes mellitus), and mycobacteria.[31] Bone and joint infection accounts for almost 2% of all instances of tuberculosis, including 10% to 35% of extrapulmonary tuberculosis. Musculoskeletal tuberculosis involves the spine in approximately half of all patients.[35] Spinal tuberculosis, also called Pott disease, most often affects the lumbar and lower thoracic region; upper thoracic or cervical disease is less common but potentially more disabling (**Figure 10**).

The organisms associated with vertebral osteomyelitis vary by geographic region. *Brucella melitensis* is an important pathogen in Middle Eastern and Mediterranean countries[36] (**Figure 11**). *Burkholderia pseudomallei* should be considered in patients from an equatorial region. *Salmonella* species and *Entamoeba histolytica* are occasionally responsible in Africa or South America. In addition, a patient who is immunosuppressed may be especially susceptible to certain pathogens including *Aspergillus* species, *Candida* species, and the M avium complex.

Table 3

Microorganisms Isolated From Patients With Bacterial Osteomyelitis

Patient Characteristics	Microorganisms
Any type of osteomyelitis	S aureus
Hematogenous osteomyelitis Age younger than 1 year	S aureus S agalactiae E coli
Hematogenous osteomyelitis Age 1 to 10 years	S aureus S pyogenes M tuberculosis Bartonella henselae
Hematogenous osteomyelitis Age older than 10 years	S aureus
Infection associated with foreign body or implant	Coagulase-negative staphylococci Propionibacterium species S aureus Corynebacterium species
Nosocomial infection	Enterobacteriaceae Pseudomonas species
Sickle cell disease	Salmonella species S pneumoniae
HIV infection	B henselae Bartonella quintana
Bite wound	P multocida E corrodens
Immunocompromise	Aspergillus species Candida species Mycobacterium avium complex
Association with tuberculosis-prevalent population	M tuberculosis
Association with pathogen-endemic population	Brucella species Coxiella burnetii B dermatitidis C immitis
Open bone fracture	Polymicrobial (S aureus, gram-negative bacilli, Clostridium species, Bacillus species)
Illicit intravenous drug use	S aureus P aeruginosa Enterobacteriaceae Candida species
Vertebral osteomyelitis	S aureus Brucella species E coli Salmonella species Enterobacteriaceae P aeruginosa M tuberculosis
Diabetic foot infection	S aureus P aeruginosa Streptococcus species Enterococcus species Coagulase-negative staphylococci Gram-negative aerobic bacilli Anaerobes

(Adapted with permission from Lew DP, Waldvogel FA: Osteomyelitis. *Lancet* 2004;364:369-379.)

1: General Considerations

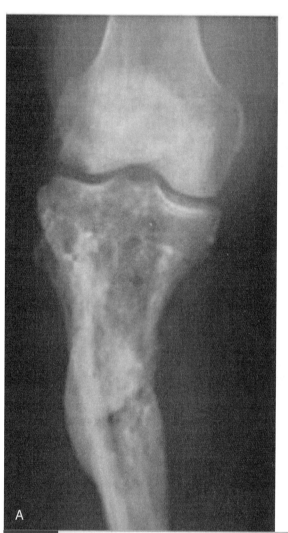
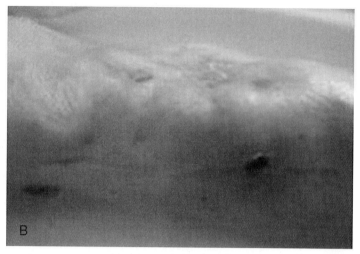
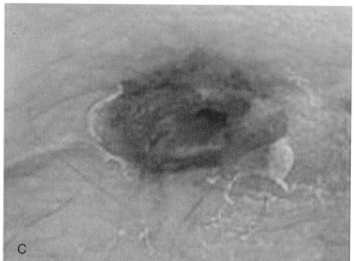

Figure 8	**A,** AP radiograph showing the femur of a patient with chronic osteomyelitis, with lucency and sclerotic areas. **B** and **C,** Photographs of the leg showing chronic fistulae to the skin. Diagnosis and therapy required microbiologic culturing of the infected bone after fistulae débridement.

Prosthesis-Related Infections

Infection of a prosthetic joint typically is caused by coagulase-negative staphylococci, S aureus, Propionibacterium acnes, or other microorganisms that produce biofilm, although virtually any microorganism can cause a prosthetic joint infection. Adherence of Staphylococcus epidermidis to the surface of a device involves rapid attachment mediated by specific adhesions or nonspecific factors such as surface tension, hydrophobicity, and electrostatic forces. Adherence of S aureus is more dependent on the presence of host-tissue ligands such as fibronectin, fibrinogen, and collagen. The microorganisms most commonly cultured from a prosthetic joint are coagulase-negative staphylococci (found in 30% to 40% of patients), S aureus (12% to 23%), mixed flora (10% to 11%), streptococci (9% to 10%), gram-negative bacilli (3% to 6%), enterococci (3% to 7%), and anaerobes (2% to 4%). No microorganisms were found in cultures from approximately 11% of patients with an apparent infection.[37] A virulent microorganism such as S aureus grown in culture from a prosthetic joint usually indicates infection. In contrast, a low-virulence microorganism such as coagulase-negative staphylococci or P acnes, as typically found in normal skin flora, may be a pathogen or a contaminant.[38] The location of the prosthesis must be considered in determining the importance of an isolated microorganism. P acnes is rarely the cause of infection after hip or knee arthroplasty but is a relatively common cause of infection after shoulder arthroplasty.[39]

The distribution of organisms varies with the length of time since implantation as well as the source of infection. Most early-onset infections (occurring within 3 months of surgery) result from contamination of the surgical wound by bacteria either from the patient's skin or from people or objects in the operating room.

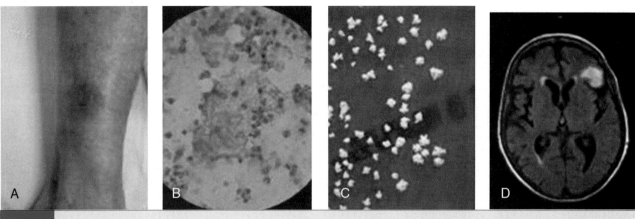

Figure 9   Disseminated nocardiosis occurred in a patient who had received a liver transplant. (*Nocardia* species tend to become disseminated in patients who are immunocompromised.) **A,** The patient had erythema and pain in the right lower extremity after traumatic laceration from a tree branch contaminated with soil. Osteomyelitis was diagnosed. **B,** Staining of a surgical specimen (100× magnification) revealed gram-positive beaded branching filaments. **C,** Culturing identified *Nocardia asteroides.* **D,** MRI revealed two frontal abscesses.

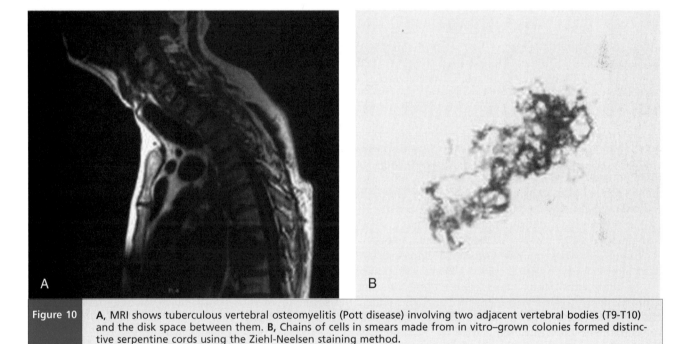

Figure 10   **A,** MRI shows tuberculous vertebral osteomyelitis (Pott disease) involving two adjacent vertebral bodies (T9-T10) and the disk space between them. **B,** Chains of cells in smears made from in vitro–grown colonies formed distinctive serpentine cords using the Ziehl-Neelsen staining method.

More than three fourths of early-onset infections are caused by a virulent microorganism such as *S aureus.*[38] Patients with postsurgical wound dehiscence may develop a prosthesis infection through contiguous spread of organisms such as gram-negative rods from the superficial wound to deeper structures. Most polymicrobial infections are early-onset infections.[40] A delayed-onset infection (occurring 3 to 24 months after surgery) also is usually acquired during implantation. As is consistent with the indolent character of a delayed infection, the cause usually is a less virulent organism such as a coagulase-negative staphylococcus or *P acnes.*[38] A late-onset infection (occurring more than 24 months af-

ter surgery) usually is caused by hematogenous seeding of the surface of the bioprosthetic material and damaged joint tissues. In approximately half of these patients, *S aureus* is the cause.[41] Small-colony variants of *S aureus* have been identified after the failure of treatment with a standard antimicrobial regimen.[42] These strains appear to emerge in patients initially infected with normally growing *S aureus.* The infection can be difficult to diagnose because of the slow-growing nature of the organisms and their auxotrophic phenotype.

Recent studies have found that prosthetic joint infection can be caused by zoonotic microorganisms, fungi, mycobacteria, or other unusual microorganisms.[43] In

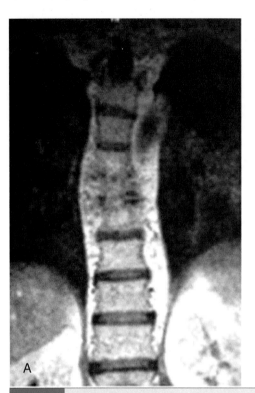
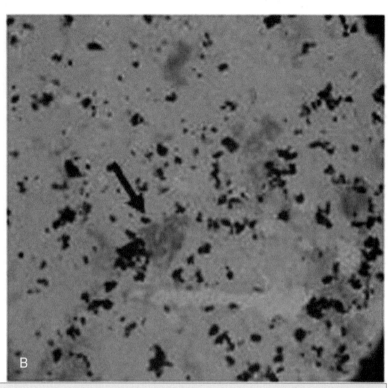

Figure 11 **A,** MRI shows brucellar spondylodiskitis involving T7 through T9. **B,** Gram stain of a positive blood culture (100× magnification) shows gram-negative coccobacilli *(arrow)* identified as *B melitensis*. This organism can be hazardous to laboratory workers, and the laboratory should be notified if it is suspected.

determining the etiology of a prosthetic joint infection, it is crucial to maintain a high index of suspicion for these unusual microorganisms and to request appropriate laboratory tests. Prosthetic joint infection caused by *Brucella* species was reported in four patients after total hip arthroplasty and six patients after total knee arthroplasty;[43] all 10 patients had occupational exposure to *Brucella* species or had consumed unpasteurized dairy products. *F tularensis* caused chronic infection of a total knee arthroplasty in a patient with rheumatoid arthritis being treated with methotrexate; the patient had a wood tick bite before the total knee arthroplasty.[44] Prosthetic joint infection caused by *Y enterocolitica* was reported in two patients who were older than 65 years and had hemarthrosis associated with anticoagulation therapy.[45,46] Infection of a total hip or knee arthroplasty caused by *Campylobacter jejuni, Campylobacter lari, Campylobacter fetus,* or *Campylobacter upsaliensis* also has been reported, usually in a patient who is immunocompromised.[43] Prosthetic joint infection with *L monocytogenes* usually occurs in patients with a malignancy, diabetes mellitus, renal disease, or liver disease, as well as patients who are older than 65 years or are receiving immunosuppressive therapy. However, prosthetic joint infection with *L monocytogenes* can occur in patients who are not immunocompromised. In 19 reports of prosthetic joint infection caused by *P multocida,* most involved total knee arthroplasty in a patient who was immunocompromised as a result

of diabetes mellitus, rheumatoid arthritis, or acute leukemia.[43] Almost all of the patients had a history of an animal bite or other animal contact with the lower extremity containing the prosthetic joint. *M hominis* was reported as the cause of prosthetic joint infection in two patients.[47] Hematogenous infection of a joint prosthesis by *S pneumoniae* was reported.[48] *Corynebacterium* species also can cause prosthetic joint infection.[49] *T whippelii* was reported as the cause of a prosthetic joint infection 2 years after successful antimicrobial treatment of the gastrointestinal manifestations of Whipple disease.[50]

Prosthetic joint infection with *M tuberculosis* usually involves the hip or knee and results from local reactivation or, less often, hematogenous spread of infection. A retrospective study of 2,116 episodes of prosthetic joint infection over a 22-year period found that only 7 (0.3%) were caused by *M tuberculosis*, and a coinfecting bacterial pathogen was detected in 5 of the 7 infections.[51] Rheumatoid arthritis, long-term steroid use, and pulmonary disease predispose a patient to prosthetic joint infection with *M tuberculosis*. Most prosthetic joint infections caused by *M fortuitum* occur during the early postsurgical period. In contrast, *M chelonae* has been reported as a cause of late prosthetic joint infection.[43] Complex prosthetic joint infection caused by *M avium* was reported in two patients; one patient was HIV positive, and the other had received a renal transplant.[52]

Prosthetic knee infection caused by *A fumigatus* was reported in two patients; one patient was being treated with steroids, and the other had an osteosarcoma.[53] Other unusual causes of fungal prosthetic joint infection include *Rhodotorula minuta*, *Histoplasma capsulatum*, and *S schenckii*. Although prosthetic joint infection with *Candida* species is rare, it is increasingly reported.[43]

Infection with *Echinococcus* species was reported as a complication of total hip arthroplasty in a patient with rheumatoid arthritis; cysts were present at the time of surgery.[54]

Diabetic Foot Infection

Patients with diabetes are at particularly high risk of infection with microorganisms including *S aureus*, group B streptococci, *Klebsiella* species, *Candida* species, Zygomycetes, and *M tuberculosis*. Diabetic foot infection is responsible for substantial morbidity, psychosocial disruption, and financial cost. The infection may be a primary diabetic foot condition or a complication of an existing lesion. Additional information on diabetic foot infections is presented in chapter 20.

Although not all neuropathic foot ulcers become infected, they are a common portal of entry for infection on the plantar surface of the foot. Infection is suggested by the presence of local inflammation, purulent drainage, sinus tract formation, or crepitus. Cellulitis can vary in severity from a mild localized process to a limb-threatening necrotizing process with fasciitis or gangrene. Most mild infections are caused by aerobic gram-positive cocci, such as *S aureus* or streptococci. Deeper, limb-threatening infections usually are polymicrobial and can be caused by aerobic gram-positive cocci, gram-negative bacilli (such as *E coli*, *Klebsiella* species, or *Proteus* species), or anaerobes (*Bacteroides* species, *Peptostreptococcus* species). Anaerobes usually are not the sole isolated organisms. Coagulase-negative staphylococci, enterococci, and *Corynebacterium* species can act as pathogens, colonizers, or contaminants. If they are cultured with typically virulent organisms, their pathogenicity can be difficult to discern. A superficial swabbing of a diabetic foot ulcer frequently does not capture the organisms responsible for deeper infection. In a patient with a chronic ulcer or a patient previously treated with antimicrobial agents, the infection usually is polymicrobial and may be caused by *Enterococcus* species, *P aeruginosa*, Enterobacteriaceae, anaerobes, or a combination of these organisms.[55]

Several *Candida* species can cause a diabetic foot infection.[56] The most common is *Candida parapsilosis*, followed in order of descending frequency by *Candida tropicalis*; *C albicans* and *Candida glabrata*; and *Candida krusei*, *Candida kefyr*, *Candida famata*, and *Candida lipolytica*. Mixed fungal-bacterial infections are found twice as frequently as purely fungal infections.

Mixed infections tend to be more severe, causing wet gangrene of a single toe or the whole foot or a deep abscess of the plantar space.

Puncture Wounds to the Plantar Surface of the Foot

Infections complicating a plantar puncture wound can be caused by a variety of microorganisms, including *S aureus* and group A β-hemolytic streptococci. The infecting microorganism varies with the circumstances of the injury. *P aeruginosa* or other gram-negative bacteria are commonly isolated in patients with a plantar puncture that occurred while they were wearing athletic shoes. The moist inner sole of the shoe provides a suitable environment for growth of this organism. A plantar puncture that occurred in a barnyard may lead to infection caused by bowel flora of farm animals; an injury that occurred in fresh water raises the possibility of infection with *Aeromonas* species. Osteomyelitis after a puncture injury most likely was caused by *S aureus* in a person with diabetes or by *P aeruginosa* in other patients.

Orthopaedic Surgical Site Infections

Surgical site infection, as defined by the Centers for Disease Control and Prevention, includes one or more of the following features: purulent exudate draining from a surgical site, a positive culture (fluid or tissue) obtained from a primarily closed surgical site, a surgeon's clinical diagnosis of infection, and a culture-positive surgical site that requires reopening.[57] Most surgical site infections occur during surgery via direct inoculation of endogenous patient flora. In a clean procedure, normal skin flora are the most common cause. As with prosthetic joint infection, *S aureus* is the organism usually responsible for early-onset infection, and coagulase-negative staphylococci are involved in most indolent, delayed-onset infections. The percentage of surgical site infections caused by antibiotic-resistant pathogens such as MRSA or vancomycin-resistant enterococci has increased during the past decade.[58] In addition, fungi, particularly *C albicans*, have been isolated from an increasing percentage of surgical site infections. Exogenous sources of infection include contamination of the surgical site by flora from the operating room environment or personnel, including group A streptococci or gram-negative bacilli. Rare outbreaks or clusters of surgical site infection caused by unusual pathogens such as *Mycobacterium abscessus* have been traced to contaminated dressings, bandages, irrigants, or disinfectant solutions.[59] *C septicum* and other *Clostridium* species can be transmitted from a contaminated musculoskeletal allograft harvested from cadaver tissue.[60]

Bite Wounds

Approximately half of all people living in the United States sustain a human or animal bite wound during their lifetime. Bite wounds account for approximately 1% of all emergency department visits and expenditures of more than $30 million annually.[61] The most serious complication of a bite wound is infection with organisms that can originate from the biter or the person who was bitten. The relative risk varies with the species of the bite-inflicting animal, the bite location, patient-related factors, and the adequacy of local wound care. Additional information on bite wounds is presented in chapter 15.

Human bite wounds have long been associated with severe infections. Normal human mouth and skin flora are the usual pathogens in human bite wound infections. The organisms recovered from other animal bite wounds are similar, except that *P multocida* is rare in human bite wounds. *E corrodens*, a gram-negative bacterium, is a common constituent of human mouth flora but is rarely recovered from an animal bite wound. Aerobic gram-positive cocci and anaerobes also are more frequently found in a human bite wound than in an animal bite wound. A multicenter prospective study of 50 patients with an infected human bite wound found a median of four isolates per wound culture (three aerobes and one anaerobe).[62] Both aerobes and anaerobes were isolated from 54% of wounds, aerobes alone were isolated from 44%, and anaerobes alone were isolated from 2%. The isolates included *Streptococcus anginosus* (52%), *S aureus* (30%), *E corrodens* (30%), *Fusobacterium nucleatum* (32%), *Prevotella melaninogenica* (22%), and *Candida* species (8%). Numerous other infectious organisms can be transmitted through a human bite wound, including those responsible for hepatitis B and C, syphilis, and herpes simplex. The risk of transmitting HIV through saliva is extremely low, even if blood is present in the saliva. Tetanus has been found to result from a human bite wound.[62]

Most infections caused by mammalian bites are polymicrobial, with mixed aerobic and anaerobic species. Dogs account for 80% to 90% of all bite injuries in the United States. The possibility of rabies exposure should be considered in most bite injuries, especially after an unprovoked attack or a bite by an animal that appeared ill or stray. Rabies can be transmitted through a bite, scratch, or abrasion or through contact with saliva via the mucous membranes or a skin break.[63] The pathogens recovered from dog and cat bite wounds are similar. *Pasteurella* species are the most common, with *Pasteurella canis* predominating in dog bite wounds and *P multocida* and *Pasteurella septica* most common in cat bite wounds. Staphylococci, streptococci, and *Bacteroides* species are common in both dog and cat bite wounds. The anaerobes typically found in infected dog and cat bite wounds include *Bacteroides* species, *Peptostreptococcus* species, *Actinomyces* species, *Fuso-*

bacterium species, *Porphyromonas* species, and *Veillonella parvula*.

Rat bite fever, caused by *S moniliformis*, is a systemic illness characterized by fever, rigors, and polyarthralgia. If left untreated, rat bite fever has a 10% mortality rate. The nonspecific initial appearance of the disease and the difficulty of culturing its causative organism can result in a significant delay or failure of diagnosis.[64] *Spirillum minus* also has been implicated in infected rat bite wounds.

The aerobes most frequently isolated from the mouths and gingival scrapings of 10 south Louisiana alligators were *A hydrophila*, *Proteus vulgaris*, several *Pseudomonas* species, and *Citrobacter freundii*; the anaerobes included *Clostridium* species, *Bacteroides* species, *Fusobacterium varium*, and *Peptococcus prevotii*. Fungi also were recovered. Iguanas frequently carry unusual subtypes of fecal *Salmonella* species, which are an important cause of salmonellosis in children younger than 5 years. *V vulnificus* and other *Vibrio* species, *E rhusiopathiae*, and *M marinum* are often isolated from shark bite wounds.

Summary

The microbiology of a musculoskeletal infection must be established to guide specific treatment. Musculoskeletal infections can be caused by diverse microorganisms that can invade soft tissue, muscle, and bone from contiguous sites or by hematogenous spread from a distant site. Classifying these infections by epidemiologic features, anatomic location, and clinical manifestations can be useful in determining the best methods for sampling and culturing. Some types of musculoskeletal infections are uncommon, such as myositis. Others are considered a medical emergency, such as clostridial myonecrosis or infectious arthritis; are difficult to treat, such as osteomyelitis; or are associated with great morbidity and medical cost, such as prosthetic joint infections.

Annotated References

1. Swartz MN: Cellulitis. *N Engl J Med* 2004;350: 904-912.

   This review of cellulitis includes a case study, the evidence supporting different treatment strategies, a discussion of formal guidelines, and clinical recommendations.

2. Moran GJ, Krishnadasan A, Gorwitz RJ, et al: Methicillin-resistant *S. aureus* infections among patients in the emergency department. *N Engl J Med* 2006;355: 666-674.

   MRSA was the most common identifiable cause of skin and soft-tissue infection among emergency department patients in 11 US cities. Whenever antimicrobial therapy is indicated for the treatment of skin or soft-tissue infection, clinicians should consider obtaining cultures and modifying empirical therapy to provide MRSA coverage.

3. Aabideen KK, Munshi V, Kumar VB, Dean F: Orbital cellulitis in children: A review of 17 cases in the UK. *Eur J Pediatr* 2006;165(suppl 1):53.

A retrospective study of all children admitted with orbital cellulitis to two British hospitals between 1996 and 2004 found that orbital cellulitis can be treated completely, without any sequelae. The *H influenzae* type b vaccine has eliminated *H influenzae* as a significant cause of orbital cellulitis in children.

4. Chuang YC, Yuan CY, Liu CY, Lan CK, Huang AH: *Vibrio vulnificus* infection in Taiwan: Report of 28 cases and review of clinical manifestations and treatment. *Clin Infect Dis* 1992;15:271-276.

5. Kiehlbauch JA, Tauxe RV, Baker CN, Wachsmuth IK: *Helicobacter cinaedi*-associated bacteremia and cellulitis in immunocompromised patients. *Ann Intern Med* 1994;121:90-93.

6. Horrevorts AM, Huysmans FT, Koopman RJ, Meis JF: Cellulitis as first clinical presentation of disseminated cryptococcosis in renal transplant recipients. *Scand J Infect Dis* 1994;26:623-626.

7. Nucci M, Anaissie E: Cutaneous infection by *Fusarium* species in healthy and immunocompromised hosts: Implications for diagnosis and management. *Clin Infect Dis* 2002;35:909-920.

8. Wong CH, Song C, Ong YS, Tan BK, Tan KC, Foo CL: Abdominal wall necrotizing fasciitis: It is still "Meleney's Minefield." *Plast Reconstr Surg* 2006;117: 147e-150e.

A 66-year-old woman with poorly controlled diabetes mellitus was admitted for right loin pain of 7 days' duration and vomiting. Necrotizing fasciitis was diagnosed. Seven wound débridements were required to achieve control of the infection. Wound coverage was achieved with split-thickness skin grafting. In many clinical series, delayed recognition or diagnosis of necrotizing fasciitis with consequent delayed surgical débridement has been shown to increase mortality.

9. Stevens DL: Streptococcal toxic shock syndrome associated with necrotizing fasciitis. *Annu Rev Med* 2000;51: 271-288.

10. Marinella MA: Group C streptococcal sepsis complicating Fournier gangrene. *South Med J* 2005;98:921-923.

In a young man with diabetes, Fournier gangrene was associated with group C streptococcal bacteremia. This association had not been previously reported. Patients typically have systemic toxicity and significant inflammatory changes in the scrotum and perineum. Fournier gangrene usually is polymicrobic and requires urgent surgical débridement and broad-spectrum antibiotic therapy.

11. Miller LG, Perdreau-Remington F, Rieg G, et al: Necrotizing fasciitis caused by community-associated methicillin-resistant *Staphylococcus aureus* in Los Angeles. *N Engl J Med* 2005;352:1445-1453.

The records of 843 patients with wound-cultured MSRA were reviewed after treatment in 2003 and 2004. Fourteen had community-acquired necrotizing fasciitis, necrotizing myositis, or both. Necrotizing fasciitis caused by community-associated MRSA is an emerging clinical entity.

12. Baevsky RH, Ishida JT, Lieberman SA: Group A beta-hemolytic streptococcal glossal necrotizing myositis: Case report and review. *MedGenMed* 2005;7:8.

The first known instance of glossal necrotizing myositis caused by a group A streptococcus was in an 8-year-old girl receiving long-term nonsteroidal anti-inflammatory drugs, immunomodulators, and steroids for juvenile rheumatoid arthritis. Treatment with partial glossectomy and parenteral antimicrobial therapy led to full recovery after a critical course.

13. Berk DR, Ahmed A: Bullous cellulitis and myonecrosis secondary to *Escherichia coli* in a patient with cirrhosis. *Clin Exp Dermatol* 2006;31:592-593.

Bullous or crepitant cellulitis in an immunocompromised patient, especially a patient with cirrhosis, should raise suspicion of *E coli*, particularly after failure of traditional antimicrobial coverage.

14. Slaven EM, Lopez FA, Hart SM, Sanders CV: Myonecrosis caused by *Edwardsiella tarda*: A case report and case series of extraintestinal E. tarda infections. *Clin Infect Dis* 2001;32:1430-1433.

15. Small LN, Ross JJ: Suppurative tenosynovitis and septic bursitis. *Infect Dis Clin North Am* 2005;19:991-1005.

Empiric antibiotic coverage for suppurative tenosynovitis and septic bursitis should be directed toward staphylococci and streptococci. The patient's characteristics and epidemiologic exposures may suggest an unusual causative organism such as *N gonorrhoeae*, *P multocida*, *Prototheca* species, a nontuberculous mycobacterium, or a fungus.

16. Zimmermann B III, Mikolich DJ, Ho G Jr: Septic bursitis. *Semin Arthritis Rheum* 1995;24:391-410.

17. Le Dantec L, Maury F, Flipo RM, et al: Peripheral pyogenic arthritis: A study of one hundred seventy-nine cases. *Rev Rhum Engl Ed* 1996;63:103-110.

18. Goldenberg DL: Septic arthritis. *Lancet* 1998;351: 197-202.

19. Ross JJ, Shamsuddin H: Sternoclavicular septic arthritis: Review of 180 cases. *Medicine (Baltimore)* 2004;83: 139-148.

In 180 patients with sternoclavicular septic arthritis, *S aureus* was responsible for 49% of infections and was the major cause in users of illicit intravenous drugs. *P aeruginosa* infection in injection drug users declined dramatically when an epidemic of pentazocine abuse ended during the 1980s.

1: General Considerations

20. Ross JJ, Saltzman CL, Carling P, Shapiro DS: Pneumococcal septic arthritis: Review of 190 cases. *Clin Infect Dis* 2003;36:319-327.

   Uncomplicated pneumococcal septic arthritis was treatable with arthrocentesis and 4 weeks of antimicrobial therapy. Pneumococcal prosthetic joint infection usually could be treated without prosthesis removal. One death from septic arthritis caused by a β-lactam–resistant strain of *S pneumoniae* was reported.

21. Ryan MJ, Kavanagh R, Wall PG, Hazleman BL: Bacterial joint infections in England and Wales: Analysis of bacterial isolates over a four year period. *Br J Rheumatol* 1997;36:370-373.

22. Gardam M, Lim S: Mycobacterial osteomyelitis and arthritis. *Infect Dis Clin North Am* 2005;19:819-830.

   Physicians can expect to see more mycobacterial bone and joint disease in North America as a result of increased travel, immigration, and immunosuppressive medication use. A long-standing, untreated mycobacterial infection typically causes significant bone destruction and loss of function. Treatment requires prolonged antimicrobial therapy, often in conjunction with surgical intervention.

23. Dalton PA, Munckhof WJ, Walters DW: *Scedosporium prolificans*: An uncommon cause of septic arthritis. *ANZ J Surg* 2006;76:661-663.

   S prolificans is an emerging fungal pathogen that has a predilection for bone and cartilaginous surfaces and is resistant to many commonly prescribed antifungal agents. Septic arthritis caused by *S prolificans* was successfully treated with a combination of surgery and new antifungal agents.

24. Sankaran-Kutty M, Sadat-Ali M, Kutty MK: Septic arthritis in sickle cell disease. *Int Orthop* 1988;12:255-257.

25. Franssila R, Hedman K: Infection and musculoskeletal conditions: Viral causes of arthritis. *Best Pract Res Clin Rheumatol* 2006;20:1139-1157.

   Postinfection arthritis is a typical manifestation of arthritogenic alphaviruses, rubella virus, and human parvovirus B19. Arthritis also occurs after infection by HIV, cytomegalovirus, hepatitis B virus, hepatitis C virus, or Epstein-Barr virus. Prolonged arthritis in particular results from alphaviruses and human parvovirus B19.

26. Lew DP, Waldvogel FA: Osteomyelitis. *Lancet* 2004;364:369-379.

   Different types of osteomyelitis require different medical and surgical strategies. A multidisciplinary approach usually is required, particularly for complex osteomyelitis with soft-tissue loss, and should involve expertise in infectious diseases as well as orthopaedic, plastic, and vascular surgery.

27. Zuluaga AF, Galvis W, Saldarriaga JG, Agudelo M, Salazar BE, Vesga O: Etiologic diagnosis of chronic osteomyelitis: A prospective study. *Arch Intern Med* 2006;166:95-100.

   Nonbone and bone specimens were taken for complete microbiologic analysis from patients with chronic osteomyelitis at the conclusion of antimicrobial therapy. Diagnosis and therapy required microbiologic culturing of infected bone; nonbone specimens were not valid for this purpose. Bone cultures allowed agent identification in 94% of patients, including anaerobic bacteria in 14%. Cultures of nonbone and bone specimens gave identical results in 30% of patients, with slightly better concordance in chronic osteomyelitis caused by *S aureus* (42%) than by all other bacterial species (22%).

28. Lew DP, Waldvogel FA: Osteomyelitis. *N Engl J Med* 1997;336:999-1007.

29. Lavery LA, Walker SC, Harkless LB, Felder-Johnson K: Infected puncture wounds in diabetic and nondiabetic adults. *Diabetes Care* 1995;18:1588-1591.

30. Wong M, Isaacs D, Howman-Giles R, Uren R: Clinical and diagnostic features of osteomyelitis occurring in the first three months of life. *Pediatr Infect Dis J* 1995;14:1047-1053.

31. Patzakis MJ, Rao S, Wilkins J, Moore TM, Harvey PJ: Analysis of 61 cases of vertebral osteomyelitis. *Clin Orthop Relat Res* 1991;264:178-183.

32. Piehl FC, Davis RJ, Prugh SI: Osteomyelitis in sickle cell disease. *J Pediatr Orthop* 1993;13:225-227.

33. Thanni LOA: Bacterial osteomyelitis in major sickling haemoglobinopathies: Geographic difference in pathogen prevalence. *Afr Health Sci* 2006;6:236-239.

   A meta-analysis of 15 publications found 281 isolates. In sub-Saharan Africa, 46% of the pathogens were *Salmonella*, and 29% were staphylococci; in the United States, the corresponding figures were 70% and 26%.

34. Torda AJ, Gottlieb T, Bradbury R: Pyogenic vertebral osteomyelitis: Analysis of 20 cases and review. *Clin Infect Dis* 1995;20:320-328.

35. Vohra R, Kang HS, Dogra S, Saggar RR, Sharma R: Tuberculous osteomyelitis. *J Bone Joint Surg Br* 1997;79:562-566.

36. Colmenero JD, Cisneros JM, Orjuela DL, et al: Clinical course and prognosis of Brucella spondylitis. *Infection* 1992;20:38-42.

37. Segawa H, Tsukayama DT, Kyle RF, Becker DA, Gustilo RB: Infection after total knee arthroplasty: A retrospective study of the treatment of eighty-one infections. *J Bone Joint Surg Am* 1999;81:1434-1445.

38. Zimmerli W, Trampuz A, Ochsner PE: Prosthetic-joint infections. *N Engl J Med* 2004;351:1645-1654.

   Prosthetic joint infection causes significant morbidity and substantial health care expenditures. Perioperative antimicrobial prophylaxis and a laminar airflow surgical environment have reduced the risk of intrasurgical infection to less than 1% in hip and shoulder replacement and 2% in knee replacement.

39. Sperling JW, Kozak TK, Hanssen AD, Cofield RH: Infection after shoulder arthroplasty. *Clin Orthop Relat Res* 2001;382:206-216.

40. Moran E, Masters S, Berendt AR, McLardy-Smith P, Byren I, Atkins BL: Guiding empirical antibiotic therapy in orthopaedics: The microbiology of prosthetic joint infection managed by debridement, irrigation and prosthesis retention. *J Infect* 2007;55:1-7.

Retrospective review of patients with prosthetic joint infection admitted to one institution from 1998 to 2003 found that most infections involved staphylococci. MRSA was infrequently isolated. Polymicrobial infection usually was early onset.

41. Murdoch DR, Roberts SA, Fowler Jr VG Jr, et al: Infection of orthopedic prostheses after *Staphylococcus aureus* bacteremia. *Clin Infect Dis* 2001;32:647-649.

42. Sendi P, Rohrbach M, Graber P, Frei R, Ochsner PE, Zimmerli W: *Staphylococcus aureus* small colony variants in prosthetic joint infection. *Clin Infect Dis* 2006;43:961-967.

Poor response to adequate antimicrobial and surgical treatment in implant-associated staphylococcal infection should lead to active investigation of small-colony variants. In a case series, two-stage exchange without spacer implantation, combined with antimicrobial therapy and an implant-free interval of 6 to 8 weeks, produced successful outcomes at a mean 24-month follow-up.

43. Marculescu CE, Berbari EF, Cockerill FR III, Osmon DR: Fungi, mycobacteria, zoonotic and other organisms in prosthetic joint infection. *Clin Orthop Relat Res* 2006;451:64-72.

A diagnosis of prosthetic joint infection caused by a zoonotic microorganism, a fungus, a mycobacterium, or another unusual microorganism typically necessitates specialized diagnostic tests and antimicrobials. Collaboration with an infectious disease specialist is advisable.

44. Cooper CL, Van Caeseele P, Canvin J, Nicolle LE: Chronic prosthetic device infection with *Francisella tularensis*. *Clin Infect Dis* 1999;29:1589-1591.

45. Oni JA, Kangesu T: *Yersinia enterocolitica* infection of a prosthetic knee joint. *Br J Clin Pract* 1991;45:225.

46. Iglesias L, Garcia-Arenzana JM, Valiente A, Gomariz M, Perez-Trallero E: *Yersinia enterocolitica* O:3 infection of a prosthetic knee joint related to recurrent hemarthrosis. *Scand J Infect Dis* 2002;34:132-133.

47. Madoff S, Hooper DC: Nongenitourinary infections caused by *Mycoplasma hominis* in adults. *Rev Infect Dis* 1988;10:602-613.

48. Bertani A, Drouin C, Demortiere E, Gonzalez JF, Candoni P, Di Schino M: A prosthetic joint infection caused by *Streptococcus pneumoniae*: A case report and review of the literature. *Rev Chir Orthop Reparatrice Appar Mot* 2006;92:610-614.

A total knee prosthesis infected with *S pneumoniae* was removed from an 82-year-old woman in poor health. The variability in treatment of these rare infections probably is related to their occurrence in seriously ill patients. Mortality is high, and a specific treatment cannot be proposed.

49. Tleyjeh IM, Qutub MO, Bakleh M, Sohail MR, Virk A: *Corynebacterium jeikeium* prosthetic joint infection: Case report and literature review. *Scand J Infect Dis* 2005;37:151-153.

Corynebacterium prosthetic joint infection was successfully treated with partial prosthesis removal and long-term antibiotic administration. This extremely rare infection is commonly treated with resection arthroplasty.

50. Fresard A, Guglielminotti C, Berthelot P, et al: Prosthetic joint infection caused by *Tropheryma whippelii* (Whipple's bacillus). *Clin Infect Dis* 1996;22:575-576.

51. Berbari EF, Hanssen AD, Duffy MC, Steckelberg JM, Osmon DR: Prosthetic joint infection due to *Mycobacterium tuberculosis*: A case series and review of the literature. *Am J Orthop* 1998;27:219-227.

52. McLaughlin JR, Tierney M, Harris WH: *Mycobacterium avium intracellulare* infection of hip arthroplasties in an AIDS patient. *J Bone Joint Surg Br* 1994;76:498-499.

53. Baumann PA, Cunningham B, Patel NS, Finn HA: *Aspergillus fumigatus* infection in a mega prosthetic total knee arthroplasty: Salvage by staged reimplantation with 5-year follow-up. *J Arthroplasty* 2001;16:498-503.

54. Voutsinas S, Sayakos J, Smyrnis P: *Echinococcus* infestation complicating total hip replacement: A case report. *J Bone Joint Surg Am* 1987;69:1456-1458.

55. Joseph WS, Axler DA: Microbiology and antimicrobial therapy of diabetic foot infections. *Clin Podiatr Med Surg* 1990;7:467-481.

56. Mlinaric Missoni E, Vukelic M, de Soy D, Belicza M, Vazic Babic V, Missoni E: Fungal infection in diabetic foot ulcers. *Diabet Med* 2005;22:1124-1125.

A low incidence of fungal infection (4.3%) was found in diabetic foot ulcers. These infections tend to develop in chronic, nonhealing foot ulcers. *Candida* species appear to play a secondary role in diabetic foot ulcers.

57. Mangram AJ, Horan TC, Pearson ML, Silver LC, Jarvis WR: Hospital Infection Control Practices Advisory Committee: Guideline for Prevention of Surgical Site Infection, 1999. http://www.cdc.gov/ncidod/dhqp/gl_surgicalsite.html. Accessed January 30, 2009.

58. Schaberg DR, Culver DH, Gaynes RP: Major trends in the microbial etiology of nosocomial infection. *Am J Med* 1991;91:72S-75S.

59. Tiwari TS, Ray B, Jost KC Jr, et al: Forty years of disinfectant failure: Outbreak of postinjection

Mycobacterium abscessus infection caused by contamination of benzalkonium chloride. *Clin Infect Dis* 2003; 36: 954-962.

Six postinjection joint infections caused by *M abscessus* were reported to the Texas Department of Health during July 1999. Investigation identified 12 patients who had received an intra-articular or periarticular steroid injection from the same physician. *M abscessus* was cultured from joint fluid or a periarticular soft-tissue specimen in 10 patients. Discontinuation of benzalkonium chloride as an antiseptic was recommended.

60. Kainer MA, Linden JV, Whaley DN, et al: *Clostridium* infections associated with musculoskeletal-tissue allografts. *N Engl J Med* 2004;350:2564-2571.

Clostridium infections were traced to allograft implantation. Interim recommendations were provided to enhance tissue-transplantation safety. Tissue banks were advised to validate processes and culturing methods, and the use of sterilization methods that do not adversely affect the functioning of transplanted tissue was emphasized.

61. Griego RD, Rosen T, Orengo IF, Wolf JE: Dog, cat, and human bites: A review. *J Am Acad Dermatol* 1995;33: 1019-1029.

62. Talan DA, Abrahamian FM, Moran GJ, Citron DM, Tan JO, Goldstein EJ: Clinical presentation and bacteriologic analysis of infected human bites in patients presenting to emergency departments. *Clin Infect Dis* 2003;37:1481-1489.

This multicenter prospective study of 50 patients with an infected human bite identified the responsible organisms as well as the treatment.

63. Jackson AC, Fenton MB: Human rabies and bat bites. *Lancet* 2001;357:1714.

64. Sakalkale R, Mansell C, Whalley D, Wisnewski-Smith K, Harte D, Reeve P: Rat-bite fever: A cautionary tale. *N Z Med J* 2007;120:U2545.

In the first reported instance of streptobacillary rat bite fever in New Zealand, a young man developed a high fever, hypotension, tender axillary lymphadenopathy, and systemic sepsis 1 week after a rat bite. Blood culturing of *S moniliformis* confirmed the diagnosis.

Chapter 3

Biofilm, Biomaterials, and Bacterial Adherence

Charalampos G. Zalavras, MD, PhD   John W. Costerton, PhD, FRCS

Introduction

Bacteria in a natural ecosystem are rarely encountered in the individual floating or planktonic state. Instead, bacteria are predominantly found in biofilms.[1] A biofilm is a highly structured community of bacterial cells that adopts a distinct phenotype,[2] communicates through cell-cell signals,[3] and adheres to an inert or living surface. The cells are enclosed in a self-produced polymeric matrix that is primarily composed of polysaccharides and is colloquially known as slime.[4,5] The bacteria in a chronic infection grow in biofilms attached to native tissues or a foreign body such as an implanted medical device. An understanding of bacterial adherence and biofilm formation is important for the diagnosis, treatment, and prevention of chronic bacterial infection.[5]

Biofilm Development

A biofilm develops as a sequential process from attachment to microcolony formation, maturation, and, finally, detachment.[1,4,6] (Figure 1). The initial stages in the development of a biofilm are the adherence of bacteria to an inert or living surface and the formation of microcolonies (as discussed below with reference to biomaterials). The attached bacteria then undergo maturation into a differentiated biofilm based on the activation of genes required for the synthesis of extracellular polysaccharide. Biofilm cells thus become embedded in the biofilm matrix. Bacterial cell-cell signaling (quorum sensing) is a key event in biofilm development. Bacteria produce and release chemical signaling molecules, which increase in concentration as a function of cell density.[3] The signaling molecules are simple acyl-homoserine lactones in gram-negative bacteria[7] and simple cyclic octapeptides in gram-positive bacteria.[8] When the concentration of signaling molecules (and therefore the bacterial population) exceeds a threshold, distinct patterns of gene expression are promoted and biofilm formation is initiated. Bacterial cells can be released from the biofilm and revert to planktonic status. Pieces of biofilm also can become detached and disperse to initiate the colonization of new

surfaces. Detachment does not appear to be random but instead is mediated by chemical signals in the biofilm.

Bacterial Adherence and Biomaterials

The first and critical stage in biofilm formation is bacterial adherence to a substratum, which can be a biomaterial, foreign body, or host tissue. Bacterial adherence occurs in two phases.[9,10] In the initial phase, an instantaneous and reversible attachment takes place based on physical factors that are determined by the characteristics of the biomaterial, the microorganism, and the ambient fluid. In the subsequent phase, a time-dependent and irreversible attachment occurs as determined by molecular and cellular processes.

The Physical Phase

Microorganisms are attracted to the surface of the substratum by physical forces including van der Waals attraction forces, hydrophobic interactions, and gravitational forces. These forces are able to overcome the repulsing negative electrostatic charge created by the bacterial wall and the biomaterial surface. Chemical interactions such as ionic, hydrogen, and covalent bonding also occur when the microorganisms are in close proximity to the substratum.

The Molecular and Cellular Phase

The attachment of the microorganisms to the substratum is consolidated by several molecular and cellular events: interaction between molecules on the substratum and the microbial surface, interaction between the substratum and microbial appendages, and bacterial secretion of extracellular polymeric substance.

When a biomaterial is implanted, its surface becomes coated with a film of plasma and extracellular matrix molecules, such as fibronectin, fibrinogen, collagen, laminin, or extracellular matrix-binding protein. These adhesive matrix molecules facilitate the attachment of bacteria via specific receptors on the bacterial surface, which are called bacterial adhesins or microbial surface components recognizing adhesive matrix

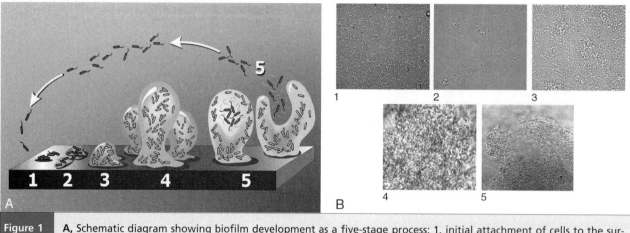

Figure 1 **A,** Schematic diagram showing biofilm development as a five-stage process: 1, initial attachment of cells to the surface; 2, production of extracellular polysaccharide resulting in firmly adhered, irreversible attachment; 3, early development of the biofilm architecture; 4, maturation of the biofilm architecture; 5, dispersion of single cells from the biofilm. **B,** The five-stage development process as represented by photomicrographs of *Pseudomonas aeruginosa* grown under continuous-flow conditions on a glass substratum. (Adapted with permission from Stoodley P, Sauer K, Davies DG, Costerton JW: Biofilms as complex differentiated communities. *Annu Rev Microbiol* 2002; 56:187-209.)

molecules (MSCRAMM). For example, fibronectin-binding proteins, fibrinogen-binding proteins, collagen-binding adhesin, and other microbial surface components are found in *Staphylococcus aureus*.[11]

Microbial fimbriae (pili) and flagella facilitate microbial attachment onto the biomaterial surface, especially if the organism is gram negative. Fimbriae are polymers that are constructed of pilin protein subunits, have a regular filamentous form, and are important adhesive structures. In *P aeruginosa,* attachment and microcolony formation depend on type IV pili and flagella-mediated motility.[12]

The extracellular polymeric substance, composed mainly of polysaccharides, consolidates adhesion of the microbes on the substratum surface and characterizes biofilm formation. The polysaccharide intercellular adhesin, which is secreted by both *S aureus* and *Staphylococcus epidermidis,* is an important component of the glycocalyx substance.[13]

Biomaterial Characteristics Affecting Bacterial Adherence

Bacterial adherence is influenced by the chemical composition of the biomaterial (Table 1). In vitro studies found that the rate of bacterial adherence is higher on titanium alloys than on stainless steel[14-16] and is higher on stainless steel than on pure titanium.[17] An in vivo study in rabbits found a higher infection rate when a stainless steel implant was used rather than a pure titanium implant.[18] An in vitro study found that *S aureus* adhered less well to tantalum than to other metals; no difference was found in the adherence of *S epidermidis* to different metals.[15]

The surface morphology of the biomaterial may have a role in bacterial adherence, although the details are unknown. An in vivo study in rabbits found that the concentration of *S aureus* required to infect a porous-coated titanium implant was 2.5 times less than the concentration required to infect a polished-surface titanium implant.[19] An in vitro study found greater adherence of *S aureus* to microrough titanium alloy than to electropolished titanium alloy.[16] However, another study found no correlation between the roughness of the surface and bacterial adhesion.[15]

Characteristics of Biofilms

The mature biofilm is not a homogeneous, amorphous structure. It has a specific architecture and can be thought of as a self-assembling, multicellular community.[20] Distinct colonies composed of bacterial cells (15% of the total volume) and extracellular matrix (85% of the volume) form mushroom-shaped structures separated by water channels that carry fluid into different areas of the biofilm.

The biofilm community is a protected form of bacterial growth that allows survival in a hostile environment. Compared with planktonic cells, sessile biofilm cells are less susceptible to antibiotic agents and host immune responses. These cells have several protective mechanisms.[5,21,22] Antibiotic agents and antibodies are not able to completely penetrate the biofilm because the biofilm matrix retards or blocks their diffusion. Biofilm cells secrete catalase, which protects them from hydrogen peroxide; the altered chemical microenvironment deactivates the products of the oxidative burst of phagocytes. Biofilm cells also are protected by metabolic variability; slow-growing or nongrowing biofilm cells are not susceptible to the effect of antibiotics, which target metabolically active bacteria. Finally, resistant phenotypes can develop as an active adaptive response to stress. Environmental stressors such as alteration in pH, osmolarity, or temperature can promote

Table 1

Studies of Interaction Between Bacteria and Biomaterial Surfaces

Study	Study Type	Bacteria	Findings
Ha et al[14] (2005)	In vitro	S epidermidis (biofilm forming)	More adherence on titanium alloy than on stainless steel
		M tuberculosis	Less adherence than for S epidermidis
Schildhauer et al[15] (2006)	In vitro	S aureus	More adherence on titanium alloy than on pure titanium or stainless steel (grit blasted, polished, or tantalum coated)
		S epidermidis	No differences in adherence to surfaces
Harris et al[16] (2007)	In vitro	S aureus	More adherence on microrough titanium alloy than on electropolished biomaterial surfaces (titanium alloy, pure titanium, or stainless steel)
Sheehan et al[17] (2004)	In vivo	S aureus	More adherence on stainless steel than on pure titanium
		S epidermidis	More adherence on stainless steel than on pure titanium; less adherence than for S aureus
Arens et al[18] (1996)	In vivo	S aureus	More infection on stainless steel than on pure titanium implants
Cordero et al[19] (1994)	In vivo	S aureus	Lower bacterial concentration needed to produce infection on porous-coated titanium than on electropolished titanium implants

the expression of stress-response genes and thereby lead to the development of a distinct phenotype that offers resistance to the environmental challenge.

Biofilms in Chronic Musculoskeletal Infection

The phenomenon of bacterial growth in biofilm communities can explain some intriguing features of chronic bacterial infection. Systemic symptoms and signs develop only when bacteria enter the planktonic phase and gain access to the circulatory system. Traditional microbiologic culturing methods fail to detect biofilm bacteria and therefore are of limited value in the diagnosis of a chronic infection. The protection that biofilm formation offers to bacteria explains the persistent nature of chronic bacterial infection.[5] Host defense mechanisms and antibiotic therapy are effective only against planktonic cells; they can suppress an acute exacerbation but cannot cure chronic infection (Figure 2).

The association between musculoskeletal prosthetic infection and biofilm formation was revealed using scanning and transmission electron microscopy.[23] Tissue and biomaterials from patients with an infection associated with the presence of a medical device or implant were directly examined. The causative bacteria were found to grow in biofilms adhering to the surface

of biomaterials and tissues in 19 of the 25 infections (76%), including 10 of the 17 orthopaedic implant-related infections (59%).[24] Animal model studies of osteomyelitis associated with a foreign body also found biofilm formation to be a feature of the infection.[25-27]

The concepts of biofilm science must be applied to the diagnosis, treatment, and prevention of chronic orthopaedic infection. In chronic osteomyelitis and implant-associated infections, bacteria grow in biofilms attached to the surface of dead bone or foreign material. This protective mode of growth shields the bacteria from antibiotic agents and host defense mechanisms and enables the infection to persist.[5,21,22,28]

Diagnosis

Chronic biofilm infection is challenging to diagnose because the inflammatory response is attenuated compared with that of an infection caused by planktonic bacteria. A biofilm infection may elicit no symptoms for months or years.[29,30] Traditional microbiologic diagnostic techniques depend on isolation and culture of planktonic bacteria, but biofilm cells grow poorly, if at all, on agar plates.[29,30] Culturing for a biofilm infection therefore may produce inaccurate results, and its diagnostic usefulness is questionable.[29,31-33] Negative culture results do not rule out the presence of pathogens growing in biofilms.

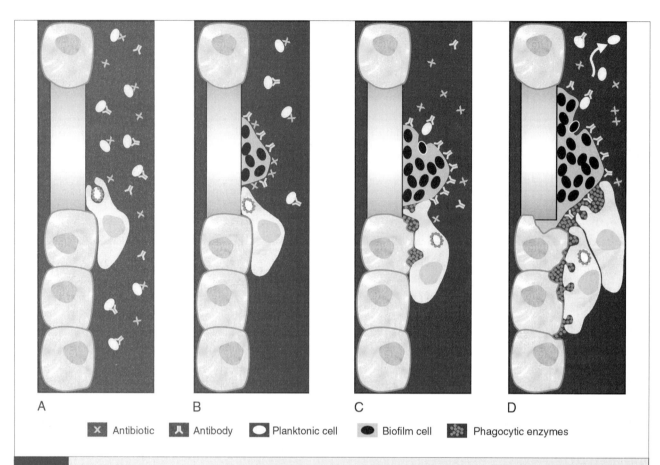

| | Antibiotic | | Antibody | | Planktonic cell | | Biofilm cell | | Phagocytic enzymes |

Figure 2   Schematic diagram showing the development of a medical biofilm. **A,** Planktonic bacteria can be cleared by antibodies and phagocytes and are susceptible to antibiotics. **B,** Adherent bacterial cells preferentially form biofilms on inert surfaces; these sessile communities are resistant to antibodies, phagocytes, and antibiotics. **C,** Phagocytes are attracted to the biofilms; phagocytosis is frustrated, but phagocytic enzymes are released. **D,** Phagocytic enzymes damage tissue around the biofilm, and planktonic bacteria are released from the biofilm; the result can be dissemination and acute infection in neighboring tissue. (Adapted with permission from Costerton JW, Stewart PS, Greenberg EP: Bacterial biofilms: A common cause of persistent infections. *Science* 1999;284:1320.)

Routine tissue sample culturing was positive in 5 of 120 patients (4%) who underwent total hip revision surgery, and culturing after sonication of retrieved implants was positive in 26 patients (22%).[32] Immunofluorescence microscopy of sonicated samples identified bacteria in 71 of 113 patients (63%).[31] Another study also found that culturing of samples obtained by sonication of prostheses was more sensitive than conventional periprosthetic tissue culturing in diagnosing prosthetic hip or knee infection.[34] Bacterial biofilms were detected by molecular methods on 8 of 10 acetabular cups removed because of aseptic loosening; cultures from removed devices or hip aspirates were negative.[29] Bacteria also were found on clinically uninfected hip prostheses after revision surgery necessitated by aseptic loosening.[35]

Novel microscopic, molecular, and immunologic assay methods have been developed to detect biofilm infection, and they are promising for clinical application.[29,36] Fluorescence in situ hybridization (FISH) uses ribosomal RNA (rRNA)-targeted probes conjugated to fluorescent stains to allow visualization of biofilm bacteria. Nonspecific FISH probes can be used to identify all bacterial cells, in broad categories, as well as their spatial relationships to physical surfaces and host eukaryotic cells. Species-specific 16S rRNA-targeted FISH probes can be used to identify cells of known bacterial species and their spatial relationships. FISH probes also can be used to evaluate the viability of microorganisms within a biofilm, based on the integrity of the cell membrane, by differentially staining microbial cells.

The surface proteins produced by biofilm bacteria are distinct from those found on the surface of planktonic cells of the same species.[5] The immunologic interaction between biofilm bacteria and the host can be used for diagnosis.[37] Staphylococcal slime polysaccharide antigen is a surface epitope produced by biofilm cells of *S aureus* and *S epidermidis* but not by comparable planktonic cells. In patients who had received a vascular graft, enzyme-linked immunosorbent assay revealed very high sensitivity and specificity for detection of antibodies to this epitope.[37] The immunologic response to biofilm antigens has been used for in vitro immunofluorescent visualization of S aureus biofilms.[38]

Treatment

Antibiotic therapy is effective against the planktonic bacteria that are released from a biofilm and cause acute symptoms. However, antibiotic therapy is not effective against sessile bacteria in a biofilm. Possible therapeutic approaches have been investigated in vitro and in vivo. A high-dosage combined administration of antibiotic agents resulted in the in vitro eradication of young P aeruginosa or S aureus biofilm cells but did not eradicate old biofilm cells.[39,40] Combined administration of clarithromycin and tobramycin enhanced the in vitro killing of established P aeruginosa biofilms, although 25% of the biofilm cells survived.[41] Combined antibiotic therapy that included rifampin was more effective than single-agent therapy against in vitro staphylococcal biofilms.[42]

Enzymes, electric current, ultrasonography, and quorum-sensing inhibitors all have been effectively used with antibiotic therapy in experimental studies. However, no clinical data are available on their efficacy. The enzyme serratiopeptidase enhanced the activity of ofloxacin against sessile P aeruginosa and S epidermidis bacteria in vitro and inhibited biofilm formation.[43] In vivo, the local addition of serratiopeptidase significantly improved the activity of systemic ofloxacin against S epidermidis.[44] The enzyme dispersin B was shown to rapidly remove S epidermidis biofilms from plastic surfaces in vitro.[45] In an animal study, ultrasonic application enhanced the action of gentamicin against Escherichia coli biofilms but not against P aeruginosa biofilms.[46]

RNAIII-inhibiting peptide (RIP) is a quorum-sensing inhibitor that blocks toxin production and biofilm formation by S aureus or S epidermidis.[8,47] In vivo studies on murine models found that RIP acts synergistically with antibiotics against S aureus biofilms.[48,49]

Complete surgical débridement is the cornerstone of treatment for chronic biofilm-associated infection of the musculoskeletal system.[20,50] All dead bone should be débrided, and all foreign material should be removed. The attached biofilm is thereby removed, initiating a new "race for the surface" between host cells and microorganisms.

Prevention

Several interventions may be useful in preventing orthopaedic biofilm infection, including surface cleaning of orthopaedic implants, surface modification of biomaterials, killing of planktonic cells before biofilm can develop, and inhibition of bacterial cell communication.

Surface Cleaning of Orthopaedic Implants

The presence on an implant of residual organic debris, especially residual biofilm matrix, accelerates the process of planktonic cell attraction and biofilm formation at least tenfold.[5] Orthopaedic implants are manufactured by machining techniques that favor biofilm development. Current sterilization techniques kill the bacteria in these biofilms but do not remove the matrix residue. These deposits can be removed before implantation as a preventive measure. Combined administration of enzymes and chemical agents (an alkaline detergent and sodium hypochlorite solution) was found to eradicate biofilm both in vitro and in a clinically used dialysis machine.[51]

Surface Modification of Biomaterials

The chemical composition and surface morphology of biomaterials contribute to bacterial adherence. However, the properties that promote bacterial adherence to the biomaterial also promote the adherence of host eukaryotic cells. Host cell adherence is necessary for integration of the implant and is particularly important, for example, in cementless arthroplasty or dental implantation.

Several methods have been investigated for modifying biomaterial surface properties to decrease bacterial surface adherence. Bacterial adhesion has been reduced in vitro by incorporating antibiotics[52,53] or silver[54] into the biomaterial surface or by coating the surface with a polymerlike carbon[55] or polyethylene glycol.[56] To resist bacterial adhesion but promote host cell adhesion, biomaterial surfaces have been experimentally modified using a polyethylene glycol coating; or a hyaluronic acid–chitosan polyelectrolyte multilayer (to reduce adhesion of both bacteria and host cells), with arginine-glycine-aspartic acid peptide (to promote the adhesion of host cells but not bacteria).[56-58]

Planktonic Cell Killing Before Biofilm Development

Materials and coatings that release antibiotics into the surrounding tissues and fluids may kill planktonic bacteria before they can initiate biofilm formation on the biomaterial. These materials can thereby prevent the colonization of implants during the early postsurgical period.[52,53] However, the presence of a subinhibitory concentration of antibiotics after the initial rapid release may favor the development of resistant bacterial strains. A polymer hydrogel matrix coated with ordered methylene chains achieved on-demand delivery of antibiotics in vitro. Ciprofloxacin was retained inside the polymer and released in response to low-intensity ultrasonography, reducing the accumulation of P aeruginosa biofilms.[59]

Quorum-Sensing Inhibition

Bacterial cell-cell signaling (quorum sensing) is critical to biofilm formation and offers a new target for preventing biofilm infection. Natural and synthetic molecules that inhibit quorum sensing were found to prevent biofilm formation.[47,60] Synthetic furanones inhibit acyl-homoserine lactone-mediated quorum sensing. They were found to reduce the virulence of P aeruginosa, increase biofilm susceptibility to tobramycin in vitro, and increase biofilm susceptibility to immune mechanisms in vivo.[60] In murine models of device-related biofilm infections, synthetic RIP prevented biofilm formation by *S aureus* or *S epidermidis*, especially when combined with antibiotics.[47,61]

Summary

An understanding of biofilm infection and the complex interaction between bacteria and biomaterials is leading to new perspectives in the diagnosis, treatment, and prevention of chronic musculoskeletal infection. Additional research is required to investigate the efficacy, safety, and feasibility of new techniques in clinical application.

Annotated References

1. Costerton JW, Lewandowski Z, Caldwell DE, Korber DR, Lappin-Scott HM: Microbial biofilms. *Annu Rev Microbiol* 1995;49:711-745.

2. Sauer K, Camper AK, Ehrlich GD, Costerton JW, Davies DG: Pseudomonas aeruginosa displays multiple phenotypes during development as a biofilm. *J Bacteriol* 2002;184:1140-1154.

3. Davies DG, Parsek MR, Pearson JP, Iglewski BH, Costerton JW, Greenberg EP: The involvement of cell-to-cell signals in the development of a bacterial biofilm. *Science* 1998;280:295-298.

4. Stoodley P, Sauer K, Davies DG, Costerton JW: Biofilms as complex differentiated communities. *Annu Rev Microbiol* 2002;56:187-209.

5. Costerton JW, Stewart PS, Greenberg EP: Bacterial biofilms: A common cause of persistent infections. *Science* 1999;284:1318-1322.

6. Costerton JW: Introduction to biofilm. *Int J Antimicrob Agents* 1999;11:217-221.

7. Fuqua WC, Winans SC, Greenberg EP: Quorum sensing in bacteria: The LuxR-LuxI family of cell density-responsive transcriptional regulators. *J Bacteriol* 1994; 176:269-275.

8. Balaban N, Goldkorn T, Nhan RT, et al: Autoinducer of virulence as a target for vaccine and therapy against Staphylococcus aureus. *Science* 1998;280: 438-440.

9. Gristina AG: Biomaterial-centered infection: Microbial adhesion versus tissue integration. *Science* 1987;237: 1588-1595.

10. An YH, Friedman RJ: Concise review of mechanisms of bacterial adhesion to biomaterial surfaces. *J Biomed Mater Res* 1998;43:338-348.

11. Gotz F: Staphylococcus and biofilms. *Mol Microbiol* 2002;43:1367-1378.

12. O'Toole GA, Kolter R: Flagellar and twitching motility are necessary for Pseudomonas aeruginosa biofilm development. *Mol Microbiol* 1998;30:295-304.

13. Olson ME, Garvin KL, Fey PD, Rupp ME: Adherence of Staphylococcus epidermidis to biomaterials is augmented by PIA. *Clin Orthop Relat Res* 2006;451:21-24.

   In an in vitro study, polysaccharide intercellular adhesin was found to be critical in the adherence of *S epidermidis* to orthopaedic biomaterials.

14. Ha KY, Chung YG, Ryoo SJ: Adherence and biofilm formation of Staphylococcus epidermidis and Mycobacterium tuberculosis on various spinal implants. *Spine* 2005;30:38-43.

   In vitro biomaterial adherence and biofilm formation was lower for *Mycobacterium tuberculosis* than for *S epidermidis*. *S epidermidis* biofilm formation was higher on titanium alloy than on stainless steel.

15. Schildhauer TA, Robie B, Muhr G, Koller M: Bacterial adherence to tantalum versus commonly used orthopedic metallic implant materials. *J Orthop Trauma* 2006; 20:476-484.

   The in vitro adherence of *S aureus* varied by biomaterial; adherence was lowest for tantalum and highest for titanium alloy. No differences were observed in *S epidermidis* adherence. Surface roughness did not influence bacterial adhesion.

16. Harris LG, Meredith DO, Eschbach L, Richards RG: Staphylococcus aureus adhesion to standard microrough and electropolished implant materials. *J Mater Sci Mater Med* 2007;18:1151-1156.

   An in vitro study found greater adhesion of *S aureus* to standard microrough titanium alloy than to other biomaterials. Electropolishing of the titanium alloy decreased bacterial adherence.

17. Sheehan E, McKenna J, Mulhall KJ, Marks P, McCormack D: Adhesion of Staphylococcus to orthopaedic metals: An in vivo study. *J Orthop Res* 2004;22:39-43.

   S aureus and *S epidermidis* both had greater adherence to stainless steel than to pure titanium implants in a rabbit model. *S epidermidis* had a lower ability to adhere to metals than *S aureus*.

18. Arens S, Schlegel U, Printzen G, Ziegler WJ, Perren SM, Hansis M: Influence of materials for fixation implants on local infection: An experimental study of steel versus titanium DCP in rabbits. *J Bone Joint Surg Br* 1996;78: 647-651.

19. Cordero J, Munuera L, Folgueira MD: Influence of metal implants on infection: An experimental study in rabbits. *J Bone Joint Surg Br* 1994;76:717-720.

20. Costerton W, Veeh R, Shirtliff M, Pasmore M, Post C, Ehrlich G: The application of biofilm science to the

study and control of chronic bacterial infections. *J Clin Invest* 2003;112:1466-1477.

Key concepts of biofilm structure and function are presented, with a discussion of the application of biofilm characteristics to the diagnosis and treatment of chronic infection. Level of evidence: V.

21. Fux CA, Costerton JW, Stewart PS, Stoodley P: Survival strategies of infectious biofilms. *Trends Microbiol* 2005; 13:34-40.

    The protective mechanisms that shield biofilms from antibiotic agents and host defenses are described.

22. Stewart PS, Costerton JW: Antibiotic resistance of bacteria in biofilms. *Lancet* 2001;358:135-138.

23. Gristina AG, Costerton JW: Bacterial adherence and the glycocalyx and their role in musculoskeletal infection. *Orthop Clin North Am* 1984;15:517-535.

24. Gristina AG, Costerton JW: Bacterial adherence to biomaterials and tissue: The significance of its role in clinical sepsis. *J Bone Joint Surg Am* 1985;67:264-273.

25. Mayberry-Carson KJ, Tober-Meyer B, Smith JK, Lambe DW Jr, Costerton JW: Bacterial adherence and glycocalyx formation in osteomyelitis experimentally induced with Staphylococcus aureus. *Infect Immun* 1984; 43:825-833.

26. Lambe DW Jr, Ferguson KP, Mayberry-Carson KJ, Tober-Meyer B, Costerton JW: Foreign-body-associated experimental osteomyelitis induced with Bacteroides fragilis and Staphylococcus epidermidis in rabbits. *Clin Orthop Relat Res* 1991;266:285-294.

27. Buxton TB, Horner J, Hinton A, Rissing JP: In vivo glycocalyx expression by Staphylococcus aureus phage type 52/52A/80 in S. aureus osteomyelitis. *J Infect Dis* 1987;156:942-946.

28. Brady RA, Leid JG, Calhoun JH, Costerton JW, Shirtliff ME: Osteomyelitis and the role of biofilms in chronic infection. *FEMS Immunol Med Microbiol* 2008; 52:13-22.

    This review of the molecular mechanisms of bacterial attachment to surfaces, biofilm development, and maturation is focused on *S aureus*.

29. Costerton JW: Biofilm theory can guide the treatment of device-related orthopaedic infections. *Clin Orthop Relat Res* 2005;437:7-11.

    Improved understanding of device-related infection based on the biofilm theory can be translated into clinical application. Level of evidence: V.

30. Fux CA, Stoodley P, Hall-Stoodley L, Costerton JW: Bacterial biofilms: A diagnostic and therapeutic challenge. *Expert Rev Anti Infect Ther* 2003;1:667-683.

    Antibiotic agents and host defenses are resisted by biofilms through mechanisms including the action of the matrix, the heterogenicity of bacterial metabolic activity within the biofilm, and the active response of bacteria to environmental stress.

31. Tunney MM, Patrick S, Curran MD, et al: Detection of prosthetic hip infection at revision arthroplasty by immunofluorescence microscopy and PCR amplification of the bacterial 16S rRNA gene. *J Clin Microbiol* 1999;37: 3281-3290.

32. Tunney MM, Patrick S, Gorman SP, et al: Improved detection of infection in hip replacements: A currently underestimated problem. *J Bone Joint Surg Br* 1998;80: 568-572.

33. Dobbins JJ, Seligson D, Raff MJ: Bacterial colonization of orthopedic fixation devices in the absence of clinical infection. *J Infect Dis* 1988;158:203-205.

34. Trampuz A, Piper KE, Jacobson MJ, et al: Sonication of removed hip and knee prostheses for diagnosis of infection. *N Engl J Med* 2007;357:654-663.

    In a prospective study of 331 patients with a hip or knee prosthesis, culturing of samples obtained by sonication of removed implants was found to be more sensitive than conventional culturing of periprosthetic tissue in the diagnosis of infection, especially if antibiotics were administered during the 2 weeks before surgery. Level of evidence: I.

35. Dempsey KE, Riggio MP, Lennon A, et al: Identification of bacteria on the surface of clinically infected and non-infected prosthetic hip joints removed during revision arthroplasties by 16S rRNA gene sequencing and by microbiological culture. *Arthritis Res Ther* 2007;9:R46.

    Bacteria were identified using molecular methods in all five patients who underwent revision hip arthroplasty necessitated by aseptic loosening and had negative presurgical and perisurgical cultures. Level of evidence: II.

36. Donlan RM: New approaches for the characterization of prosthetic joint biofilms. *Clin Orthop Relat Res* 2005;437:12-19.

    New methods are reviewed for using fluorescent stain technology to evaluate the structure and composition of biofilm communities.

37. Selan L, Passariello C: Microbiological diagnosis of aortofemoral graft infections. *Eur J Vasc Endovasc Surg* 1997;14(suppl A):10-12.

38. Brady RA, Leid JG, Kofonow J, Costerton JW, Shirtliff ME: Immunoglobulins to surface-associated biofilm immunogens provide a novel means of visualization of methicillin-resistant Staphylococcus aureus biofilms. *Appl Environ Microbiol* 2007;73:6612-6619.

    An in vitro study found that antibodies to specific cell-wall antigens of biofilm-producing *S aureus* are useful in viewing biofilm growth and architecture using immunofluorescence confocal microscopy.

39. Anwar H, Costerton JW: Enhanced activity of combination of tobramycin and piperacillin for eradication of sessile biofilm cells of Pseudomonas aeruginosa. *Antimicrob Agents Chemother* 1990;34:1666-1671.

40. Anwar H, Strap JL, Chen K, Costerton JW: Dynamic interactions of biofilms of mucoid Pseudomonas aeruginosa with tobramycin and piperacillin. *Antimicrob Agents Chemother* 1992;36:1208-1214.

41. Tre-Hardy M, Vanderbist F, Traore H, Devleeschouwer MJ: In vitro activity of antibiotic combinations against Pseudomonas aeruginosa biofilm and planktonic cultures. *Int J Antimicrob Agents* 2008;31:329-336.

    Combined administration of clarithromycin and tobramycin had a synergistic effect and enhanced the killing of established *P aeruginosa* biofilms in vitro. However, 25% of biofilm cells survived.

42. Saginur R, Stdenis M, Ferris W, et al: Multiple combination bactericidal testing of staphylococcal biofilms from implant-associated infections. *Antimicrob Agents Chemother* 2006;50:55-61.

    An in vitro study found that combined antibiotic therapy including rifampin was more effective than single-agent therapy against staphylococcal biofilms.

43. Selan L, Berlutti F, Passariello C, Comodi-Ballanti MR, Thaller MC: Proteolytic enzymes: A new treatment strategy for prosthetic infections? *Antimicrob Agents Chemother* 1993;37:2618-2621.

44. Mecikoglu M, Saygi B, Yildirim Y, Karadag-Saygi E, Ramadan SS, Esemenli T: The effect of proteolytic enzyme serratiopeptidase in the treatment of experimental implant-related infection. *J Bone Joint Surg Am* 2006; 88:1208-1214.

    In a murine infection model, the local addition of serratiopeptidase was found to significantly improve the activity of systemic ofloxacin against biofilm-producing *S epidermidis*.

45. Kaplan JB, Ragunath C, Velliyagounder K, Fine DH, Ramasubbu N: Enzymatic detachment of Staphylococcus epidermidis biofilms. *Antimicrob Agents Chemother* 2004;48:2633-2636.

    An in vitro study found that dispersin B, an enzyme produced by oral bacterium *Actinobacillus actinomycetemcomitans*, rapidly removed *S epidermidis* biofilms from plastic surfaces. Surface precoating with dispersin B prevented *S epidermidis* biofilm formation.

46. Carmen JC, Roeder BL, Nelson JL, et al: Treatment of biofilm infections on implants with low-frequency ultrasound and antibiotics. *Am J Infect Control* 2005;33: 78-82.

    An in vivo study of rabbits found that combined ultrasonography and gentamicin administered for 48 hours reduced the viability of *E coli* biofilms to an almost undetectable level but had no significant effect against *P aeruginosa* biofilms.

47. Balaban N, Giacometti A, Cirioni O, et al: Use of the quorum-sensing inhibitor RNAIII-inhibiting peptide to prevent biofilm formation in vivo by drug-resistant Staphylococcus epidermidis. *J Infect Dis* 2003;187: 625-630.

    In a murine model, RIP inhibited the in vitro adhesion of *S epidermidis* to host cells and plastic as well as Dacron grafts. The combination of RIP with antibiotic prophylaxis (local mupirocin, local quinupristin-dalfopristin, or systemic teicoplanin) led to 100% bacterial inhibition.

48. Balaban N, Cirioni O, Giacometti A, et al: Treatment of Staphylococcus aureus biofilm infection by the quorum-sensing inhibitor RIP. *Antimicrob Agents Chemother* 2007;51:2226-2229.

    In a murine Dacron graft infection model, RIP had synergistic action with antibiotic agents against established *S aureus* biofilms and significantly reduced bacterial load.

49. Cirioni O, Giacometti A, Ghiselli R, et al: RNAIII-inhibiting peptide significantly reduces bacterial load and enhances the effect of antibiotics in the treatment of central venous catheter-associated Staphylococcus aureus infections. *J Infect Dis* 2006;193:180-186.

    In a murine central venous catheter infection model, biofilm bacterial cells were as susceptible to antibiotics as planktonic cells when first treated with RIP in vitro. The combination of RIP and antibiotics significantly reduced the biofilm bacterial load in vivo.

50. Patzakis MJ, Zalavras CG: Chronic posttraumatic osteomyelitis and infected nonunion of the tibia: Current management concepts. *J Am Acad Orthop Surg* 2005; 13:417-427.

    The principles of diagnosing and treating chronic osteomyelitis are reviewed, with an emphasis on the importance of radical débridement. Level of evidence: V.

51. Marion K, Pasmore M, Freney J, et al: A new procedure allowing the complete removal and prevention of hemodialysis biofilms. *Blood Purif* 2005;23:339-348.

    A new antibiofilm procedure using enzymes and detergents was able to detach adherent biofilm cells, both in vitro and in a clinically used dialysis machine. This procedure may improve the disinfection of medical devices.

52. Aviv M, Berdicevsky I, Zilberman M: Gentamicin-loaded bioresorbable films for prevention of bacterial infections associated with orthopedic implants. *J Biomed Mater Res A* 2007;83:10-19.

    Poly-L-lactic acid and poly (D,L-lactic-coglycolic acid) films containing gentamicin resulted in drug concentration in the surrounding medium exceeding the minimal inhibitory concentration against bacterial species involved in orthopaedic infections.

53. Antoci V Jr, King SB, Jose B, et al: Vancomycin covalently bonded to titanium alloy prevents bacterial colonization. *J Orthop Res* 2007;25:858-866.

    A titanium alloy surface was engineered with covalently bound vancomycin. The vancomycin-modified surface was stable in aqueous solutions over extended periods and prevented bacterial colonization in vitro.

54. Chen W, Liu Y, Courtney HS, et al: In vitro antibacterial and biological properties of magnetron co-sputtered silver-containing hydroxyapatite coating. *Biomaterials* 2006;27:5512-5517.

A silver-containing hydroxyapatite coating significantly reduced bacterial adhesion in vitro compared with titanium and hydroxyapatite surfaces. There was no significant difference in cytotoxicity in vivo.

55. Wang J, Huang N, Yang P, et al: The effects of amorphous carbon films deposited on polyethylene terephthalate on bacterial adhesion. *Biomaterials* 2004;25:3163-3170.

Amorphous carbon films deposited on polyethylene terephthalate reduced the adhesion of *S epidermidis* and *S aureus* to 14% and 35%, respectively, compared with adhesion to an untreated control surface.

56. Harris LG, Tosatti S, Wieland M, Textor M, Richards RG: Staphylococcus aureus adhesion to titanium oxide surfaces coated with non-functionalized and peptide-functionalized poly(L-lysine)-grafted-poly(ethylene glycol) copolymers. *Biomaterials* 2004;25:4135-4148.

Titanium surfaces coated with poly(L-lysine)-grafted-poly(ethylene glycol) copolymers exhibited reduced *S aureus* adhesion in vitro. Functionalization of the surface by adding the arginine-glycine-aspartic acid peptide to promote host cell adhesion did not increase *S aureus* adhesion compared with the nonfunctionalized coating.

57. Chua PH, Neoh KG, Kang ET, Wang W: Surface functionalization of titanium with hyaluronic acid/chitosan polyelectrolyte multilayers and RGD for promoting osteoblast functions and inhibiting bacterial adhesion. *Biomaterials* 2008;29:1412-1421.

Titanium coated with hyaluronic acid–chitosan polyelectrolyte multilayers and arginine-glycine-aspartic acid peptide was found to be a highly effective antibacterial surface that enhanced osteoblast adhesion, proliferation, and alkaline phosphatase production.

58. Maddikeri RR, Tosatti S, Schuler M, et al: Reduced medical infection related bacterial strains adhesion on bioactive RGD modified titanium surfaces: A first step toward cell selective surfaces. *J Biomed Mater Res A* 2008;84:425-435.

Adhesion of *S epidermidis*, *Streptococcus mutans*, and *P aeruginosa* was reduced in vitro 88% to 98% on titanium surfaces coated with poly(L-lysine)-grafted-poly(ethylene glycol), with or without arginine-glycine-aspartic acid peptide, compared with uncoated surfaces.

59. Norris P, Noble M, Francolini I, et al: Ultrasonically controlled release of ciprofloxacin from self-assembled coatings on poly(2-hydroxyethyl methacrylate) hydrogels for Pseudomonas aeruginosa biofilm prevention. *Antimicrob Agents Chemother* 2005;49:4272-4279.

Biofilm accumulation on ciprofloxacin-loaded hydrogels with ultrasonography-induced drug delivery was significantly lower than biofilm growth in control experiments.

60. Hentzer M, Wu H, Andersen JB, et al: Attenuation of Pseudomonas aeruginosa virulence by quorum sensing inhibitors. *EMBO J* 2003;22:3803-3815.

A synthetic derivate of natural furanone compounds was found to act as a potent antagonist of *P aeruginosa* quorum sensing, increasing biofilm susceptibility to tobramycin in vitro and immune mechanisms in a murine pulmonary infection model.

61. Giacometti A, Cirioni O, Gov Y, et al: RNA III inhibiting peptide inhibits in vivo biofilm formation by drug-resistant Staphylococcus aureus. *Antimicrob Agents Chemother* 2003;47:1979-1983.

S aureus biofilm formation was inhibited by RIP in a murine Dacron graft model.

1: General Considerations

Chapter 4

Procedure-Related Reduction of the Risk of Infection

*George Cierny III, MD   Nalini Rao, MD, FACP, FSHEA

1: General Considerations

Introduction

Surgical site infection (SSI) is the third most common type of nosocomial infection, accounting for 38% of all infections in the 27 million patients who undergo surgery in the United States each year.[1] These infections are associated with substantial morbidity, mortality, and expense. Critical bacterial burden is by far the most significant of the many factors that influence surgical wound healing and determine the potential for infection and its incidence.

Classification and Monitoring

Since 1986, nosocomial infection rates have been identified as an indicator of quality of care and a reliable measure of institutional quality assurance. The 2006 Institute of Medicine report *Rewarding Provider Performance: Aligning Incentives in Medicare*[2] recommended pay-for-performance programs as a means of aligning performance improvement incentives. The US Centers for Medicare and Medicaid Services soon adopted the pay-for-performance approach for provider reimbursement under Medicare. More than half of all commercial health maintenance organizations now use a pay-for-performance system, despite widespread concern as to the choice and validity of the measures used to determine improvement.

The American public has come to believe that every surgical infection is preventable. An increasing number of health plans now include the rate of SSIs in the hospital and physician profiles available to patients, for the purpose of encouraging patients to seek care from providers with favorable profiles. As the number of provider categories, the number of measures, and the financial risks increase, clinicians increasingly are held accountable for their actions and omissions. Ortho-

*George Cierny III, MD or the department with which he is affiliated has received miscellaneous nonincome support, commercially derived honoraria, or other nonresearch-related funding from Kimberly-Clark; has received royalties from Wright Medical; and holds stock or stock options in Royer Biomedical.

paedic surgeons have come under particular scrutiny as the use of surgical implants, the complexity of surgical procedures, and the percentage of patients with a significant comorbidity have increased. However, the high cost of health care, increased patient awareness, legal issues, and pressure from insurance companies may cause medical practice to be defined less by patient safety and outcomes than by evidence-based or possibly unrealistic best practice scenarios.

Classification Systems

In 1964, the US National Research Council introduced a system for classifying surgical wounds into four sequential categories (clean, clean contaminated, contaminated, and dirty) based on critical bacterial burden and increasing risk of SSI.[3] Subsequent improvements in treatment and outcomes led to a decreased risk of SSI[4,5] (Table 1). However, investigation revealed considerable variation within each wound class associated with the type, nature, and length of the surgical procedure[6] as well as extrinsic and intrinsic factors influencing the incidence of SSI.

The risk index of the Study on the Efficacy of Nosocomial Infection Control, known as the SENIC index, was introduced in 1985. The SENIC index considers patient and wound characteristics, including the presence of comorbidities, the anatomic site, and the duration of the procedure.[5] This index proved twice as effective in predicting the incidence of SSI as the US National Research Council's original classification. However, a wide range of infection risk once again was observed within each wound category.

Investigators at the US Centers for Disease Control and Prevention (CDC) currently use a risk index created as part of the National Nosocomial Infections Surveillance (NNIS) system.[6] The NNIS risk index is based on three independent and equally weighted variables, which are used to assign a three-point score.[6,7] One point is assigned to each of the following, if present: a contaminated or dirty wound; severe systemic disease, as indicated by a score of 3 or higher on the American Society of Anesthesiologists physical status classification[8-10] (Table 2); and excessive duration of surgery, defined as surgical time exceeding the 75th percentile for the specific procedure.[11] For total hip arthroplasty

Table 1

Surgical Wound Classification System of the US National Research Council, With Initial (1980) and Improved (1991) Risk of Infection

Category	Characteristics	Risk of Infection, 1980*	Risk of Infection, 1991†
Clean	No inflammation Respiratory, alimentary, genitourinary tracts not entered No break in aseptic surgical technique	2%-5%	< 2.1%
Clean contaminated	Healed but previously infected wound Respiratory, alimentary, genitourinary tracts entered with no significant spillage Break in aseptic surgical technique	6%-9%	3.3%
Contaminated	Acute inflammation (no pus) Open trauma wound < 4 hr old Visible wound contamination (gross intrasurgical spillage from a hollow viscous	13%-20%	6.4%
Dirty	Acute inflammation (pus) Open trauma wound ≥ 4 hr old Previously perforated viscous	40%	7.1%

*Data from Cruse PJ, Ford R: The epidemilogy of wound infection: A 10-year prospective study of 62,939 wounds. *Surg Clin North Am*1980;60:27-40.
† Data from Culver DH, Horan TC, Gaynes RP, et al: Surgical wound infection rates by wound class, operative procedure, and patient risk index: The National Nosocomial Infections Surveillance System. *Am J Med*1991;91:152S-157S.

Table 2

American Society of Anesthesiologists Physical Status Classification

Score	Patient Physical Status
1	Normal, healthy
2	Mild systemic disease
3	Severe systemic disease
4	Severe systemic disease that is a constant threat to life
5	Moribund; not expected to survive without surgical procedure
6	Declared brain dead; organs being removed for donation

(Adapted with permission from American Society of Anesthesiologists: ASA Physical Status Classification System. http://www.asahq.org/clinical/physicalstatus.htm. Accessed June 11, 2008.)

procedures requiring less than 2 hours, an NNIS risk index of 0, 1, or 2 to 3 was correlated with an SSI rate of 0.86%, 1.65%, or 2.5%, respectively.[12] Refinement of the NNIS risk index is needed to incorporate anatomic and site-specific outliers to the formula.[12,13]

Monitoring

The CDC developed the NNIS system during the early 1970s to monitor the incidence of health care–associated infections as well as the associated risk factors and pathogens. The NNIS system helps profession-als and hospitals stay abreast of the rapidly expanding science and practice of infection prevention and control and improve their management of endemic and epidemic episodes of nosocomial infection. In 1992, the CDC introduced the term "surgical site infection" to distinguish infection of a surgical incision from infection of a traumatic wound.[14] SSI is defined as an incisional (superficial) or deep infection occurring within 30 days of surgery or within 1 year of the introduction of a surgical implant.

The Biology of Surgical Site Infection

Unacceptable SSI rates still sometimes occur, despite the best efforts of infection prevention practitioners and improvements in surgical technique, antibiotic prophylaxis, instrument sterilization methods, and operating room practices. Bacteria can gain access to a surgical wound from several sources. Endogenous contamination arises from the patient's skin or nares; the gastrointestinal, genitourinary, bronchial, or sinusoidal tract; or a concomitant remote-site infection. Exogenous contamination comes from airborne or transient pathogens transferred from instruments, implants, or personnel.

Most SSIs are caused by commensal organisms from the patient's skin or transient organisms disseminated from health care personnel or surgical instruments.[15] Normal resident skin flora inhabit even the deepest layers of the dermis and are difficult to remove; these commensal organisms include *Staphylococcus*, diphtheroid, *Pseudomonas,* and *Propionibacterium* species. Transient organisms are not consistently present but are easily exchanged between individuals. Studies have identified operating room personnel as the source of contamination in 98% of SSIs, with 30% of the contaminants airborne and 70% transferred through surgical instruments or other contact.[16-19]

Although microorganisms gain access to all surgical wounds, only a small percentage of surgical patients develop a clinical infection. The presence of organisms in a wound is less important than the level of bacterial growth during the hours or days after the surgery. Whether an infection develops depends on the number and virulence of the bacteria in the wound, the status or viability of the wound, and the ability of host defenses to eliminate the bacteria.

Best Practices for Reducing Pathogen Load

Aseptic practice must include procedures to reduce the number of microorganisms present and prevent them from reaching the wound. In addition, operating room practices must prevent the accidental transfer of microorganisms from people, places, or equipment. Surgical best practices encompass both the principles of asepsis and measures to safeguard efficient wound healing using the host's natural defenses.

Coexisting Remote-Site Infection

Any open or inflamed presurgical wound is a potential source of hematogenous or contiguous surgical wound contamination and should be treated and resolved before elective surgery is undertaken.[9,20,21] Because systemic disease can be caused by infectious oral microbes, a patient with an immunologic or nutritional deficiency should be in good dental health before an elective surgical procedure.[22]

Colonization With Virulent Microflora

Presurgical nares colonization with *Staphylococcus aureus* is present in 20% to 30% of all healthy patients and is strongly associated with skin colonization.[23] However, some carriers may have negative nasal cultures. High-density nasal colonization is the single most important risk factor for developing SSI with *S aureus* after hip or knee replacement surgery.[24] Carriers of *S aureus* in the anterior nares were found to have five times the risk of developing SSI than patients without colonization.[25] Patients with nasal colonization who were treated with 2% mupirocin nasal ointment for 5 days before surgery had a rate of endogenous infection with *S aureus* two to nine times lower than comparable untreated patients.[26,27] Presurgical screening, colonization-directed prophylaxis, and decolonization protocols have led to significantly lower rates of SSI caused by *S aureus.*

Presurgical Length of Stay

A patient may be exposed to transient strains of nosocomial pathogens during hospitalization, leading to a change in skin flora and an increased risk of infection.[4,28] Length of stay in a health care facility is significantly associated with SSI risk.[10,29,30] A patient who has had a prolonged stay in a health care facility should be evaluated for comorbid conditions, cultured for potential colonization with virulent pathogens, and given a prophylactic antibiotic tailored to the antibiogram of both sending and receiving facilities.[10]

Antibiotic Prophylaxis

Routine use of prophylactic antibiotics has led to a dramatic reduction in infection rates for most types of wounds.[6] Prospective double-blind studies supported the use of antibiotic prophylaxis for clean and clean-contaminated orthopaedic procedures. The antibiotic should be carefully selected by considering current recommendations as well as timing, dosage, patient allergies, and possible pathogen resistance to antimicrobial agents. Prophylactic antibiotics should be administered over a short period of time to avoid opportunistic nosocomial infection, including late SSI caused by hematogenous seeding of implants or surgical hematomas[31-33] (see chapter 19).

Hair Removal

The risk of SSI was found to be significantly higher when hair was removed before surgery using a razor than when hair was not removed or was removed using electric clippers immediately before the incision.[34] Razor shaving produces microscopic cuts in the epidermis, exposing deep-seated microorganisms and increasing the risk of bacteremia or direct wound contamination.

Antimicrobial Skin Preparation

The CDC recommends showering with chlorhexidine gluconate before elective surgery as a means of reducing microbial colony counts on the skin. However, this practice has not been proved to decrease the incidence of SSI.[1,35]

For presurgical preparation, a 4% concentration of chlorhexidine gluconate has been shown to be more effective than povidone-iodine or triclocarban soap and water in reducing rates of intrasurgical wound contamination.[36] Povidone-iodine and 4% chlorhexidine gluconate are equally effective for decreasing the initial bacterial skin contamination of both the patient and the surgeon. However, 4% chlorhexidine gluconate is effective for a longer period of time ($P < 0.0001$) and has a greater cumulative effect with prolonged use;[37-39] it also is less toxic, more stable in an open wound, and less irritating to the skin. Repeated scrubbing with alcohol alone or with chlorhexidine gluconate and alcohol was found to be more effective in reducing bacteria than traditional povidone-iodine and chlorhexidine gluconate scrubbing regimens.[40]

1: General Considerations

Barrier Draping

Although the use of either antiseptic-impregnated, adhesive surgical drapes or a postpreparation microbiologic sealant (InteguSeal, Kimberly-Clark, Roswell, GA) can reduce skin bacterial counts, no published controlled clinical study has documented a decreased incidence of SSI.[41]

Glove perforation routinely occurs during most orthopaedic procedures, and, therefore, double gloves should be used. The number of perforations is directly correlated with procedure duration; almost all gloves were found to be punctured after a procedure longer than 3 hours.[42]

Ventilation and Clean Air System

The amount of airborne contamination can be significantly reduced by controlling movement into and within the operating room and by using personal isolation suits.[43] The design and efficiency of the operating room ventilation system, measured in air exchanges per hour, and staff compliance with air flow procedures also are important.[44] Although clean air technology has not been proved to independently decrease the incidence of deep SSI, it was found to significantly decrease rates of bacterial wound contamination, prolonged wound discharge, and superficial infection of the surgical site.[45,46] The CDC recommends that an orthopaedic implantation procedure be performed in an operating room equipped with an ultraclean air system, and the National Institutes of Health concluded that a laminar airflow system is the best option.

Duration of Surgery

The risk of SSI is proportional to the duration of the surgical procedure and roughly doubles with every elapsed hour.[4,9,10,47] Increasing endogenous and exogenous contamination, increasing wound compromise, and the effect of intrinsic and extrinsic host defense factors are responsible. In addition, time-sensitive factors including prolonged patient immobility, patient positioning, and maintenance of sufficient padding for dependent parts and bony prominences can be affected by an unanticipated delay in completing the surgery.[48] Presurgical attention to patient positioning and padding as well as diligent postsurgical surveillance for injury can be helpful in avoiding ulceration, remote-site infection, or SSI caused by bacteremia or direct cross contamination.

Earlier Same-Site Surgery

The risk of SSI is increased if the patient has undergone an earlier surgical procedure at the site.[49,50] The factors responsible for the increased risk include the additional time required to perform a revision procedure, the presence of ischemic scar tissue, and unsuspected microbial contamination of previously implanted hardware by dormant strains in an exopolysaccharide biofilm.[9,51,52] Subclinical infection must be anticipated and pursued with tissue cultures in any revision surgery. To decrease the risk of SSI, every effort should be made to avoid tissue devitalization, hasten wound closure, and intervene aggressively as soon as any sign of wound failure or infection appears.

Suture Materials

The surgeon must consider the chemical composition of suture material, as the presence of any foreign material increases a wound's susceptibility to infection.[53] Absorbable synthetic monofilament suture is associated with a lower rate of infection than absorbable synthetic braided suture, which in turn is associated with a lower rate of infection than nonabsorbable braided suture or natural suture such as catgut or silk.[54] Antimicrobial-impregnated surgical suture materials are beneficial in preventing SSI in a critically contaminated wound.[55]

Best Practices for Avoiding Wound Contamination

Intrinsic and extrinsic factors can contribute to wound contamination even after the surgery. Bacteremia often is associated with a remote-site nosocomial infection (such as pneumonia, a urinary tract infection, or primary bloodstream infection) resulting from the use of an invasive medical device (such as a ventilator, a urinary catheter, an indwelling drain, or a central intravascular line). These devices act as a pathway for environmental microorganisms, facilitate the transfer of pathogens from one part of the body to another, and provide surfaces on which pathogens can proliferate while protected from antimicrobial agents and host defenses; they should be avoided whenever possible.

Postsurgical Drains

A retrospective analysis of more than 73,000 SSIs found that retention of a surgical drain for more than 24 hours was associated with a significantly increased risk of cross contamination with a resistant nosocomial pathogen.[31] The CDC recommends that clean procedures be performed without using a surgical drain; if a drain is necessary, a closed suction system is preferred. The drain should exit through a separate incision and, if possible, should be removed within 24 hours.[1]

Wound Dressings

A surgical wound can be contaminated directly through closed wound margins until it seals.[31] A systematic review of 111 studies found that the rate of infection under an occlusive dressing was significantly lower than the rate of infection under a nonocclusive dressing.[56]

Induced Bacteremia

A patient who is immunocompromised or immunosuppressed or has undergone a prosthetic joint replacement is at an increased risk of developing a prosthesis-related joint infection caused by the hematogenous spread of microorganisms. Patients with pins, plates, screws, or other orthopaedic hardware at sites other than a synovial joint are not at increased risk of hematogenous seeding. The American Academy of Orthopaedic Surgeons recommends that clinicians consider antibiotic prophylaxis for all patients with a joint replacement before any invasive procedure that could cause bacteremia.[57]

Best Surgical Practices for Enhancing the Wound Environment

The local host defenses for controlling or eliminating the proliferation of contaminating pathogens include a physiologic responsiveness to injury fueled by adequate tissue perfusion. The primary defense against surgical pathogens is oxidative killing by neutrophils. Local factors that compromise tissue perfusion, cellular responsiveness, and wound closure are associated with wound-healing disturbances and an increased risk of SSI.[58] Before surgical intervention, every effort should be made to reverse or counter site-specific factors affecting outcomes (**Table 3**).

Wound Oxygenation

Transcutaneous measurement of tissue oxygen tension at the proposed surgical site can reveal ischemia predictive of a postsurgical healing disturbance.[59] A study of patients with diabetes and chronic ischemia found healing of major and minor amputations in 91% of patients whose tissue oxygen tension value was higher than 30 mm Hg; in comparison, the rate of healing was 50% for patients with a value lower than 30 mm Hg. Reversal of tissue hypoxia both restored the ability to heal normally and decreased the incidence of SSI.[60]

Normothermia

Intrasurgical hypothermia causes vasoconstriction, reduction in blood flow to the surgical site, and increased susceptibility to SSI. The use of presurgical and intrasurgical warming decreases the rate of SSI in clean and clean-contaminated procedures.[61,62]

Pain Control

Surgical and postsurgical pain evokes profound neuroendocrine cytokine activity, which in turn evokes a regional arteriolar vasoconstriction and thereby reduces tissue perfusion, tissue oxygen tension, collagen deposition, and wound tensile strength.[63] Poorly controlled surgical pain is associated with an increased risk of SSI.[64]

Hyperbaric Oxygen Therapy

Hyperbaric oxygen therapy is the only method proved to reverse the effects of ionizing radiation. The sensitivity of endothelial cells and myofibroblasts to the effects of radiation causes progressive and permanent fibrosis, capillary loss, and regional ischemia resulting from obliterating endarteritis. In hyperbaric oxygen therapy,

Table 3
Local Wound Factors Associated With Increased Risk of Surgical Site Infection
Anatomic site (superficial joint [elbow, knee], unprotected bone [tibia, sternum], area at risk of contamination [sacrum, coccyx])
Chronic edema
Earlier infection
Earlier surgery
Excessive scarring
Ischemia
Obesity
Radiation injury
Soft-tissue deficit
Vascular disease

a steep oxygen gradient is created between normal and injured tissues, catalyzing the release of platelet- and macrophage-derived angiogenesis factors, which stimulates fibroblast proliferation and collagen synthesis to promote ingrowth of new blood vessels.[65,66] Presurgical treatment with hyperbaric oxygen enhances the potential for normal wound healing in previously irradiated tissues and reduces the incidence of SSI.[67,68]

Surgical Wound Hematoma

A rapidly expanding hematoma in the surgical wound can be an important contributor to the development of SSI.[69] The lesion can block the influx of antibiotics into the surgical site, cause wound-healing disturbances through tissue devitalization, and lead to prolonged wound drainage.[70] The presence of an expansile hematoma mandates débridement and wound revision.

Prolonged Wound Drainage

Serous drainage from a postsurgical wound initially can be treated with compressive and occlusive dressings to prevent retrograde introduction of bacteria. Prolonged drainage requires a biopsy for culturing as well as formal débridement and wound revision.[71] Drainage exceeding 5 days' duration is associated with a threefold to fourfold increase in the risk of developing a deep SSI.[70,72-74]

Blood Transfusion

Several prospective randomized studies have associated intrasurgical or postsurgical blood transfusion with SSI.[75] However, presurgical blood transfusion was not associated with increased risk. This discrepancy suggests that the deleterious effect of intrasurgical or postsurgical transfusion may in part be a surrogate for risk factors such as hypovolemia, decreased tissue perfusion, low oxygen tension, and prolonged surgical time.

Table 4

Systemic Factors Associated With Increased Risk of Surgical Site Infection

Advanced age
Alcoholism
Coagulopathies
Colonization with pathogens resistant to antimicrobial agents
Diabetes mellitus
Hemoglobinopathy
Hypoxia
Immune deficiency
Malignancy
Malnutrition
Nicotine use
Obesity
Organ failure
Parenteral drug abuse
Skin colonization with bacterial pathogens

Best Surgical Practices for Treating Patients With Comorbidities

A patient's predisposition to SSI is strongly influenced by risk factors inherent in underlying health conditions (Table 4). Compromised health is associated with a high incidence of skin or wound breakdown, frequent episodes of bacteremia, immune deficiencies, multiple-joint surgical procedures, poor nutritional status, and increased risk of bleeding. The overall effect is cumulative, and the baseline risk of developing SSI increases with each adverse medical condition.[58,76,77] The presence of three or more comorbidities in patients with a periprosthetic total joint infection of the hip or knee led to a 22% mortality rate and a 100% rate of treatment failure.[58] Elective orthopaedic reconstruction is contraindicated if the patient has a neutrophil count lower than 1,000, a CD4 (T cell) count lower than 200, or an active remote site of infection; or is an intravenous drug abuser.[76,77]

The treatment of patients with comorbidities requires specific precautions.[78] If surgical intervention is necessary, a low-risk procedure of short duration should be chosen. The exposure should be straightforward, with the use of foreign materials limited.[79] If an implant is required, concomitant use of an antibiotic-impregnated depot will help to clear any transient wound contamination (see chapter 9).[80] The outcome can be further safeguarded by postsurgical surveillance for conditions amenable to early intervention, including superficial skin necrosis, prolonged wound drainage, an expansile hematoma, and early signs of sepsis.

Table 5

Methodology for Prevention of Surgical Site Infection

Reduce Pathogen Load
Avoidance of additional surgery
Avoidance of shaving
Clean air systems
Decolonization
Glove changes
Isolation suits
Limited operating room traffic
Limited surgical time
Limited use of postsurgical drains
Occlusive wound dressings
Pressure sore prevention
Prevention or treatment of remote infection
Prophylactic antibiotics
Refreshed instrument basins
Suction tip replacement
Surgical barriers
Surgical preparation
Surgical scrubs
Suture material selection
Wound irrigation

Avoid Wound Contamination and Enhance the Wound Environment
Early intervention for complications
Hematoma decompression
Hemostasis
Hyperbaric oxygen
Implant selection
Limited surgical time
Normothermia
Pain control
Soft-tissue flaps
Supplemental oxygen
Surgical technique
Vacuum-assisted wound closure
Vascular bypass
Wound surveillance

Treat Patients With Comorbidities
Antibiotic desensitization
Detoxification (alcohol, tobacco, drugs)
Glucose control
Low-risk procedures
Nutrition
Reverse coagulopathies
Systems maintenance

Glucose Control

In patients with diabetes who underwent a gastrointestinal or coronary artery bypass graft procedure, a glucose level above 220 mg/dL led to a fivefold increase in the SSI rate. Patients whose glucose level was kept within the normal range had the same SSI rates as patients who did not have diabetes.[81] An elevated intrasurgical or postsurgical glucose level is a risk factor for SSI.[1,9,81-83]

Tobacco Use

Tobacco use is an important risk factor for serious postsurgical complications.[9] A study of 811 consecutive patients after hip or knee arthroplasty found that smoking tobacco was the most important risk factor for developing a postsurgical complication, especially a complication related to wound healing.[84,85] The CDC recommends that patients abstain from using all tobacco products for at least 30 days before elective surgery to reduce the risk of SSI.[1]

Nutritional Status

The association of malnutrition and surgical morbidity is well recognized.[9,86-88] Malnourished patients are at increased risk of developing deep SSI after a major surgical procedure.[89] Perisurgical nutritional support decreases the risk of septic postsurgical complications.[90-92]

Renal Status

Chronic renal failure increases the risk of SSI.[9,93] A patient who is dependent on hemodialysis should receive such a treatment the day before major surgery to minimize the effects of fluid and electrolyte shifts and to correct abnormalities inherent in renal disease.[94]

Summary

To decrease the risk of SSI, caregivers must limit patient exposure to exogenous and endogenous pathogens; establish and maintain a vital, resilient wound; and work to prevent, accommodate, and minimize systemic factors affecting the overall immunity of the host. Infection occurs when the number and virulence of a pathogen are sufficient to overwhelm the wound and the physiologic capability of the host to respond (**Table 5**).

Annotated References

1. Mangram AJ, Horan TC, Pearson ML, Silver LC, Jarvis WR, Hospital Infection Control Practices Advisory Committee: Guideline for prevention of surgical site infection, 1999. *Am J Infect Control* 1999;27:97-134.

2. Institute of Medicine: *Rewarding Provider Performance: Aligning Incentives in Medicare.* Washington, DC, National Academies Press, 2006.

3. Berard F, Gandon J: Postoperative wound infections: The influence of ultraviolet irradiation of the operating room and of various other factors. *Ann Surg* 1964;160: 1-192.

4. Cruse PJ, Ford R: The epidemiology of wound infection: A 10-year prospective study of 62,939 wounds. *Surg Clin North Am* 1980;60:27-40.

5. Culver DH, Horan TC, Gaynes RP, et al: Surgical wound infection rates by wound class, operative procedure, and patient risk index: The National Nosocomial Infections Surveillance System. *Am J Med* 1991;91: 152S-157S.

6. Haley RW, Culver DH, Morgan WM, White JW, Emori TG, Hooton TM: Identifying patients at high risk of surgical wound infection: A simple multivariate index of patient susceptibility and wound contamination. *Am J Epidemiol* 1985;121:206-215.

7. Gherini S, Vaughn BK, Lombardi AV, Mallory TH: Delayed wound healing and nutritional deficiencies after total hip arthroplasty. *Clin Orthop Relat Res* 1993;293: 188-195.

8. Garibaldi RA, Cushing D, Lerer T: Risk factors for postoperative infection. *Am J Med* 1991;91:158S-163S.

9. Peersman G, Laskin R, Davis J, Peterson M: Infection in total knee replacement: A retrospective review of 6489 total knee replacements. *Clin Orthop Relat Res* 2001; 392:15-23.

10. Ridgeway S, Wilson J, Charlet A, Kafatos G, Pearson A, Coello R: Infection of the surgical site after arthroplasty of the hip. *J Bone Joint Surg Br* 2005;187:844-850.

    The risk of infection after primary total hip replacement was greater if the surgery was nonelective, the wound was not classified as clean, the American Society of Anesthesiologists score was 3 or higher, and the patient had a presurgical hospitalization of 3 or more days. The risk increased with advancing age, body mass index greater than 30, and surgical duration of more than 2 hours. Patients in the highest NNIS risk index groups were significantly more likely than other patients to develop SSI.

11. Gaynes RP, Culver DH, Horan TC, Edwards JR, Richards C, Tolson JS: Surgical site infection (SSI) rates in the United States, 1992-1998: The National Nosocomial Infections Surveillance System basic SSI risk index. *Clin Infect Dis* 2001;33(suppl 2):S69-S77.

12. National Nosocomial Infections Surveillance System: National Nosocomial Infections Surveillance (NNIS) System Report: Data summary from January 1992 through June 2004 issued October 2004. *Am J Infect Control* 2004;32:470-485.

    This summary of data collected and reported by the 300 hospitals participating in the NNIS system includes a record for every patient undergoing selected procedures, with SSI risk factors.

13. Ferraz EM, Bacelar TS, Aguiar JL, Ferraz AA, Pagnossin G, Batista JE: Wound infection rates in clean sur-

1: General Considerations

gery: A potentially misleading risk classification. *Infect Control Hosp Epidemiol* 1992;13:457-462.

14. Horan TC, Gaynes RP, Martone WJ, Jarvis WR, Emori TG: CDC definitions of nosocomial surgical site infections, 1992: A modification of CDC definitions of surgical wound infections. *Infect Control Hosp Epidemiol* 1992;13:606-608.

15. Malangoni M: *Critical Issues in Operating Room Management.* Philadelphia, PA, Lippincott-Raven, 1997.

16. Hoborn J: Wet strike-through and transfer of bacteria through operating barrier materials. *Hyg & Med* 1990; 15:15-20.

17. Werner HP, Hoborn J, Schön K, Petri E: Influence of drape permeability on wound contamination during mastectomy. *Eur J Surg* 1991;157:379-383.

18. Whyte W, Hambraeus A, Laurell G, Hoborn J: The relative importance of the routes and sources of wound contamination during general surgery: I. Non-airborne. *J Hosp Infect* 1991;18:93-107.

19. Whyte W, Hambraeus A, Laurell G, Hoborn J: The relative importance of the routes and sources of wound contamination during general surgery: II. Airborne. *J Hosp Infect* 1992;22:41-54.

20. Edwards LD: The epidemiology of 2056 remote site infections and 1966 surgical wound infections occurring in 1865 patients: A four year study of 40,923 operations at Rush-Presbyterian-St. Luke's Hospital, Chicago. *Ann Surg* 1976;184:758-766.

21. Valentine RJ, Weigelt JA, Dryer D, Rodgers C: Effect of remote infections on clean wound infection rates. *Am J Infect Control* 1986;14:64-67.

22. Pallasch TJ, Slots J: Antibiotic prophylaxis and the medically compromised patient. *Periodontol 2000* 1996;10: 107-138.

23. Wenzel RP, Perl TM: The significance of nasal carriage of Staphylococcus aureus and the incidence of postoperative wound infections. *J Hosp Infect* 1995;31:13-24.

24. Kalmeijer MD, van Nieuwland-Bollen E, Bogaers-Hofman D, de Baere GA: Nasal carriage of *Staphylococcus aureus* is a major risk factor for surgical site infections in orthopaedic surgery. *Infect Control Hosp Epidemiol* 2000;21:319-323.

25. Perl TM: Prevention of Staphylococcus aureus infections among surgical patients: Beyond traditional perioperative prophylaxis. *Surgery* 2003;134:S10-S17.

    S aureus carriers have a twofold to ninefold increased risk of developing surgical site or intravenous catheter infection. Mupirocin ointment is 97% effective in reducing S aureus nasal carriage.

26. Hacek DM, Robb WJ, Paule SM, Kudrna JC, Stamos VP, Peterson LR: Staphylococcus aureus nasal de-colonization in joint replacement surgery reduces infection. *Clin Orthop Relat Res* 2008;466:1349-1355.

    A molecular diagnostic surveillance program taking only 2 hours to complete was used to detect S aureus carriers before hip or knee surgery, with subsequent decolonization of carriers using mupirocin twice a day for 5 days before surgery.

27. Rao N, Cannella B, Schnebel JA, Crossett LS, Yates AJ Jr, McGough R III: A preoperative decolonization protocol for Staphylococcus aureus prevents orthopaedic infections. *Clin Orthop Relat Res* 2008;466: 1343-1348.

    Presurgical eradication of S aureus in known nasal carriers decreased the risk of SSI after total joint arthroplasty. The rates of SSI caused by S aureus in carriers were 0% and 3.5% in the treated and control patients, respectively (P = 0.016), with control carrier numbers projected on the basis of a 25% population incidence.

28. Larson EL, Cronquist AB, Whittier S, Lai L, Lyle CT, Della Latta P: Differences in skin flora between inpatients and chronically ill outpatients. *Heart Lung* 2000; 29:298-305.

29. Altemeier WA, Culbertson WR, Hummel RP: Surgical considerations of endogenous infections: Sources, types and methods of control. *Surg Clin North Am* 1968;48: 227-240.

30. Kowli SS, Nayak MH, Mehta AP, Bhalerao RA: Hospital infections. *Indian J Surg* 1985;48:475-486.

31. Manian FA, Meyer PL, Setzer J, Senkel D: Surgical site infections associated with methicillin-resistant Staphylococcus aureus: Do postoperative factors play a role? *Clin Infect Dis* 2003;36:863-868.12652387

    Patients infected with methicillin-resistant S aureus were retrospectively compared with patients infected with other organisms. Only discharge to a long-term care facility and duration of postsurgical antibiotic treatment were significantly associated with an increased risk of SSI on multivariate analysis.

32. Bratzler DW, Hunt DR: The surgical infection prevention and surgical care improvement projects: National initiatives to improve outcomes for patients having surgery. *Clin Infect Dis* 2006;43:322-330.

33. Gould CV, McDonald LC: Bench to bedside review: Clostridium difficile colitis. *Crit Care* 2008;12:203.

    The incidence and severity of *Clostridium difficile* disease have greatly increased with the emergence of highly virulent strains resistant to fluoroquinolones and cephalosporins. Short-term antibiotic prophylaxis, careful selection of agents, and early testing for C difficile are recommended. Hospitals are the major source of infection.

34. Tanner J, Woodings D, Moncaster K: Preoperative hair removal to reduce surgical site infection. *Cochrane Database Syst Rev* 2006;2:CD004122.

    Eleven randomized, controlled trials studied presurgical hair removal and SSI. There was no statistically significant difference between no hair removal and depilatory cream or razor use. More SSIs appeared after shaving than after clipping or depilatory cream use.

35. Hayek LJ, Emerson JM, Gardner AM: A placebo-controlled trial of the effect of two preoperative baths or showers with chlorhexidine detergent on postoperative wound infection rates. *J Hosp Infect* 1987;10: 165-172.

36. Garibaldi RA: Prevention of intraoperative wound contamination with chlorhexidine shower and scrub. *J Hosp Infect* 1988;11:5-9.

37. Aly R, Maibach HI: Comparative antibacterial efficacy of a 2-minute surgical scrub with chlorhexidine gluconate, povidone-iodine, and chloroxylenol sponge-brushes. *Am J Infect Control* 1988;16:173-177.

38. Ostrander RV, Botte MJ, Brage ME: Efficacy of surgical preparation solutions in foot and ankle surgery. *J Bone Joint Surg Am* 2005;87:980-985.

A prospective study of 125 consecutive patients evaluated the efficacy of three skin preparation solutions for presurgical elimination of bacterial pathogens: Dura-Prep (0.7% iodine and 74% isopropyl alcohol; 3M, St. Paul, MN), Techni-Care (3% chloroxylenol; Care-Tech, St. Louis, MO), and ChloraPrep (2% chlorhexidine gluconate and 70% isopropyl alcohol; Cardinal Health, Dublin, OH) were most effective (P < 0.0001).

39. Culligan PJ, Kubik K, Murphy M, Blackwell L, Snyder J: A randomized trial that compared povidone iodine and chlorhexidine as antiseptics for vaginal hysterectomy. *Am J Obstet Gynecol* 2005;192:422-425.

Chlorhexidine gluconate was more effective than providine iodine in decreasing bacterial colony counts in several tissue specimens taken at fixed time intervals during routine vaginal hysterectomies (P = 0.003).

40. Pereira LJ, Lee GM, Wade KJ: An evaluation of five protocols for surgical hand washing in relation to skin condition and microbial counts. *J Hosp Infect* 1997;36: 49-65.

41. Johnston DH, Fairclough JA, Brown EM, Morris R: Rate of bacterial recolonization of the skin after preparation: Four methods compared. *Br J Surg* 1987;74:64.

42. Sanders R, Fortin P, Ross E, Helfet D: Outer gloves in orthopaedic procedures: Cloth compared to latex. *J Bone Joint Surg Am* 1990;72:914-917.

43. Owers KL, James E, Bannister GC: Source of bacterial shedding in laminar flow theatres. *J Hosp Infect* 2004; 58:230-232.

Microbiological swabbing of facial areas not covered by theater clothing in 20 staff members found significantly more colonies cultured from the ears (P = 0.047, Freidman's test) than the forehead or eyebrows. Exhaust helmets or mandatory ear coverage is supported for scrub staff in arthroplastic surgery.

44. Laufman H: Surgical hazard control: Effective architecture and engineering. *Arch Surg* 1973;107:552-559.

45. Knobben BA, van Horn JR, van der Mei HC, Busscher HJ: Evaluation of measures to decrease intraoperative bacterial contamination in orthopaedic implant surgery. *J Hosp Infect* 2006;62:174-180.

At 18-month follow-up of 207 patients after total hip or knee replacement, laminar air system and staff behavior modifications were found to significantly decrease contamination (P = 0.001), prolonged wound discharge (P = 0.002), and superficial SSI (P = 0.004). Deep periprosthetic infection was not significantly decreased (P = 0.359).

46. Ritter MA, Olberding EM, Malinzak RA: Ultraviolet lighting during orthopaedic surgery and the rate of infection. *J Bone Joint Surg Am* 2007;89:1935-1940.

Joint arthroplasty was performed using horizontal laminar air flow without ultraviolet lighting or standard-exchange ventilation with ultraviolet lighting and appropriate safety precautions. The odds of infection were 3.1 times greater after procedures performed without ultraviolet lighting (P < 0.0001).

47. Haley RW, Culver DH, Morgan WM, White JW, Emori TG, Hooton TM: Identifying patients at high risk of surgical wound infection: A simple multivariate index of patient susceptibility and wound contamination. *Am J Epidemiol* 1985;121:206-215.

48. Schoonhoven L, Defloor T, Grypdonck MHF: Incidence of pressure ulcers due to surgery. *J Clin Nurs* 2002;11: 479-487.

49. Wimmer C, Gluch H, Franzreb M, Ogon M: Predisposing factors for infection in spine surgery: A survey of 850 spinal procedures. *J Spinal Disord* 1998;11: 124-128.

50. Lee J, Singletary R, Schmader K, Anderson DJ, Bolognesi M, Kaye KS: Surgical site infection in the elderly following orthopaedic surgery: Risk factors and outcomes. *J Bone Joint Surg Am* 2006;88:1705-1712.

In a multicenter risk factor and outcomes study of 15,218 orthopaedic procedures (mean patient age, 74.7 years), 171 patients developed SSI. Admission from a health care facility (odds ratio = 4.35, P = 0.003) and earlier same-site surgery (odds ratio = 2.98, P = 0.006) were the only independent predictors of SSI.

51. Dobbins JJ, Seligson D, Raff MJ: Bacterial colonization of orthopedic devices in the absence of clinical infection. *J Infect Dis* 1988;158:203-205.

52. Nelson CL, McLaren AC, McLaren SG, Johnson JW, Smeltzer MS: Is aseptic loosening truly aseptic? *Clin Orthop Relat Res* 2005;437:25-30.

Relatively mild ultrasonic intensity (60 Hz for 30 minutes) was used to disrupt bacterial adherence to surgically removed hardware. Infestations as low as 50 colony-forming units per implant were reported in patients with no clinical or laboratory evidence of infection.

1: General Considerations

53. Elek SD, Conen PE: The virulence of Staphylococcus pyogenes for man: A study of the problems of wound infection. *Br J Exp Pathol* 1957;38:573-586.

54. Chu CC, Williams DF: Effects of physical configuration and chemical structure of suture materials on bacterial adhesion: A possible link to wound infection. *Am J Surg* 1984;147:197-204.

55. Marco F, Vallez R, Gonzalez P, Ortega L, de la Lama J, Lopez-Duran L: Study of the efficacy of coated Vicryl plus antibacterial suture in an animal model of orthopedic surgery. *Surg Infect (Larchmt)* 2007;8:359-366.

    In a validated rat model, *Staphylococcus epidermidis* (100,000 colony-forming units/mL) was used to contaminate a deep surgical steel suture in wounds closed with treated or untreated Vicryl sutures. After 16 days, positive culture counts were significantly lower in retrieved specimens from wounds closed with Vicryl with triclosan (*P* = 0.005).

56. Hutchinson JJ, McGuckin M: Occlusive dressings: A microbiologic and clinical review. *Am J Infect Control* 1990;18:257-268.

57. American Academy of Orthopaedic Surgeons: Antibiotic prophylaxis for bacteremia in patients with joint replacements. Rosemont, IL, American Academy of Orthopaedic Surgeons, 2009. http://www.aaos.org/about/papers/advistmt/1033.asp. Accessed May 20, 2009.

    The current information statement relates to all patients with a joint replacement who are undergoing an invasive procedure.

58. Cierny G III, DiPasquale D: Periprosthetic total joint infections: Staging, treatment and outcomes. *Clin Orthop Relat Res* 2002;403:23-28.

59. Burgess EM, Matsen FA III, Wyss CR, Simmons CW: Segmental trans-cutaneous measurements of PO2 in patients requiring below-knee amputations for peripheral vascular insufficiency. *J Bone Joint Surg Am* 1982;64:378-382.

60. Bunt TJ, Holloway GA: TcPO2 as an accurate predictor of therapy in limb salvage. *Ann Vasc Surg* 1996;10:224-227.

61. Mahoney CB, Odom J: Maintaining intraoperative normothermia: A meta-analysis of outcomes with costs. *AANA J* 1999;67:155-163.

62. Melling AC, Ali B, Scott EM, Leaper DJ: Effects of preoperative warming on the incidence of wound infection after clean surgery: A randomized controlled trial. *Lancet* 2001;358:876-880.

63. Hopf HW, Hunt TK, West JM, Blomquist P, Goodson WH III, Jensen JA: Wound tissue oxygen tension predicts the risk of wound infection in surgical patients. *Arch Surg* 1997;132:997-1005.

64. Akca O, Melischek M, Scheck T, et al: Postoperative pain and subcutaneous oxygen tension. *Lancet* 1999;354:41-42.

65. Wu L, Pierce GF, Ladin DA, Zhao LL, Rogers D, Mustoe TA: Effects of oxygen on wound responses to growth factors: Kaposi's FGF, but not basic FGF stimulates repair in ischemic wounds. *Growth Factors* 1995;12:29-35.

66. Gleadle JM, Ratcliffe PJ: Hypoxia and the regulation of gene expression. *Mol Med Today* 1998;4:122-129.

67. Marx RE, Johnson RP, Kline SN: Prevention of osteoradionecrosis: A randomized prospective clinical trial of hyperbaric oxygen versus penicillin. *J Am Dent Assoc* 1985;111:49-54.

68. Myers RA, Marx RE: Use of hyperbaric oxygen in postradiation head and neck surgery. *NCI Monogr* 1990;9:151-157.

69. Nelson CL: Prevention of sepsis. *Clin Orthop Relat Res* 1987;222:66-72.

70. Cheung EV, Sperling JW, Cofield RH: Infection associated with hematoma formation after shoulder arthroplasty. *Clin Orthop Relat Res* 2008;466:1363-1367.

    Positive cultures were obtained from 66% of shoulders after surgery for hematoma following arthroplasty. The organisms included *Propionibacterium acnes, S epidermidis, Streptococcus* species, and *Peptostreptococcus* species. A 42% rate of unsatisfactory results was associated with this complication, including a 17% rate of deep infection. Level of evidence: IV.

71. Jaberi FM, Parvizi J, Haytmanek BS, et al: Procrastination of wound drainage and malnutrition affects the final outcome of total joint arthroplasty. *Clin Orthop Relat Res* 2008;466:1368-1371.

    A stepwise logistic regression-adjusted analysis determined predictors of irrigation and débridement failure in 300 patients with refractory wound drainage after total hip or knee arthroplasty. Malnutrition (*P* = 0.002) and days from initial surgery to irrigation and débridement (*P* = 0.02) were significant risk factors.

72. Nelson CL, Bergfeld JA, Schwartz J, Kolczun M: Antibiotics in human hematoma and wound fluid. *Clin Orthop Relat Res* 1975;108:138-144.

73. Surin VV, Sundholm K, Bäckman L: Infection after total hip replacement with special reference to a discharge from the wound. *J Bone Joint Surg Br* 1983;65:412-418.

74. Weiss AP, Krackow KA: Persistent wound drainage after primary total knee arthroplasty. *J Arthroplasty* 1993;8:285-289.

75. Jensen LS, Anderson AJ, Christiansen PM, et al: Postoperative infection and natural killer cell function following blood transfusion in patients undergoing elective colorectal surgery. *Br J Surg* 1992;79:513-516.

76. McPherson EJ, Tontz WT, Patzakis M, et al: Outcome of infected total knees utilizing a staging system for

prosthetic joint infection. *Am J Orthop* 1999;28: 161-165.

77. Lai K, Bohm ER, Burnell C, Hedden DR: Presence of medical co-morbidities in patients with infected primary hip or knee arthroplasties. *J Arthroplasty* 2007;22: 651-656.

    A retrospective case-control study examined medical co-morbidities and SSI risk after total hip or knee arthroplasty. Diabetes mellitus and total number of medical conditions were associated with significantly higher risk of infection. Optimization of medical comorbidities before surgery is recommended.

78. Bongartz T, Sutton AJ, Sweeting MJ, Buchan I, Matteson EL, Montori V: Anti-TNP antibody therapy in rheumatoid arthritis and the risk of serious infections and malignancies: Systematic review and meta-analysis of rare harmful effects in randomized controlled trials. *JAMA* 2006;295:2275-2285.

    A formal meta-analysis with pooled sparse adverse effects data from randomized, placebo-controlled studies with a total of 5,005 patients found that the pooled odds ratio for malignancy was 3.3 (95% confidence interval, 1.2-9.1) and for serious infection was 2.2 (95% confidence interval, 1.3-3.1), indicating an increased incidence of both disease states.

79. Cierny G III, DiPasquale D: Treatment of chronic infection. *J Am Acad Orthop Surg* 2006;14:S105-S110.

    This is a 15-year chronological history of one center's experience in treating segmental, osseous, and composite defects in 1,966 adult patients with chronic osteomyelitis. Identification of a subset of low-risk surgical procedures closes the outcomes gap between healthy and compromised patients.

80. Jiranek WA, Hanssen AD, Greenwald AS: Antibiotic-loaded bone cement for infection prophylaxis in total joint replacement. *J Bone Joint Surg Am* 2006;88:2487-2500.

    The US Food and Drug Administration approves commercially available, low-dose antibiotic-loaded bone cement only for use in the second stage of a revision total joint arthoplasty. High-dose antibiotic-loaded bone cement, which is required for treating an established musculoskeletal infection, must be hand mixed using antibiotics and acrylic substrates.

81. Lilienfeld DE, Vlahov D, Tenney JH, McLaughlin JS: Obesity and diabetes as risk factors for postoperative wound infections after cardiac surgery. *Am J Infect Control* 1988;16:3-6.

82. Furnary AP, Zerr KJ, Grunkemeier GL, Starr A: Continuous intravenous insulin infusion reduces the incidence of deep sternal wound infection in diabetic patients af-

ter cardiac surgical procedures. *Ann Thorac Surg* 1999; 67:352-360.

83. Zerr KJ, Furnary AP, Grunkemeier GL, Bookin S, Kanhere V, Starr A: Glucose control lowers the risk of wound infection in diabetics after open heart operations. *Ann Thorac Surg* 1997;63:356-361.

84. Ridderstolpe L, Gill H, Granfeldt H, Ahlfeldt H, Rutberg H: Superficial and deep sternal wound complications: Incidence, risk factors and mortality. *Eur J Cardiothorac Surg* 2001;20:1168-1175.

85. Møller AM, Villebro N, Pedersen T, Tønnesen H: Effect of preoperative smoking intervention on postoperative complications: A randomised clinical trial. *Lancet* 2002; 359:114-117.

86. Green KA, Wilde AH, Stulberg BN: Preoperative nutritional status of total joint patients: Relationship to postoperative wound complications. *J Arthroplasty* 1991;6: 321-325.

87. Gherini S, Vaughn BK, Lombardi AV Jr, Mallory TH: Delayed wound healing and nutritional deficiencies after total hip arthroplasty. *Clin Orthop Relat Res* 1993; 293:188-195.

88. Klein JD, Garfin SR: Nutritional status in the patient with spine infection. *Orthop Clin North Am* 1996;27: 33-36.

89. Marin LA, Salido JA, Lopez A, Silva A: Preoperative nutritional evaluation as a prognostic tool for wound healing. *Acta Orthop Scand* 2002;73:2-5.

90. Sizer T: *Standards and Guidelines for the Nutritional Support of Patients in Hospitals.* Maidenhead, Berks, England, British Association for Parenteral and Enteral Nutrition, 1996.

91. Torosian MH: Perioperative nutrition support for patients undergoing gastrointestinal surgery: Critical analysis and recommendations. *World J Surg* 1999;23: 565-569.

92. Heys SD, Ogston KN: Peri-operative nutritional support: Controversies and debates. *Int J Surg Investig* 2000;2:107-115.

93. Bradley JR, Evans DB, Calne RY: Long-term survival in haemodialysis patients. *Lancet* 1987;1:295-296.

94. Sunday JM, Guille JT, Torg JS: Complications of joint arthroplasty in patients with end-stage renal disease on hemodialysis. *Clin Orthop Relat Res* 2002;397: 350-355.

1: General Considerations

Section 2

Diagnostic Modalities

SECTION EDITOR:

ROBIN PATEL, MD

Chapter 5

Clinical and Laboratory Evaluation

*Carl A. Deirmengian, MD   *Robin Patel, MD

Introduction

Accurate diagnosis of bone and joint infection is critical to providing high-quality patient care. An infected extremity is best evaluated through a combination of clinical examination, patient history, and laboratory evaluation. A systematic multiorgan examination is required for identifying or ruling out the presence of infection elsewhere in the body as well as for accurately interpreting laboratory data. Identification of one or more causative microorganisms and their in vitro antimicrobial susceptibility is essential to directing the optimal medical therapy.

Clinical Evaluation

Most of the direct clinical information used in diagnosis is obtained from the local examination. The components of the examination can be thought of as the individual elements of a clinical picture. No formula can identify and interpret the clinical signs; they must be evaluated together in the context of the patient's clinical history and the suspected diagnosis. The pattern-recognition skills necessary for the clinical identification of an infection are developed through experience.

The Four Cardinal Signs of Inflammation

The Roman encyclopedist Aulus Cornelius Celsus is credited with describing the four cardinal signs of inflammation: calor, dolor, tumor, and rubor (temperature, pain, swelling, and erythema, respectively). The presence of these signs is highly suggestive of infection, which is an especially potent form of inflammation.

Bacteria at the site of infection release a specific set of antigens that are recognized by local immune cells. The characteristic response of the immune cells leads to local and systemic changes including increased local blood flow and vascular permeability, which generate the cardinal signs of inflammation.

Temperature

Cellulitis, septic arthritis, osteomyelitis, and other local infections are almost invariably associated with locally increased temperature. Early surgical studies established that increases in temperature at the site of infection are related to blood temperature and flow rather than exothermic reaction.[1] The clinical examination should include a manual comparison of the temperature in the affected area to the temperature on the contralateral side or in nearby tissues. Temperature elevation is not a conclusive sign of infection because many aseptic forms of inflammation also cause local warmth.

Pain

The local immune response to infection generates a series of compounds that stimulate the pain response. Although many forms of inflammation cause pain, the pain associated with infection tends to be especially severe. For example, gout and osteoarthritis both cause tenderness when the joint is taken through an arc of motion; in contrast, an infected joint is usually exquisitely tender when the joint is taken through even a very small arc of motion. For this reason, the phrase "pain with micromotion" is used in describing an especially painful and possibly infected joint.

The anatomic origin of the pain should be determined, if possible. Testing of specific anatomic tissues can be extremely useful in isolating the origin of the pain and thus contributing to the diagnosis. For example, cellulitis of the skin over the knee causes significant tenderness to light skin touch but less discomfort with gentle knee motion; in septic arthritis, the skin over the knee is usually less tender, but gentle knee motion leads to severe pain.

The patient's general medical condition and history must be considered when evaluating pain. In a patient with diabetes, neuropathy may be masking the pain. An acute or chronic spinal condition also can blunt or mask pain.

Swelling

Vascular permeability at the site of inflammation results in a release of fluid into the interstitial tissue space. On a T2-weighted MRI study, this local fluid is

*Carl A. Deirmengian, MD or the department with which he is affiliated has received research or institutional support from the Orthopaedic Research and Education Foundation and is a consultant for or an employee of Zimmer. Robin Patel, MD or the department with which she is affiliated has received research or institutional support from the Orthopaedic Research and Education Foundation. Robin Patel, MD has filed a patent application for an implant sonication apparatus and technique but has foregone the right to receive royalties.

2: Diagnostic Modalities

responsible for an increased tissue signal indicating local inflammation; the response associated with infection is generally more significant than that of other forms of inflammation.

Clinical examination of the tissues can help in identifying the extent and location of edema, which can greatly facilitate the formulation of a differential diagnosis. For example, the presence of generalized, bilateral lower extremity edema usually indicates systemic fluid retention. Generalized, unilateral edema from the thigh to the toes suggests a deep vein thrombosis. For example, circumferential edema around the knee suggests a localized pathology; a saclike swelling anterior to the patella results from prepatellar bursitis.

Erythema
The magnitude, location, and pattern of erythema all contribute to the clinical evaluation. Increased local blood flow from inflammation results in redness at the site of inflammation. Pressure applied to an area of redness caused by increased blood flow usually results in blanching as blood is removed from the area of point pressure. Blood soon returns to the blanched area, reinstating the erythematous appearance.

Other Local Clinical Signs
Joint Effusion
Fluid accumulation in the synovial space can be caused by many inflammatory joint conditions. In a joint with a deep capsule, such as the hip, an effusion is difficult to detect clinically. An effusion can easily be identified in a joint with a more superficial capsule, such as the knee or elbow.

Fluid-filled bursae must be differentiated from joint effusions. In the elbow or knee, the superficial bursae often are found to be inflamed or fluid filled. An inflamed olecranon bursa can be palpated as a discrete mass posterior to the olecranon. An inflamed prepatellar bursa is found as a discrete mass superficial to the patella. Many etiologies can lead to joint effusion. However, the presence or absence of an effusion can significantly aid in the differential diagnosis. For example, a knee with pain on motion but without effusion is unlikely to be affected by septic arthritis.

Drainage
Drainage refers to the fluid that flows from a wound or surgical incision. Drainage from deep tissue implies the presence of a route between the skin and deep tissue, possibly representing contamination and infection. The quantity and quality of the drainage are significant. Purulent fluid is thick, heterogeneous, off-white in color, and highly cellular. Purulent fluid often is infected and seldom is aseptic. Serous fluid is thin, homogeneous, slightly yellow in color, and acellular. Serous drainage can be either infected or aseptic.

Usually the amount of serous drainage from a surgical wound steadily decreases during the first 1 to 3 days after a surgical procedure. Persistent drainage or an increasing volume of drainage suggests the presence of infection.

A sinus is a chronic communication between the skin and deeper tissue. Sinuses vary in size from a small circular skin defect to a larger hole. They almost always represent a deep infection. A sinus located near a joint should be assumed to communicate with the joint unless proved otherwise. A sinus located at the site of earlier surgery is highly suggestive of a deep, chronic infection.

Systemic Clinical Signs
A systematic examination of multiple organ systems can be useful in identifying the underlying cause of a local infection. In addition, the discovery of another infection can alter the interpretation of systemic laboratory tests. Every patient with a suspected musculoskeletal infection should undergo a systematic examination of other systems. If systemic signs and symptoms of infection are present but the local examination does not suggest infection, the possible presence of an infection elsewhere in the body should be considered.

Pulmonary System
Pulmonary conditions such as pneumonia or bronchitis can cause fever and alter laboratory values, indicating the presence of infection. The possibility of an infectious pulmonary condition should be considered in the diagnosis of musculoskeletal infection. The examination should include observation of coughing, difficulty in breathing, mucus production, and oxygen saturation.

Urinary Tract
The patient should be questioned about urinary symptoms, and urine should be analyzed for evidence of infection. Systemic signs and laboratory values suggesting a postsurgical wound infection often are caused by a urinary tract infection. The urinary tract also can be the underlying bacterial source of a musculoskeletal infection.

Gastrointestinal System
The patient should be questioned about gastrointestinal symptoms, and the feces should be analyzed for evidence of infection. In the setting of antibiotic use, *Clostridium difficile* colitis is a common cause of fever and an elevated white blood cell count, which may incorrectly influence the clinical diagnosis of musculoskeletal infection.

Cardiovascular System
The patient's heart and blood vessels should be examined for evidence of disease. The presence of a murmur may indicate endocarditis, which can cause periprosthetic infection. Local vasculitis or thrombosis also can cause systemic fever or local signs and symptoms that could confound the diagnosis.

Table 1

Sample Leukocyte Counts and Likelihood Ratios for the Diagnosis of Septic Arthritis

Leukocyte Count	Likelihood Ratio	Range (95% Confidence Interval)
< 25 × 10³/μL	0.32	0.23-0.43
≥ 25 × 10³/μL	2.90	2.50-3.40
> 50 × 10³/μL	7.70	5.70-11.00
> 100 × 10³/μL	28.00	12.00-66.00

Laboratory Evaluation

The optimal medical therapy for a patient with infection requires the identification of causative microorganisms and their in vitro antimicrobial susceptibility. If possible, antimicrobial agents should be withheld until specimens are collected for culturing.

Septic Arthritis in a Native Joint

The erythrocyte sedimentation rate (ESR) and C-reactive protein (CRP) level often are elevated in a patient with septic arthritis. The white blood cell count and procalcitonin level may be elevated or normal.

Synovial fluid aspiration is the most important test for the diagnosis of septic arthritis. Fluoroscopic- or CT-guided aspiration is recommended for joints in which aspiration is difficult, such as the hip. If polyarticular infection is suspected, aspiration should be performed for all potentially infected joints. Synovial fluid should be sent for leukocyte count, Gram staining, and aerobic and anaerobic culturing. Septic arthritis and acute crystal-induced arthritis can occur simultaneously, and a diagnosis of crystalline arthritis therefore does not exclude the possibility of infection.[2]

The American Rheumatologic Association specifies a synovial fluid leukocyte count higher than 50 × 10³/μL for the diagnosis of septic arthritis.[3] This criterion has recently been questioned. One study found that 18 × 10³/μL is a more appropriate criterion.[4] Another recent study found that the summary likelihood ratio for the diagnosis of septic arthritis increases with the synovial fluid leukocyte count[5] (Table 1). A synovial fluid leukocyte differential count of at least 90% neutrophils suggests the presence of septic arthritis with a likelihood ratio of 3.4; a count of less than 90% neutrophils lowers the likelihood ratio to 0.34.

The sensitivity of synovial fluid culturing for diagnosing nongonococcal septic arthritis is 75% to 90%, and the sensitivity of synovial fluid Gram staining is 50% to 75%.[6] The method used to culture synovial fluid is important. The BACTEC Peds Plus/F vial used in conjunction with the BACTEC 9240 instrument (Becton Dickinson, Sparks, MD) is more sensitive and specific than conventional agar plate methods for detecting microorganisms in synovial fluid.[7] In addition to synovial fluid, bacteria for culturing should be obtained from blood, any wound contiguous to the affected joint, and any skin lesions. Fungal and mycobacterial staining and culturing sometimes are appropriate, as is serologic testing for parvovirus B19 or *Borrelia burgdorferi*. In a patient with a positive *B burgdorferi* serology and suspected Lyme arthritis, a polymerase chain reaction of synovial fluid for *B burgdorferi* DNA may be helpful, although this type of testing is not routinely available. Testing for fungal and mycobacterial pathogens as well as *Brucella* species may be useful in diagnosing chronic arthritis.

Tuberculin skin testing has a positive result in approximately 90% of patients with tuberculous arthritis, and interferon-γ release tests such as QuantiFERON (Cellestis, Carnegie, Victoria, Australia) should be equally successful. In a patient with tuberculous arthritis, the synovial fluid typically has a leukocyte count of 10 to 20 × 10³/μL. Acid-fast stains of synovial fluid are rarely positive. However, mycobacterial culturing yields *Mycobacterium tuberculosis* in approximately 80% of patients. Synovial biopsy culturing is the most sensitive test for diagnosing tuberculous arthritis, yielding a positive finding in approximately 90% of patients. Synovial biopsy characteristically reveals granulomas. Antimicrobial susceptibility testing of *M tuberculosis* should always be performed to help in determining the optimal therapy.

Synovial fluid from a patient with gonococcal arthritis usually has a leukocyte count of 50 to 100 × 10³/μL, with a neutrophil predominance. Joint aspirate from a patient with disseminated gonococcal infection without frank suppurative arthritis may have a lower leukocyte count. Approximately one quarter of patients with suppurative gonococcal arthritis have a positive synovial fluid Gram stain. *Neisseria gonorrhoeae* can be cultured from synovial fluid for approximately one half of patients with gonococcal arthritis and one quarter of those with disseminated gonococcal infection. Among patients with disseminated gonococcal infection or gonococcal arthritis, *N gonorrhoeae* is more likely to be isolated from or detected in mucosal sites such as the cervix, urethra, rectum, or oropharynx than from synovial fluid or blood. Nucleic acid amplification tests using urine or urethral or cervical swabs should be considered for a patient suspected of having gonococcal arthritis.

Table 2

Synovial Fluid Characteristics and Arthritis-Related Laboratory Findings

Characteristic	Finding				
	Normal (No Arthritis)	Noninflammatory Arthritis*	Inflammatory Arthritis†	Septic Arthritis (Native Joint)‡	Prosthetic Hip or Knee Infection§
Appearance	Clear	Clear	Opaque or translucent	Opaque Yellow or green	Clear or opaque
WBC/mm³	< 1,000	< 1,000	5,000–75,000	> 50,000	> 1,100-3,000
Polymorphonuclear cells	< 25%	< 25%	> 50%	> 75%	> 64%-80%
Culture	Negative	Negative	Negative	Positive	Positive

WBC = white blood cell count.
*Associated conditions: Degenerative joint disease, trauma, pigmented villonodular synovitis, neuropathy, systemic lupus erythematosus, acute rheumatic fever.
†Associated conditions: Rheumatoid arthritis, crystal-induced arthritis, seronegative arthropathy, systemic lupus erythematosus, acute rheumatic fever.
‡An immunocompromised patient may not have an elevated synovial WBC. A normal or noninflammatory WBC does not preclude active septic arthritis.
§Data are unavailable for other types of prosthetic joints. Underlying inflammatory arthritis may cause false-positive results.

The findings of synovial fluid analysis are summarized in Table 2.

Osteomyelitis
Presurgical Evaluation
In a patient with osteomyelitis, the ESR and CRP level are often elevated; the white blood cell count and procalcitonin level may be elevated or normal. In a patient with a diabetic foot infection, an ESR higher than 70 mm/h predicts the presence of an underlying bone infection.[8]

Cultures from a foot ulcer or draining sinus tract may not indicate an infectious process in bone, and a bone biopsy is therefore recommended. Nonetheless, obtaining swab cultures from an ulcer or draining sinus tract has two potential benefits. Detection of a resistant organism such as a vancomycin-resistant *Enterococcus* species may indicate the need for a specific infection-control measure. Isolation of *Staphylococcus aureus* from a superficial tissue culture is strongly correlated with its presence in deep tissues. (This relationship is not found in other organisms.) Swab specimens taken from a decubitus ulcer or another surface ulcer are inappropriate for anaerobic culturing.

Intrasurgical and Interventional Radiographic Evaluation
Aerobic and anaerobic culturing should be performed on material obtained through punch biopsy, fluid aspiration, or curettage from deep tissue at the margin of a decubitus or other surface ulcer. The sensitivity of CT-guided percutaneous biopsy and aspiration is 50% for the diagnosis of vertebral osteomyelitis. If the results of aspiration are inconclusive, a repeat aspiration is warranted. Open vertebral biopsy may be needed if percutaneous biopsy does not yield a diagnostic result or the patient has not responded to empiric antimicrobial chemotherapy (administered in the absence of a microbiologic diagnosis of vertebral osteomyelitis).

Cultures should be obtained for *Brucella* species, mycobacteria, and fungi if the aerobic and anaerobic bacterial culture results are negative. The possibility of tuberculous osteomyelitis should be considered after a bone biopsy finding of granulomatous inflammation, if epidemiologically and clinically appropriate. Acid-fast staining and mycobacterial culturing of bone biopsy specimens are also appropriate, and tuberculin skin testing or interferon-γ release testing can be helpful. In a child, the diagnosis of acute hematogenous osteomyelitis often is made based on compatible radiographic and clinical findings as well as positive blood cultures.

Prosthetic Joint Infection
Presurgical Evaluation
The laboratory evaluation for prosthetic joint infection differs from the evaluation for septic arthritis of a native joint. The key presurgical laboratory tests include ESR, CRP level, and a synovial fluid leukocyte count, differential, and culture.

In a retrospective analysis of laboratory test results before total knee or hip arthroplasty revision or resection in 227 patients, an ESR higher than 30 mm/h was 66% sensitive and 90% specific for the diagnosis of prosthetic joint infection; a CRP level higher than 1.0 mg/dL was 77% sensitive and 84% specific[9] (Figure 1). The combination of a normal ESR and a normal CRP level predicted the absence of a prosthetic hip or knee infection in 92% of the patients studied. However, conditions such as rheumatoid arthritis can cause an elevation in ESR or CRP level. ESR and CRP level appear to be insensitive for the diagnosis of prosthetic shoulder infection. The presurgical leukocyte count is insensitive as a marker of underlying prosthetic joint infection.

Procalcitonin, a precursor of calcitonin, is elevated in some patients with systemic bacterial infection. Nonorthopaedic studies suggest that both procalcitonin and interleukin-6 levels are elevated in patients with sys-

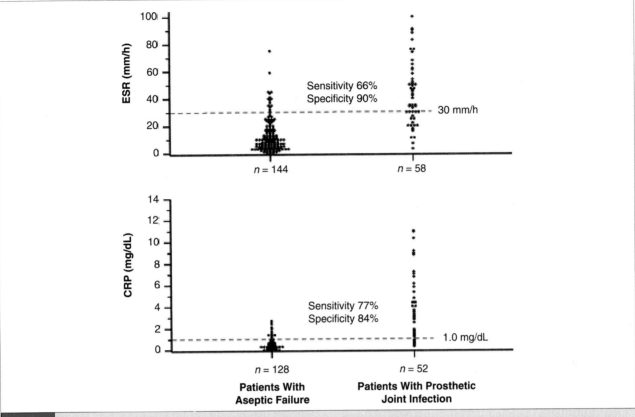

Figure 1 Presurgical ESR and CRP level of patients undergoing knee or hip arthroplasty revision or resection (*N* = 227), as related to sensitivity and specificity at the criterion level. (Adapted with permission from the Mayo Foundation for Medical Education and Research.)

temic bacterial infections.[10] Interleukin-6 and tumor necrosis factor–α are released by monocytes in response to infection. A recent study of 78 patients undergoing revision surgery for total knee or hip replacement evaluated procalcitonin, interleukin-6, tumor necrosis factor–α, and CRP levels as markers of prosthetic joint infection. CRP (at a level higher than 3.2 mg/dL) and interleukin-6 (at a level higher than 12 pg/mL) were found to have the greatest sensitivity (96% and 87%, respectively).[10] The combination of CRP and interleukin-6 levels identified all patients with a deep infection of an implant. Procalcitonin (at a level higher than 0.3 ng/mL) and tumor necrosis factor–α (at a level higher than 40 ng/mL) had low sensitivity (33% and 43%, respectively), although they were specific (98% and 94%, respectively).

Synovial fluid aspiration may be considered for any patient who will undergo a revision or resection knee or hip arthroplasty. The aspirated fluid should be submitted for a leukocyte count and differential as well as aerobic and anaerobic bacterial culturing. Some patients, including those with an acute periprosthetic fracture in the absence of antecedent symptoms, may not require aspiration. Synovial fluid leukocyte and differential cell counts were evaluated before revision knee arthroplasty in a prospective study of 133 patients with

no underlying inflammatory joint disease.[11] A leukocyte count higher than 1.7 × 10³/μL was 94% sensitive and 88% specific for the diagnosis of prosthetic joint infection. A differential of more than 65% neutrophils was 97% sensitive and 98% specific. *S aureus* was the only organism associated with a leukocyte count higher than 100 × 10³/μL. Synovial fluid leukocyte and differential cell counts were evaluated in a similar prospective study of 168 patients with a prosthetic knee or hip joint.[12] A synovial fluid leukocyte count higher than 1.8 × 10³/μL was 90% sensitive and 99% specific for the diagnosis of prosthetic joint infection, and a leukocyte differential of more than 73% neutrophils was 83% sensitive and 93% specific. However, these synovial fluid leukocyte and differential levels were not sensitive for the diagnosis of prosthetic shoulder infection. These criteria differ from those used in the same tests for patients with septic arthritis of a native joint.

Culturing of synovial fluid was found to be 56% to 92% sensitive for the diagnosis of prosthetic joint infection (depending on the study); specificity ranged from 94% to 98%.[13-15] Isolation of an organism that can be either a contaminant or a pathogen, such as a coagulase-negative *Staphylococcus* species, should prompt the culturing of synovial fluid from a second aspiration. Isolation of the organism from the second

2: Diagnostic Modalities

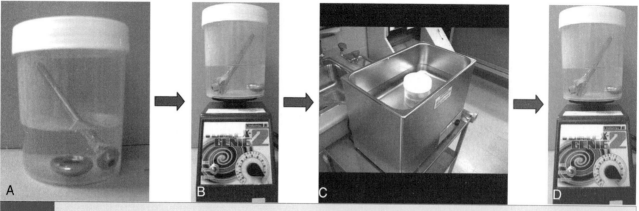

Figure 2 Orthopaedic hardware sonication to obtain fluid for culturing. Explanted joint instrumentation (a shoulder implant is shown) is placed into a sterile jar with 400 mL of Ringer solution (**A**), vortexed for 30 seconds (**B**), bath sonicated for 5 minutes at 40 kHz (**C**), and vortexed for 30 seconds (**D**). The resulting fluid is concentrated and cultured.

aspiration strongly suggests that the organism is the cause of the infection. The sensitivity of a synovial fluid Gram stain is 32%, and this test is not generally indicated.

Intrasurgical Laboratory Evaluation

Periprosthetic tissue culturing is the standard approach to intrasurgical microbiologic diagnosis of prosthetic joint infection. Intrasurgical swabbing is generally inappropriate because of its low sensitivity.[16] Because a single periprosthetic tissue culture has low specificity and sensitivity, multiple specimens should be submitted for culturing. A study using mathematical modeling to determine the ideal number of periprosthetic tissue specimens for culturing found that five or six specimens obtained during surgery must be cultured to produce an accurate diagnosis.[17] The isolation of indistinguishable microorganisms from three or more specimens was highly predictive of infection, although only 65% of patients who were found to be infected on the basis of histopathologic findings had three positive cultures. For a patient undergoing hip or knee arthroplasty revision, at least three periprosthetic tissue specimens should be submitted for bacterial culture. Gram staining of periprosthetic tissue is generally not recommended because its sensitivity is less than 12%.[17]

In a recently described technique, microorganisms are taken from the surface of an explanted hip or knee prosthesis. The explanted components are placed into a sterile jar, Ringer solution is added, and the components are vortexed and bath sonicated (**Figure 2**); aerobic and anaerobic culturing of the resulting fluid is then performed. A prospective trial compared this technique with conventional periprosthetic tissue culturing for microbiologic diagnosis of prosthetic joint infection in patients undergoing revision or resection arthroplasty of a total knee (*n* = 208) or hip prosthesis (*n* = 125).[13] Of the 333 patients, 252 had aseptic failure, and 81 had prosthetic joint infection. The sensitivities of the periprosthetic tissue and sonicate fluid cultures were 60.5% and 77.8%, respectively (*P* < 0.001), and the

specificities were 99.2% and 98.8%, respectively. In the patients who had received antimicrobial therapy during the 2 weeks before surgery, the sensitivities of the periprosthetic tissue and sonicate fluid cultures were 47.5% and 75.0%, respectively (*P* = 0.002). Similar results recently were reported for shoulder explants. The sonicate fluid culturing technique improves the microbiologic diagnosis of spinal implant infection, in comparison with culturing of the tissue surrounding the implant. Orthopaedic implants should be processed only in a solid container; sonication using a plastic bag was associated with a risk of contamination.[18]

Administration of antimicrobial therapy before revision or resection surgery is known to decrease the sensitivity of both periprosthetic tissue and sonicate fluid cultures. However, the optimal time for discontinuing therapy before surgery has not been determined. In addition, the use of antimicrobial-impregnated cement can negatively affect culture sensitivity. The ideal duration of culture incubation is undetermined, although 2 weeks is recommended for the isolation of *Propionibacterium acnes* in anaerobic cultures.

The presence of acute inflammation in a periprosthetic tissue specimen from the hip or knee was found in several studies to be both sensitive and specific for the diagnosis of prosthetic joint infection (**Table 3**), although testing for inflammation does not provide a microbiologic diagnosis. The accuracy of the test can be affected by sampling variation or the pathologist's level of experience. The criteria defining a positive result vary among studies and institutions. Histopathologic findings appear to be insensitive for the diagnosis of prosthetic shoulder infection.

Summary

The clinical examination for musculoskeletal infection is highly subjective, and it depends on multiple findings. A thorough evaluation will not only suggest possible disease etiology but also identify the anatomic location and infected tissue. Differentiation of infection

2: Diagnostic Modalities

Table 3

Studies of Intrasurgical Frozen-Section Histopathologic Findings
of Acute Inflammation in Prosthetic Joint Infection Diagnosis

Study	N	Joint(s) Studied	Number of Polymorphonuclear Leukocytes (> or ≥)	Sensitivity (%)	Specificity (%)	Positive Predictive Value (%)
Athanasou et al[19] (1995)	106	Hip, knee	1	90	96	88
Feldman et al[20] (1995)	33	Hip, knee	5	100	100	100
Lonner et al[21] (1996)	142	Hip	5	84	96	70
	33	Knee	10	84	99	89
Pace et al[22] (1997)	18	Hip, knee	5	82	93	82
Abdul-Karim et al[23] (1998)	64	Hip, knee	5	43	97	60
Banit et al[24] (2002)	55	Knee	10	100	96	82
	63	Hip	10	45	92	55
Musso et al[25] (2003)	45	Hip, knee	5	50	95	60
Ko et al[26] (2005)	40	Hip, knee	5	67	97	86
Wong et al[27] (2005)	33	Hip	5	93	77	68
		Knee	10	86	85	75
Frances Borrego et al[28] (2007)	63	Hip	10	67	90	80
	83	Knee	10	50	100	100
Nunez et al[29] (2007)	136	Hip	5	86	87	79

from other forms of inflammation is difficult because no clinical signs are specific only to infection. Each component of the clinical evaluation has characteristics that contribute to the clinical picture, and the experienced physician uses pattern recognition skills in considering the clinical components. The clinical evaluation is critical to the interpretation of the laboratory evaluation. The laboratory diagnosis of musculoskeletal infection varies depending on the type of infection and its anatomic location. The diagnostic tests for prosthetic joint infection are different from those for native bone and joint infection.[20-30]

Annotated References

1. Waterman NG, Goldberg L, Appel T: Tissue temperatures in localized pyogenic infections. *Am J Surg* 1969; 118:31-35.

2. Shah K, Spear J, Nathanson LA, McCauley J, Edlow JA: Does the presence of crystal arthritis rule out septic arthritis? *J Emerg Med* 2007;32:23-26.

This retrospective study conducted at a university tertiary care referral center examined the incidence of septic arthritis in patients with synovial fluid joint crystals. Of 265 joint aspirates containing crystals, 4 had a positive synovial culture.

3. Hasselbacher P: Arthrocentesis, synovial fluid and synovial biopsy, in Klippel JH, Weyland CM, Wortmann RL (eds): *Primer on the Rheumatologic Diseases*, ed 11. Atlanta, GA, Arthritis Foundation, 1997, pp 98-104.

4. Li SF, Cassidy C, Chang C, Gharib S, Torres J: Diagnostic utility of laboratory tests in septic arthritis. *Emerg Med J* 2007;24:75-77.

A retrospective cohort study evaluated 156 patients who had undergone arthrocentesis. The 16 patients who had a positive arthrocentesis culture or surgical findings were considered to have septic arthritis. A synovial fluid leukocyte count of at least $17.5 \times 10^3/\mu L$ was found to maximize sensitivity and specificity for the diagnosis of septic arthritis.

5. Margaretten ME, Kohlwes J, Moore D, Bent S: Does this adult patient have septic arthritis? *JAMA* 2007;297: 1478-1488.

The summary likelihood ratio for the diagnosis of septic arthritis was found to increase with the synovial fluid leukocyte count. A polymorphonuclear cell differential count of at least 90% suggested a diagnosis of septic arthritis with a likelihood ratio of 3.4 (95% CI, 2.8-4.2), and a polymorphonuclear cell differential count of less than 90% lowered the likelihood ratio to 0.34 (95% CI, 0.25-0.47).

6. Swan A, Amer H, Dieppe P: The value of synovial fluid assays in the diagnosis of joint disease: A literature survey. *Ann Rheum Dis* 2002;61:493-498.

7. Hughes JG, Vetter EA, Patel R, et al: Culture with BACTEC Peds Plus/F bottle compared with conventional methods for detection of bacteria in synovial fluid. *J Clin Microbiol* 2001;39:4468-4471.

8. Cavanagh PR, Lipsky BA, Bradbury AW, Botek G: Treatment for diabetic foot ulcers. *Lancet* 2005;366: 1725-1735.

    This discussion of the diagnosis and treatment of diabetic foot ulcers stresses that antimicrobial therapy should be guided by tissue culture results, and the goal should be to cure the infection rather than simply to heal the wound.

9. Trampuz A, Piper KE, Hanssen AD, Osmon DR, Steckelberg JM, Patel R: Erythrocyte sedimentation rate and C-reactive protein are useful preoperative predictors of the absence of prosthetic hip and knee infection. *Clin Microbiol Infect* 2005;11(suppl 2):526.

    The ESR and CRP level were examined in 227 patients before total knee or hip arthroplasty revision or resection. An ESR higher than 30 mm/h had sensitivity and specificity of 66% and 90%, respectively, for the diagnosis of prosthetic joint infection; a CRP level higher than 1.0 mg/dL had sensitivity and specificity of 77% and 84%, respectively.

10. Bottner F, Wegner A, Winkelmann W, Becker K, Erren M, Gotze C: Interleukin-6, procalcitonin and TNF-alpha: Markers of peri-prosthetic infection following total joint replacement. *J Bone Joint Surg Br* 2007;89: 94-99.

    In an evaluation of biomarkers useful in the diagnosis of prosthetic knee or hip infection, CRP and interleukin-6 levels were found to be the most sensitive; procalcitonin and tumor necrosis factor–α levels were insensitive.

11. Trampuz A, Hanssen AD, Osmon DR, Mandrekar J, Steckelberg JM, Patel R: Synovial fluid leukocyte count and differential for the diagnosis of prosthetic knee infection. *Am J Med* 2004;117:556-562.

    A synovial fluid leukocyte differential of more than 65% neutrophils and a leukocyte count higher than $1.7 \times 10^3/\mu L$ were found to be sensitive and specific for the diagnosis of prosthetic knee infection in patients without underlying inflammatory joint disease.

12. Parvizi J, Ghanem E, Menashe S, Barrack RL, Bauer TW: Periprosthetic infection: What are the diagnostic challenges? *J Bone Joint Surg Am* 2006;88(suppl 4): 138-147.

Synovial fluid leukocyte and differential cell counts were prospectively evaluated in 168 patients with a prosthetic knee or hip joint. A synovial fluid leukocyte count higher than $1.8 \times 10^3/\mu L$ was 90% sensitive and 99% specific for the diagnosis of prosthetic joint infection; a differential of more than 73% neutrophils was 83% sensitive and 93% sensitive.

13. Trampuz A, Piper KE, Jacobson MJ, et al: Sonication of removed hip and knee prostheses for diagnosis of infection. *N Engl J Med* 2007;357:654-663.

    Culturing of samples obtained by prosthesis vortexing and sonication was more sensitive than conventional periprosthetic tissue culturing for the microbiologic diagnosis of prosthetic hip and knee infection, particularly if the patient had received antimicrobial therapy within 2 weeks before surgery.

14. Spanghel MJ, Masri BA, O'Connell JX, Duncan CP: Prospective analysis of preoperative and intraoperative investigations for the diagnosis of infection at the sites of two hundred and two revision total hip arthroplasties. *J Bone Joint Surg Am* 1999;81:672-683.

15. Lachiewicz PF, Rogers GD, Thomason HC: Aspiration of the hip joint before revision total hip arthroplasty: Clinical and laboratory factors influencing attainment of a positive culture. *J Bone Joint Surg Am* 1996;78: 749-754.

16. Zimmerli W: Infection and musculoskeletal conditions: Prosthetic-joint-associated infections. *Best Pract Res Clin Rheumatol* 2006;20:1045-1063.

    Prosthetic joint infection is difficult to diagnose. The causative organism may not appear in synovial fluid and may be exclusively present as a device-associated biofilm.

17. Atkins BL, Athanasou N, Deeks JJ, et al: Prospective evaluation of criteria for microbiological diagnosis of prosthetic-joint infection at revision arthroplasty: The OSIRIS Collaborative Study Group. *J Clin Microbiol* 1998;36:2932-2939.

18. Piper KE, Jacobson MJ, Cofield RH, et al : Microbiologic diagnosis of prosthetic shoulder infection by use of implant sonication. *J Clin Microbiol* 2009 [published online ahead of print March 4, 2009].

    The sonication technique was applied to 136 shoulder explants. Sonicate fluid culture was found to be more sensitive and specific than periprosthetic tissue culture for diagnosing prosthetic infections.

19. Trampuz A, Piper KE, Hanssen AD, et al: Sonication of explanted prosthetic components in bags for diagnosis of prosthetic joint infection is associated with risk of contamination. *J Clin Microbiol* 2006;44:628-631.

    Sonication of resected hip and knee arthroplasty components in bags enabled the recovery of large numbers of bacteria from the surface of orthopaedic implants. Because of bag leakage, the method as applied in this study lacked specificity.

20. Athanasou NA, Pandey R, de Steiger R, Crook D, Smith PM: Diagnosis of infection by frozen section dur-

ing revision arthroplasty. *J Bone Joint Surg Br* 1995;77: 28-33.

21. Feldman DS, Lonner JH, Desai P, Zuckerman JD: The role of intraoperative frozen sections in revision total joint arthroplasty. *J Bone Joint Surg Am* 1995;77:1807-1813.

22. Lonner JH, Desai P, Dicesare PE, Steiner G, Zuckerman JD: The reliability of analysis of intraoperative frozen sections for identifying active infection during revision hip or knee arthroplasty. *J Bone Joint Surg Am* 1996;78:1553-1558.

23. Pace TB, Jeray KJ, Latham JT Jr: Synovial tissue examination by frozen section as an indicator of infection in hip and knee arthroplasty in community hospitals. *J Arthroplasty* 1997;12:64-69.

24. Abdul-Karim FW, McGinnis MG, Kraay M, Emancipator SN, Goldberg V: Frozen section biopsy assessment for the presence of polymorphonuclear leukocytes in patients undergoing revision of arthroplasties. *Mod Pathol* 1998;11:427-431.

25. Banit DM, Kaufer H, Hartford JM: Intraoperative frozen section analysis in revision total joint arthroplasty. *Clin Orthop Relat Res* 2002;401:230-238.

26. Musso AD, Mohanty K, Spencer-Jones R: Role of frozen section histology in diagnosis of infection during revision arthroplasty. *Postgrad Med J* 2003;79:590-593.

   This retrospective study reports the use of frozen section histology as a diagnostic tool in 45 patients with suspected prosthetic joint infection. The sensitivity and specificity of frozen section histology were 50% and 95%, respectively.

27. Ko PS, Ip D, Chow KP, Cheung F, Lee OB, Lam JJ: The role of intraoperative frozen section in decision making in revision hip and knee arthroplasties in a local community hospital. *J Arthroplasty* 2005;20:189-195.

Intrasurgical frozen sections from 40 hip and knee revision arthroplasty procedures were evaluated. The presence of five neutrophils per high-power field was found to constitute a positive result, with sensitivity of 67% and specificity of 97%.

28. Wong YC, Lee QJ, Wai YL, Ng WF: Intraoperative frozen section for detecting active infection in failed hip and knee arthroplasties. *J Arthroplasty* 2005;20:1015-1020.

   The results of intrasurgical frozen section analysis were reported for 33 patients undergoing exploration or revision hip or knee surgery, using a positive criterion of a neutrophil count higher than 5 per high-power field. Sensitivity, specificity, positive predictive value, and negative predictive value were 93%, 77%, 68%, and 95%, respectively.

29. Frances Borrego A, Martinez FM, Cebrian Parra JL, Graneda DS, Crespo RG, Lopez-Duran Stern L: Diagnosis of infection in hip and knee revision surgery: Intraoperative frozen section analysis. *Int Orthop* 2007; 31:33-37.

   This study examined intraoperative frozen section analysis and periprosthetic tissue culture in 170 patients with prosthetic revision. In the knee arthroplasty revision group, the sensitivity and specificity were 67% and 90%, respectively. In the hip arthroplasty revision group, the sensitivity and specificity were 50% and 100%, respectively.

30. Nunez LV, Buttaro MA, Morandi A, Pusso R, Piccaluga F: Frozen sections of samples taken intraoperatively for diagnosis of infection in revision hip surgery. *Acta Orthop* 2007;78:226-230.

   The diagnostic accuracy of frozen section histopathology taken during revision hip surgery was evaluated in 136 prostheses thought to be infected. The presence of five or more polymorphonuclear leukocytes per high-power field was considered a positive result. Comparison with culture results revealed an 85% sensitivity and 87% specificity.

2: Diagnostic Modalities

Chapter 6

Diagnostic Imaging of Periprosthetic Joint Infections

*Javad Parvizi, MD, FRCS   *William B. Morrison, MD   Abbas Alavi, MD

Introduction

Radiography, CT, scintigraphy, MRI, and ultrasonography can be used for imaging of joint pathology, and often they are used in combination. The advantages and limitations of each should be considered in formulating an imaging algorithm for the diagnosis of periprosthetic joint infection.

Radiography

Plain radiography is the primary modality for imaging of a potentially infected joint. The many advantages of plain radiography include the level of anatomic detail, versatility in positioning and views, widespread availability, and low cost. The development of digital or computed radiography is the most important recent advance in radiology. This technology provides linear response curves over a broader range than is allowed by film-screen radiography. Small or moderate variations in exposure are better tolerated, and, as a result, the images are of consistently higher quality. Processing algorithms can be used to optimize images specific to a body part or projection. The need to retake a radiograph is decreased substantially because of the extended dynamic range of digital radiography. Image processing and distribution are managed through a picture-archiving and communication system, which allows images to be viewed on any computer with a compact disk reader. Digital radiography allows panning, zooming, and windowing of images, thereby improving the diagnostic yield. Although the spatial resolution of digital radiography is not as high as that of film-screen radiography, experience and data accumulation have led to the conclusion that improved contrast resolution is more important than spatial resolution.[1]

AP and lateral radiographs should be taken whenever a patient has joint pain after implant placement. Radiographs are useful in determining the cause of implant failure and revealing wear, osteolysis, fracture, and additional information about the environment around the prosthesis. Radiographs can also reveal periosteal reaction, bone cysts, and focal resorption indicative of periprosthetic joint infection[2] (**Figure 1**). Early implant loosening should alert the surgeon to the possibility of a dormant underlying infection.[3] Although the characteristic radiographic appearance of infection, such as periosteal reaction, focal osteolysis, and eventual loosening of components, can be used to diagnose periprosthetic joint infection, these radiographic signs rarely appear in infected arthroplasties. The role of radiography therefore is to rule out the presence of other aseptic etiologies such as aseptic loosening or periprosthetic fracture.

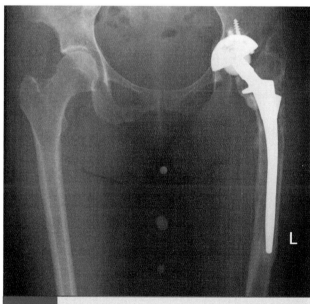

Figure 1 AP radiograph showing focal osteolysis, periosteal reaction, and loosening of the hip component, subsequently found to be caused by an infection.

*Javad Parvizi, MD, FRCS or the department with which he is affiliated has received research or institutional support from Stryker and is a consultant for or an employee of Stryker and Smith and Nephew. William B. Morrison, MD is a consultant for or an employee of ONI Medical Systems.

2: Diagnostic Modalities

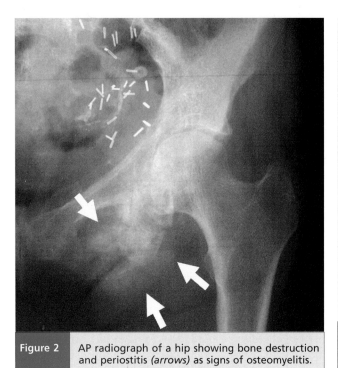

Figure 2 AP radiograph of a hip showing bone destruction and periostitis *(arrows)* as signs of osteomyelitis.

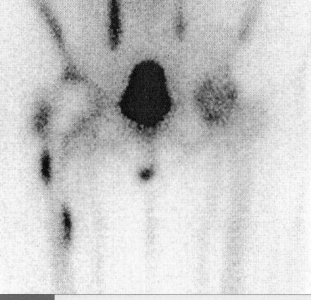

Figure 3 Bone scan of a hip with focal uptake in a patient who was confirmed to have a periprosthetic joint infection.

Radiographs are unable to detect osteomyelitis during its early stages. The earliest radiographic findings related to osteomyelitis include adjacent soft-tissue swelling, joint effusion, erosion related to adjacent septic arthritis, and rarefaction or lucency in the underlying bone. These features typically appear on radiographs only after extensive underlying osteomyelitis has developed. In the later stages of osteomyelitis, frank bone destruction and sequestered bone necrosis may be seen within the area of infection. Chronic osteomyelitis appears as a mixed destructive-sclerotic density, and a diagnosis of acute-on-chronic osteomyelitis requires radiographic visualization of bone destruction or periostitis (**Figure 2**).

Radionuclide Imaging

Traditional Methods

Radionuclide imaging is the method of choice for diagnosing periprosthetic joint infection. Three scintigraphic methods for imaging the musculoskeletal system are clinically available: the technetium Tc 99m (^{99m}Tc) methylene diphosphonate (MDP) scan (performed in a delayed fashion or in three phases producing early vascular images, midrange blood pool images, and delayed images); the gallium 67 scan; and the labeled white blood cell scan, using indium In 111 (^{111}In) or ^{99m}Tc as the radiotracer. Because ^{99m}Tc MDP accumulates in areas of bone turnover and is nonspecific, tracer uptake and the resulting hot spot may be related to a tumor, infection, arthritis, trauma, or another cause (**Figure 3**). A ^{99m}Tc MDP bone scan is often used in the initial diagnostic work-up of periprosthetic joint infection because an absence of tracer uptake effectively rules out the presence of infection. However, differentiation between a normal process and a pathologic state is complicated by the appearance of increased activity on bone marrow scintigraphy for as long as 12 months after surgery, particularly if a cementless stem was used. Many joint infections occur during the first 12 months after arthroplasty, and bone marrow scintigraphy therefore has limited value during this period.[4] Sensitivity of 33%, specificity of 86%, a positive predictive value of 30%, and a negative predictive value of 88% were found using bone marrow scintigraphy to examine 72 total joint arthroplasties.[5]

A ^{99m}Tc bone scan is rarely used alone in the diagnosis of periprosthetic joint infection. Usually a dual-tracer technique is used, such as a simultaneous ^{111}In-labeled leukocyte scan and ^{99m}Tc MDP bone scan.[6] The diagnosis of infection is based on the relative difference in the uptake of the two tracers. The combination of ^{99m}Tc and ^{111}In decreases the rate of false positive findings and improves specificity. The reported accuracy of this technique ranges from 89% to 98%.[6] In theory, labeled leukocyte tracers such as ^{111}In do not accumulate at sites of increased bone turnover, in the absence of infection. The combination of a ^{99m}Tc sulfur colloid scan and a leukocyte scan relies on a similar principle. Gallium 67 is taken up by areas of inflammation and has been used in the diagnosis of infection. However, gallium tracer also can be taken up by areas of neuropathic disease.

The combination of in vitro labeling of white blood cells with ^{111}In and ^{99m}Tc sulfur colloid marrow imaging provides the highest sensitivity and specificity and is the preferred imaging modality for assessing infection after total joint arthroplasty.[4] However, administration of a combined scan is labor intensive and associated with risks including transfusion reaction. The ^{99m}Tc tracer is injected first and allowed to accumulate in areas of high metabolic activity and increased blood flow. Leukocytes are then obtained, labeled with ^{111}In, and reinjected into the patient.[6]

All scintigraphic methods have two important limitations. Image production is delayed because of the time required for the tracer to be distributed, although the use of ^{99m}Tc (which has a shorter half-life than ^{111}In) has somewhat reduced the delay. In addition, scintigraphic methods produce low-resolution images.

Positron Emission Tomography

Because of the limitations of scintigraphic methods, interest is increasing in alternative imaging modalities, including positron emission tomography (PET). The introduction of PET and the combination of PET and CT are the most significant recent advancements in nuclear medicine. Combining PET and CT allows precise localization of areas of abnormal uptake to specific anatomic features. PET uses short-lived positron-emitting radioisotopes that must be produced by an on-site cyclotron. As a result, it has only recently come into widespread use. PET using fluorodeoxyglucose (FDG) is a high-resolution technique that identifies the energy consumption of different tissues in three dimensions.[7] FDG is advantageous as a diagnostic radiopharmaceutical agent because its uptake reflects the amount of glucose used by a given tissue and therefore indicates the tissue's metabolic rate.[8] FDG PET has been shown to have 95% sensitivity and 93% specificity in diagnosing infection around a hip prosthesis.[7,9] When FDG is taken up by a cell, it is phosphorylated to deoxyglucose-6-phosphate and trapped in the cell long enough to be imaged by PET. However, PET is generally nonspecific and targets any area of inflammation; noninfectious inflammatory conditions therefore must be ruled out.

PET may compensate for some shortcomings of conventional bone scans. FDG uptake rapidly produces in vivo labeling of inflammatory cells at the site of infection. FDG PET therefore can be used to image a substantially larger population of cells, including those residing in or traveling to the area of infection and inflammation. The scans can be completed within 2 hours of intravenous FDG injection because of its rapid uptake by inflammatory cells.[10] In the presence of infection, a massive exudation of leukocytes and other immunologically active cells can be observed because of increased vascular permeability and mediator-induced chemotaxis. These activated leukocytes and macrophages have an increased energy requirement, which is reflected by increased FDG uptake (Figure 4). Periprosthetic tissue also is affected by the immunologic reaction, and a diffuse accumulation of FDG may be found not only at the prosthesis-bone interface but also in the surrounding soft tissues. FDG uptake does not rely on leukocyte migration, as conventional bone scans do, and treatment with antibiotics is unlikely to affect the

sensitivity of PET in delineating sites of infection. A semiquantification technique called standardized uptake value can be used to assess the degree of infection revealed by PET.[11] Standardized uptake value is sometimes helpful, but it cannot be recommended as the sole criterion for interpreting a PET study.

Some institutions are using FDG PET in presurgical evaluation of patients with a suspected periprosthetic infection in the hip or another joint. In one study, combined ^{99m}Tc-^{111}In scans were found to have greater specificity than FDG PET,[12] but other studies reported superior sensitivity and specificity with the use of PET.[6] A recent prospective comparison of FDG PET to the combined ^{99m}Tc-^{111}In scan found FDG PET to have much greater sensitivity (95% versus 50%) and to be useful in differentiating periprosthetic joint infection from aseptic hip failure.[7] However, the incidence of false-positive results in FDG PET should be considered, especially in areas of particle-induced inflammation where macrophages accumulate. Specific diagnostic criteria for infection must be applied. Tracer uptake between the bone and the prosthesis, but not around the femoral neck or the soft tissues, is indicative of an infection.

Although radionuclide imaging is an exciting development, it requires extensive resources that are not readily available at many institutions. Less expensive, more cost-effective diagnostic methods remain the primary means of diagnosing a periprosthetic joint infection.

Computed Tomography

CT and MRI have relatively minor roles in diagnosing periprosthetic infection. Multidetector CT (MDCT) is an important advance in which simultaneous activation of multiple detector rows allows acquisition of interweaving helical sections. Short gantry-rotation intervals combined with multiple detectors provide increased coverage along the z-axis, allowing rapid data acquisition. The currently available scanners are configured with as many as 16 channel detectors, and 32- to 40-channel detectors will soon be available. A MDCT scanner can be used to generate images of different thicknesses from one data acquisition. The use of submillimeter slice thickness and higher photon flux can improve image quality. The minimum section thickness is approximately 0.6 mm, and images can be reconstructed at an interval of 0.5 mm. The isotropic voxels used in MDCT, measuring 0.5 mm in all directions, greatly improve spatial resolution and the quality of reconstructing algorithms, allowing exquisite multiplanar reformatting and three-dimensional imaging. The other advantages of MDCT over conventional CT include greater speed and greater total volume coverage. In the presence of joint implants, the ability to acquire high-quality images is improved (Figure 5). Metal artifacts

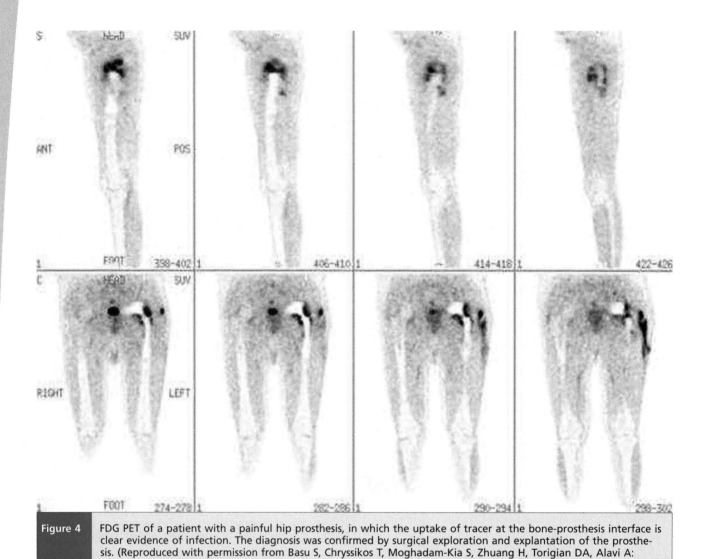

Figure 4 FDG PET of a patient with a painful hip prosthesis, in which the uptake of tracer at the bone-prosthesis interface is clear evidence of infection. The diagnosis was confirmed by surgical exploration and explantation of the prosthesis. (Reproduced with permission from Basu S, Chryssikos T, Moghadam-Kia S, Zhuang H, Torigian DA, Alavi A: Positron emission tomography as a diagnostic tool in infection. *Semin Nucl Med* 2009;39:36-51.)

caused by photopenic defects in the back projection appear on CT images as streak artifact. On MDCT images, the holes in the filtered back projection are less pronounced, and the severity of streak artifact is lessened. However, additional tissue radiation is required to obtain this improvement; the exposure time and radiation dose must be increased in the interest of maintaining a reasonable noise level.

The use of CT in diagnosing periprosthetic infection is evolving because of the capabilities of MDCT. However, significant artifact can limit image quality, and tissue characterization also is limited. CT sometimes is useful; it is rapid, widely available, and able to provide thin, high-resolution images of osseous cortical, trabecular, and articular detail.

Magnetic Resonance Imaging

MRI is the preferred imaging modality to assess bone for the presence of infection (**Figure 6**), although its role in diagnosing periprosthetic joint infection is lim-

ited. MRI studies can reveal internal derangement of joints as well as bone marrow and soft-tissue disease. Planes can be preselected to depict relevant anatomic features, and sequences can be chosen to highlight specific tissue types or anatomic detail. Although MRI techniques are evolving rapidly, a few basic sequences predominate. In a T1-weighted study, fluid appears dark, fat is bright (unless it is suppressed), and gadolinium contrast is bright. This sequence is useful for depicting anatomy, evaluating for bone marrow disease, and maximizing contrast. In a T2-weighted or short tau inversion recovery study, fluid appears bright. These images are often used to detect disease because most pathologic processes involve edema. A proton density sequence has the advantage of a high signal-to-noise ratio and is often used for high-resolution imaging. Gradient echo sequences are versatile and can be used for high-speed, high-resolution, and three-dimensional volumetric data collection. Gadolinium contrast, administered intravenously and taken up nonspecifically in areas of increased vascularity or extracellular fluid

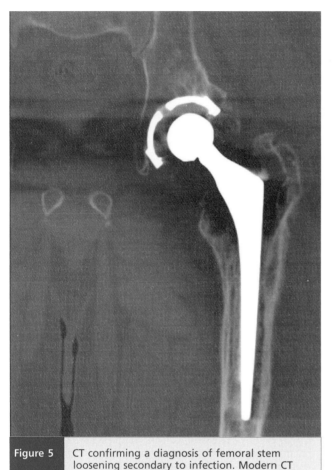

Figure 5 CT confirming a diagnosis of femoral stem loosening secondary to infection. Modern CT imaging allows clear visualization of joints with a metal prosthesis.

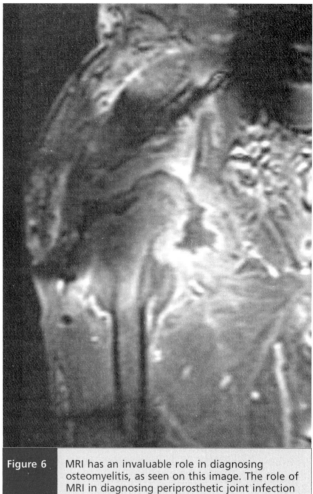

Figure 6 MRI has an invaluable role in diagnosing osteomyelitis, as seen on this image. The role of MRI in diagnosing periprosthetic joint infection remains unknown.

deposition, is useful in evaluating inflammation, neoplasia, and areas of increased or decreased vascularity. Dynamic contrast-enhanced MRI, in which multiple sequential fast-imaging studies are performed immediately after injection of a bolus of contrast, is especially useful in determining the vascularity of musculoskeletal structures such as tumors or areas of osteonecrosis.

The most important recent developments in MRI are high field-strength (3.0 Tesla) clinical systems for imaging the entire body and dedicated extremity scanners operating at 1.0 Tesla. In addition, improvements in gradients and radiofrequency coils are continuing. The time required for acquiring an MRI study is an important limitation that is being addressed by the development of parallel imaging and faster novel pulse sequences. However, the availability of MRI equipment and expertise continues to be limited.

MRI is an excellent tool for the evaluation of osteomyelitis, especially in the early stages of disease when radiography is less sensitive.[13,14] Osteomyelitis is seen on MRI as a diffuse region of bone marrow replacement with adjacent soft-tissue changes characteristic of cellulitis. Septic hip arthritis is often seen, as are sinus tracts to the skin. Osteomyelitis appears as low signal on a T1-weighted study, as edema on a T2-weighted study, and as diffuse enhancement on a postcontrast study. An abscess can be seen in the adjacent soft tissues or in bone itself as a focal area of fluid signal with thick rim enhancement.

Ultrasonography

Ultrasonography is a valuable tool for evaluating soft-tissue structures. In the diagnosis of infection, it is used to detect abscesses, joint effusions, and periosteal reactions. Ultrasonographic technology is widely available and relatively inexpensive. It can produce high-resolution, real-time dynamic images of articular and soft-tissue pathology in any plane. In addition, ultrasonography is used for real-time needle guidance in aspiration of a hip effusion or periarticular abscess. The musculoskeletal applications of ultrasonography continue to be developed.

Summary

Plain radiography still is the most valuable imaging modality. It sometimes can confirm periprosthetic joint infection and can provide information regarding other causes of failure. Triple bone scanning without white cell labeling has little value in diagnosing periprosthetic infections. PET using FDG tracer has been shown to be very useful in the diagnosis of periprosthetic infection of the hip. CT using thin-slice, high-resolution images with artifact subtraction has gained popularity as an imaging modality for diagnosing periprosthetic joint infection. MRI, although useful in diagnosing osteomyelitis, does not appear to be useful in diagnosing periprosthetic joint infection.

Annotated References

1. Ackerman SJ, Gitlin JN, Gayler RW, et al: Receiver operating characteristic analysis of fracture and pneumonia detection: Comparison of laser-digitized workstation images and conventional analog radiographs. *Radiology* 1993;186:263-268.

2. Toms AD, Davidson D, Masri BA, Duncan CP: The management of peri-prosthetic infection in total joint arthroplasty. *J Bone Joint Surg Br* 2006;88:149-155.

   Chronic infection can cause radiographic changes including periostitis, osteopenia, endosteal reaction, and rapid progressive loosening or osteolysis. Although osteolysis and loosening can have other causes, the possibility of infection always must be considered.

3. Della Valle CJ, Zuckerman JD, Di Cesare PE: Periprosthetic sepsis. *Clin Orthop Relat Res* 2004;420:26-31.

   The diagnosis of septic implant failure can be difficult, but it is imperative for optimal outcome of revision total hip arthroplasty.

4. Stumpe KD, Notzli HP, Zanetti M, et al: FDG PET for differentiation of infection and aseptic loosening in total hip replacements: Comparison with conventional radiography and three-phase bone scintigraphy. *Radiology* 2004;231:333-341.

   The results of FDG PET were similar to those of three-phase bone scintigraphy in suspected infection of total hip replacement. FDG PET was more specific but less sensitive than conventional radiography for the diagnosis of infection.

5. Levitsky KA, Hozack WJ, Balderston RA, et al: Evaluation of the painful prosthetic joint: Relative value of bone scan, sedimentation rate, and joint aspiration. *J Arthroplasty* 1991;6:237-244.

6. Palestro CJ, Swyer AJ, Kim CK, Goldsmith SJ: Infected knee prosthesis: Diagnosis with In-111 leukocyte, Tc-99m sulfur colloid, and Tc-99m MDP imaging. *Radiology* 1991;179:645-648.

7. Pill SG, Parvizi J, Tang PH, et al: Comparison of fluorodeoxyglucose positron emission tomography and (111)indium-white blood cell imaging in the diagnosis of periprosthetic infection of the hip. *J Arthroplasty* 2006;21(6 suppl 2):91-97.

   FDG PET enabled the correct diagnosis in 20 of 21 patients with infection (sensitivity, 95.2%) and ruled out infection in 66 of 71 aseptic hips (specificity, 93%); these results corresponded to a positive predictive value of 80% (20/25) and a negative predictive value of 98.5% (66/67).

8. Zhuang H, Yu JQ, Alavi A: Applications of fluorodeoxyglucose-PET imaging in the detection of infection and inflammation and other benign disorders. *Radiol Clin North Am* 2005;43:121-134.

   The glucose intake of inflammatory cells usually is relatively low in the resting state, but it increases significantly after in vivo or in vitro stimulation. Increased glucose metabolism frequently is noted in inflammatory and infectious processes.

9. Parvizi J, Ghanem E, Menashe S, Barrack RL, Bauer TW: Periprosthetic infection: What are the diagnostic challenges? *J Bone Joint Surg Am* 2006; 88(suppl 4):138-147.

   The criterion for the diagnosis of periprosthetic infection with FDG PET requires increased FDG uptake at the prosthesis-bone interface, not limited to the soft tissue or neck of the prosthesis.

10. Vanquickenborne B, Maes A, Nuyts J, et al: The value of (18)FDG-PET for the detection of infected hip prosthesis. *Eur J Nucl Med Mol Imaging* 2003;30:705-715.

    An 18-FDG PET scan can be completed within 2 hours after injection of the tracer agent because FDG accumulates rapidly in the inflammatory cells.

11. Mumme T, Reinartz P, Alfer J, Muller-Rath R, Buell U, Wirtz DC: Diagnostic values of positron emission tomography versus triple-phase bone scan in hip arthroplasty loosening. *Arch Orthop Trauma Surg* 2005;125: 322-329.

    Standardized uptake values were calculated from the lesion with the highest FDG uptake.

12. Love C, Marwin SE, Tomas MB, et al: Diagnosing infection in the failed joint replacement: A comparison of coincidence detection 18F-FDG and 111In-labeled leukocyte/99mTc-sulfur colloid marrow imaging. *J Nucl Med* 2004;45:1864-1871.

    Coincidence detection-based 18F-FDG imaging is less accurate than labeled leukocyte-marrow imaging for diagnosing infection of a failed prosthetic joint, regardless of how the images are interpreted.

13. Huang AB, Schweitzer ME, Hume E, Batte WG: Osteomyelitis of the pelvis/hips in paralyzed patients: Accuracy and clinical utility of MRI. *J Comput Assist Tomogr* 1998;22:437-443.

14. Lee SK, Suh KJ, Kim YW, et al: Septic arthritis versus transient synovitis at MR imaging: Preliminary assessment with signal intensity alterations in bone marrow. *Radiology* 1999;211:459-465.

Chapter 7

The Microbiologic and Histopathologic Diagnosis of Orthopaedic Infections

Alex C. McLaren, MD   Michael A. Saubolle, PhD, ABMM, FAAM, FIDSA
Edwin Yu, MD   J. Timothy Feltis, MD, FRCPC

Introduction

The diagnosis and treatment of infection rely heavily on identifying the infecting organism and its susceptibility to antimicrobial agents. Isolating the pathogen in culture is the time-honored standard. False-positive results often are caused by specimen contamination or propagation of bacteria from noninvasive colonization. False-negative results can occur because of the difficulty of growing some organisms, especially those from biofilm-based infections; from loss of viability during transport; or in a patient receiving antimicrobial treatment. The possibility of a false-positive or false-negative result requires that corroborating information be obtained and clinical judgment be exercised before making treatment decisions. Usually histopathologic analysis of biopsy specimens from the site of the culture can provide the necessary corroboration.

Microbiologic Diagnosis of Orthopaedic Infections

Specimen Collection and Transport

Specimens for microbiologic analysis should be obtained with the understanding that the environment is not sterile and the patient's normal flora can be pathogenic in the right conditions. Normal human flora can include coagulase-negative staphylococci, propionibacteria, micrococci, corynebacteria, commensal *Neisseria* species, and bacilli. In a patient who has been ill, has recently taken broad-spectrum antimicrobial agents, or has significant contact with a health care facility, the normal flora may be transiently replaced by nosocomial flora. Many recognized pathogens, including *Staphylococcus aureus, Pseudomonas aeruginosa,* and *Acinetobacter* and *Candida* species, can be colonized in such a patient. As many as 30% of all patients may have skin, mucous membrane, or gastrointestinal tract colonization with recognized pathogens. One such colonizer, *S aureus*, increasingly is associated with resistance to methicillin, nafcillin, and other β-lactam agents. Nose and skin carriers of *S aureus* shed the *S aureus* into the environment; some disperse as many as 10^7 staphylococcal-carrying particles into the air daily.[1,2] Normal and nosocomial bacterial flora can act as pathogens in infected implants. Meticulous technique is extremely important during the collection of bacterial specimens to prevent inadvertent culturing of ambient bacteria that could be pathogens.

Orthopaedic infections frequently involve biofilm growing on an implant surface or on devitalized bone or soft tissue. Bacterial populations in biofilm are in various stages of decreased metabolic and mitotic activity.[3,4] (Biofilms are further discussed in chapter 3.) These sessile bacteria are exceedingly difficult to grow in the laboratory.[4] In infections with active purulence, the infecting organisms are at least in part planktonic (individually free in fluid), and they can be grown readily. Sonication can increase the yield of cultures from infected implant surfaces.[5] However, purulence does not in any way indicate the absence of sessile bacteria in a biofilm.

Specimen collection from sites without clinical findings consistent with active infection has little or no clinical value. The collection of specimens from skin or from a fistula that is colonized with commensal or nosocomial flora can lead to the identification of nonetiologic microbes, an incorrect diagnosis, and inappropriate therapy.[6-8] When specimens are collected before débridement of a traumatic wound or an open fracture, the culture results do not reliably predict the microorganisms responsible if subsequent infection occurs.[8,9]

The laboratory analysis of microbiologic specimens relies heavily on appropriate sampling. It is important to collect material that contains sufficient numbers of the causative organisms to inoculate multiple culture media. If the specimen is too small, the laboratory is severely restricted in the diagnostic tests that can be performed. A sample size of several millimeters in dimension or several milliliters in volume usually is adequate.

The best specimens for microbiologic studies are tissue biopsy material, pus, exudate, or small pieces of implant material such as screws or pieces of methacrylate.[6-8,10] A specimen should be placed in a sterile, leak-proof container, such as a glass or plastic tube, or in a urine collection container with a screw-on cap.

The preferred method of sending a bacterial specimen to the laboratory is immediate transport without the use of a transport medium. Heat and desiccation are lethal to bacteria. A small amount of sterile, nonbacteriostatic saline (0.5 to 3 mL) can be used to barely cover a small tissue specimen that is at risk of drying out. Identifying and retrieving a small specimen can be difficult if it is floating in a large amount of saline. At room temperature, many bacteria have significant loss of viability within 1 to 2 hours unless they are surrounded by an adequate volume of fluid, pus, or tissue. The optimal temperature for the survival of aerobic organisms and viruses is 4° to 8°C; the survival of anaerobes is best at room temperature.[6-8]

Many clinically important anaerobes, such as the Bacteroides fragilis group, can reliably survive transport in room air. Pus, abscess material, and adequate-size tissue biopsy material retain anaerobic conditions if they are held in a suitable container and not subjected to excessive agitation. In such conditions, anaerobes can survive for 12 to 24 hours or longer. Anaerobes are reliably viable for 24 to 48 hours when held in a commercially available transport container filled with carbon dioxide. This type of container must be kept upright during specimen insertion so that the heavier carbon dioxide is not spilled out and replaced by oxygen.[6-8]

For all specimens, a transport medium should be used if laboratory processing is likely to be delayed more than 1 hour after collection. For most specimens, a commercial transport system can be used, with a medium consisting of a liquid or gel formulation in a specialized container. Unfortunately, some transport media contain dead, sterile organisms, which can cause confusion during Gram staining and with molecular amplification techniques.

Many hospitals and clinics transport specimens to an off-site central reference laboratory, which delays processing and the reporting of results. Specimens should be carefully evaluated by a microbiology technologist before they are transported off site. Rapid tests such as Gram staining should be performed at the collection location. The specimens then should be placed in a transport medium and stored in the correct conditions until expeditious transport to the central laboratory for processing. This protocol enables repeat specimen collection and manipulation of specimens, if necessary, in a timely fashion. The institution's collection and transport protocol for microbiology specimens should be followed, especially for specimens that will be processed at an off-site facility.

Blood Cultures

Blood cultures are an integral part of diagnosing bone and joint infections. All patients with suspected septic arthritis should have a blood culture before antimicrobial agents are administered because 50% to 70% of these patients have concurrent bacteremia. The importance of blood cultures in the evaluation of prosthetic joint infection is less clear. A positive blood culture in a patient with acute hematogenous osteomyelitis may obviate the need for bone biopsy if it yields a typical bone pathogen such as S aureus or Salmonella.[11] All blood cultures should be collected and transported with strict attention to the institution's blood culture policies.

Joint Fluid Cultures

Sterile technique must be used for aspiration of a native joint. Penetration through areas of overlying cellulitis should be avoided to prevent inadvertent introduction of bacteria into the synovial space. Aspiration of a prosthetic joint requires a surgical-equivalent sterile technique because of the catastrophic consequences of introducing bacteria directly onto a prosthetic surface. Surgical skin preparation, drapes, gloves, and masks should be used. Any required needle repositioning should be done without withdrawing the needle through the skin.[12] Fluid should not be injected into the joint; it may be prudent, however, to inject a small amount of contrast to document the site where the specimen was acquired. Aspiration of deep bursae and joints, including prosthetic hip joints, should be performed under image guidance.[13]

At least 1 mL of fluid obtained from the aspiration should immediately be sent to the microbiology laboratory for processing. Immediate inoculation of an aerobic blood culture bottle is a good method for improving the culture yield of fastidious organisms such as Kingella from septic arthritis in young children.[14] Immediate inoculation of blood culture vials for adult septic arthritis, especially prosthetic joint infections, may be appropriate when the nonblood use of the blood culture vials is communicated to the microbiology laboratory and the protocol from the microbiology laboratory is followed. Care must be taken to use appropriate culture bottles and prevent contamination of bottles, particularly at the injection site. Fluid inoculated into a blood culture bottle cannot be used for other studies.[15] Separate samples should be sent for cell count, Gram staining, and crystal analysis. Atypical organisms, such as fungi and mycobacteria, require specialized culture techniques, and the laboratory must specifically be instructed to culture for these organisms when indicated. Fungal and mycobacterial cultures usually detect most atypical organisms, including Nocardia species. Not all microorganisms can be cultured, and consultation with the microbiology laboratory or an infectious disease specialist is warranted when there is concern for other atypical organisms.

The yield of cultures from prosthetic joint fluid aspirate ranges from 45% to 100%, depending on whether

2: Diagnostic Modalities

the patient had received antimicrobial agents and the criteria used for diagnosing prosthetic joint infection.[8,13,16-19] Synovial fluid aspiration primarily detects planktonic bacteria rather than bacteria contained in biofilm or osteoblasts. Other investigations, such as a synovial fluid leukocyte count and differential, may have greater predictive value for an infective process.[12,19]

Surgical or Wound Specimen Cultures

Surgical fields commonly are not sterile, and multiple sites on the surgical field, including gloved hands, gowns, light handles, and suction tips, have been found to be culture positive in more than 1 in 4 cases.[17] Fomites, including airborne dust and dander, falling eyelashes, and flakes from exposed skin, are present in the operating room. Even after an extensive effort to minimize the presence of fomites by limiting traffic and using a clean-air room, body exhaust suits, and incision drapes, there is surgical wound exposure to ambient bacteria as well as bacteria from the cut edge of the skin. A meticulous sampling technique must be used to be certain that specimens contain only bacteria from the biopsy site. The biopsy site may have predominantly sessile bacteria, of which only a few, if any, will propagate in the laboratory. It could be impossible, therefore, to distinguish between a colony of contaminating coagulase-negative staphylococci and a single colony of a pathogen from biofilm. It is important to develop and follow a best practices routine for the collection and transport of surgical culture specimens.

All biopsy instruments must be unused and placed where they cannot be contaminated with ambient bacteria before they are used. It is best to bring biopsy instruments onto the surgical field immediately before the biopsy, but it is acceptable to immediately cover them with a sterile towel during setup and keep them covered until the biopsy. The instruments should be held by the handles only; the jaws that will contact the specimen should never be touched. Transport containers should be kept closed, opened only to insert the specimen, then closed tightly (preferably with a screw cap) and immediately handed off for transport to the laboratory.

To optimize the culture yield, biopsy specimens should be taken from high-probability sites, including thickened synovium, periprosthetic membrane, slime and fibrinous exudate in the interface between modular components, necrotic or purulent bone and soft tissue, intramedullary canals (proximal and distal), pieces of foreign material or devices, and sequestrum. It is important to know whether antibiotic-loaded bone cement is present in the wound and, if so, to avoid touching or disturbing it in any way before the culture specimens are obtained. Freshly disturbed antibiotic-loaded bone cement can release a burst of antibiotic even years after the original implantation and thereby compromise the culture yield.[18] A careful, stepwise execution of the procedure with good hemostasis delays

cross contamination between tissue planes, often allowing discrete specimens to be collected from multiple sites. Careful removal of an implant often allows biopsy of the underlying tissue before ambient wound fluid contaminates the site. Antibacterial irrigation should not be used before all biopsies for culture are obtained. All biopsies should be performed with different unused instruments to prevent cross contamination between specimens.

To maximize culture yield, antimicrobial agents should be withheld for 2 weeks before intraoperative culture specimens are obtained. Recent antimicrobial exposure is of less concern if sonication is available for an explanted prosthesis because the yield achieved by sonication is superior to that of cultures from periprosthetic tissue. Even if sonication is used, antimicrobial agents should be withheld for at least 4 days before a planned explantation.[5]

Tissue biopsy specimens are homogenized in the microbiology laboratory to release as many bacteria as possible into suspension for media and smear inoculation. Homogenization can be done with a commercial disposable grinding device or an automated homogenizer or by vortexing with glass beads in a fluid such as thioglycolate broth to macerate the tissue into a fine puree.[6-8] Alternatively, the tissue can be gently minced into small pieces with a fine scalpel; this technique is preferred if fungi (especially *Mucor*) are suspected because mechanical agitation can kill the organisms. The prepared specimen is inoculated into a variety of nutrient agars or broths that enhance growth.[6-8]

For biofilm infections that do not induce leukorrhea, the number of bacteria shed from the biofilm into the surrounding tissue may not be sufficient for successful culture. Furthermore, the bacteria retrieved may not be sufficiently active to grow in the laboratory. If they do grow, these bacteria may form only small colonies on agar plates, called small colony variants.[20]

A removed prosthesis can be sonicated to improve the culture yield. The equipment for sonication of an explant is inexpensive and readily available, and the protocol has been well described. Explants should be sonicated in nonbacteriostatic fluid to release and disperse adherent bacterial biofilm from the implant surface; the sonicate fluid is then centrifuged and cultured.[5]

Swabs for Specimen Collection

Swabs are a particularly poor way to obtain culture specimens. Bacteria in general and mycobacterial species in particular become attached to the swab fibers by adsorption because of their hydrophobic cell walls; swabs retain most of the bacteria that contact the fibers, and the chance of culture success is thereby limited. Swabs with wooden handles may contain elements toxic to some bacteria. The swab handle frequently is a source of contamination, and the long handle can be used to push a specimen so far down into the transport medium that it is difficult to retrieve in the laboratory.

2: Diagnostic Modalities

Swabs should not be used to sample the surface of tissue specimens; instead, the tissue should be sent to the laboratory. Swab cultures of sinus tract drainage or wound ulcers with contiguous osteomyelitis are not useful in diagnosing bone and joint infections because of their poor correlation with deep tissue specimens. Cultures from superficial swabs often yield organisms that have colonized the wound and completely miss the etiologic pathogens involved in the infection. *S aureus* isolated from a swab culture of sinus tract drainage has a predictive value of 80% or less, which is insufficient to rely on without additional diagnostic information. Swab cultures of diabetic foot ulcers with contiguous osteomyelitis do not predict the organisms involved in infection of underlying bone.[6-8,11,21,22]

Despite their poor efficacy in determining the microbial cause of an orthopaedic infection, swab cultures may be clinically relevant for purposes of epidemiology and infection control (for example, contact isolation of patients with a wound colonized with methicillin-resistant *S aureus*).[6-8]

Laboratory Procedures

To provide clear instructions to the laboratory and increase the likelihood that cultures will be successful, it is necessary to understand the procedures used to process specimens in the laboratory. Cultures of routine wound specimens generally are incubated at 35°C, in 5% to 10% carbon dioxide, and for at least 3 days. The total time required for the incubation of cultures specific to orthopaedic wounds and implants is controversial, but there is general agreement that longer periods of incubation provide higher culture yields; a period of at least 5 days is necessary, and 14 to 21 days is preferable. Any culture in broth that remains clear should not be opened for routine analysis. Only when growth is seen should Gram staining and subculturing for identification and susceptibility testing be done. Agar plates should be read every 24 hours for the first 4 or 5 days, and then every 3 or 4 days for the duration of the incubation period. Anaerobic plates should not be opened during the first 48 hours, unless they are in an anaerobic chamber. Because agar plates tend to dry out in 4 to 5 days, plates incubated for longer periods of time should be sealed with a self-adhering thermoplastic film. A negative result is reported only when the final analysis of the agar and broth cultures reveals no growth after 5 to 21 days.[6,7]

Although several types of agar plates or broth media are available, the mainstay for bacterial cultures is sheep blood agar, which facilitates the growth of almost all clinically significant bacteria found in surgical and orthopaedic infections. Chocolate agar plates (red blood cells hemolyzed by heat) can be used if a fastidious organism such as *Haemophilus influenzae, Neisseria gonorrhoeae,* or *Mycobacterium haemophilum* is suspected. When processing tissue or other specimens collected from a topical site such as skin or a superficial lymph node, blood and chocolate agar plates should be incubated at a lower temperature (25° to 30°C); some mycobacteria, such as *Mycobacterium marinum* and *M haemophilum,* require a cooler temperature and a medium that is specifically enhanced nutritionally for different mycobacteria. When culturing for anaerobes, blood agar supplemented with vitamin K and hemin or another supplemented agar also should be used. Selective media containing antimicrobial agents or chemicals, such as MacConkey agar, inhibit the overgrowth of cultures by normal or contaminating flora; usually they are not indicated for orthopaedic specimens, which rarely are contaminated by large numbers of commensal organisms.

Identification of Microorganisms

Microorganisms typically are identified using phenotypic characteristics such as growth, colony morphology, biochemical reactions, and antigenic composition. Presumptive identification can be made based on a few key morphologic characteristics. More rigorous identification is performed by determining a large number of characteristics, often with a commercial kit or automated system. Gas chromatography and high-pressure liquid chromatography can be used for identifying difficult-to-characterize organisms such as the mycobacteria. Genetic characterization was introduced as a rapid means of identification, and specific genetic probes for RNA or DNA have been introduced for identifying groups A and B streptococci, some mycobacteria (*Mycobacterium tuberculosis* complex, *Mycobacterium avium* complex, and *Mycobacterium kansasii*), and some fungi (*Histoplasma capsulatum, Coccidioides* species, *Blastomyces dermatitidis,* and *Candida* species). Immunofluorescence microscopy also is capable of identifying specific organisms. Direct detection of microorganisms in specimens by genetic amplification methods such as polymerase chain reaction (PCR), which uses specific primer sets as well as 16S rRNA sequencing, is becoming more cost-effective and more readily available in reference laboratories and larger academic institutions. However, these methods are not routinely available in most clinical laboratories.[23]

Unfortunately, many of these sophisticated methods require expensive equipment and reagents. Most of them have not been approved by the US Food and Drug Administration and therefore often are not reimbursable under Medicare or many insurance contracts. As a result, these methods are not routinely used by most clinical microbiology laboratories. Rapid, cost-effective, Food and Drug Administration–approved molecular methods will soon be available that will be able to detect and identify small numbers of organisms and characterize the genetic material responsible for resistance to antimicrobial agents within the specimens themselves.

Antimicrobial Susceptibility Testing

Susceptibility testing measures the activity of antimicrobial agents in specific in vitro growth conditions in the laboratory. In vitro susceptibility studies do not always reflect the actual clinical situation and may not appropriately predict an agent's efficacy. Clinical outcomes can depend on the pharmacokinetics of the drug delivery, the interaction between the antimicrobial agent and the microorganism, the presence or absence of foreign material at the site of infection, and the patient's immunocompetency. Microorganisms living in biofilm may be in different states of metabolism and growth, and they exist in an ecosystem protected from antimicrobial action also affecting clinical efficacy.

Agar diffusion studies using antimicrobial-impregnated disks provide semiquantitative results. Each of the three interpretive categories (susceptible, intermediate, and resistant) suggests the clinical outcome. These studies can be performed only on rapidly growing bacteria for which standards have been published.[6-8] A quantitative agar diffusion study using an epsilometer (Etest, AB Biodisk, Stockholm, Sweden), which is a paper strip containing a gradient of a single antimicrobial agent, can measure minimal inhibitory concentration (MIC) in micrograms per milliliter for rapidly and slowly growing bacteria as well as some fastidious organisms. Epsilometers are expensive, however, especially if multiple agents must be tested. MIC is more commonly measured by microdilution, typically with an automated system (VITEK 2, bioMérieux, Durham, NC; Microscan WalkAway, Dade Behring, West Sacramento, CA; Phoenix, Becton Dickinson, Sparks, MD). The MIC can be important for deciding on the best treatment of some infections, including osteomyelitis, particularly if systemic antimicrobial agents with poor bone penetration are being considered.

Genetic material or specific polypeptides can be evaluated for several markers to determine resistance to specific antimicrobial agents, but these methods are not yet widely available in clinical laboratories. Methicillin resistance in staphylococci can be predicted by the presence of penicillin-binding protein 2 (pBp2) or the *mecA* gene, which codes for it. Susceptibility to one agent often can be used to predict susceptibility to similar agents. Phenotypic or genetic measurement of resistance to methicillin in staphylococci predicts resistance to all β-lactam antimicrobial agents except ceftobiprole, which is not yet available in the United States.

Laboratories commonly perform susceptibility studies using a panel of antimicrobial agents. The antimicrobial agents in a panel often are determined by commercial availability and are not easily changed; all of the agents may not be appropriate for a particular clinical infection, even if they have in vitro activity against specific organisms.

Decisions about therapeutic antimicrobial agents almost always are based on clinical knowledge of infectious processes. The bacterial etiology, the site of infection, host factors such as allergy, and prevalent clinical responses to specific antimicrobial agents are used to determine a first-, second-, and third-line agent. In vitro susceptibility studies can confirm or refute the susceptibility of the etiologic microbe to the clinically chosen agents. Susceptibility testing can be used to refine the antimicrobial choice to a less toxic or less expensive clinically appropriate agent that will penetrate the site of infection and minimize adverse effects. Clinicians should use the antimicrobial panel report to evaluate clinically appropriate antimicrobial agents and should not arbitrarily choose an agent from the report.

Interpretation of Surgical Cultures From Prosthetic Joint Infections

Perhaps the most difficult culture results to interpret are those from prosthetic joint infections. No clearly accepted reference standard is available for clinical practice, primarily because of shortcomings in standard culture techniques. Cultures of periprosthetic tissue may miss infection on the implant surface, or small numbers of organisms shed from biofilm may have a low culture yield.[24] Culture specificity also is an issue. Many organisms involved in prosthetic joint infections are normal skin flora; when isolated, they can represent either true infection or contamination during specimen collection and processing. To differentiate a prosthetic joint infection from culture contamination, several authors evaluated the number of positive cultures taken from five or six surgical specimens at the time of revision arthroplasty.[10,13,16,18,19,25] Isolation of the same microorganism from three or more independent surgical specimens was found to be highly predictive of prosthetic joint infection. This microbiologic criterion (46% to 65% sensitivity) is quite insensitive, however. If septic loosening is suspected despite negative surgical cultures, it may be possible to find bacteria through sonication of the prosthesis, identify bacterial DNA on PCR, or even view bacteria embedded within biofilm adhering to the prosthesis (using electron microscopy).[23,24] Even a single positive surgical culture can be significant, particularly if histopathology reveals associated inflammation. Correlation with histopathology results and clinical findings is required. In a patient with no earlier antimicrobial exposure and a negative synovial fluid leukocyte count, one or two colonies of normal skin flora probably represent contamination during specimen collection or processing. The result is far more likely to be significant if the patient was heavily pretreated with antimicrobial agents and the same isolate was recovered from synovial fluid aspiration or earlier surgical cultures.

At least three periprosthetic tissue specimens should be obtained for bacterial culture.[18] The specimens should be biopsies from sites with evident inflammation or from other high-probability sites. Because of the low burden of infection typical of prosthetic joint infections, five or six biopsy specimens may be necessary to improve the diagnostic sensitivity of operative cultures. It is important to evaluate the sites of biopsy and the quality of each specimen. Cross contamination of the biopsy sites with pus or wound fluid makes multiple samples repeated assays of the same specimen, rather than multiple discrete tests. When collecting multiple

2: Diagnostic Modalities

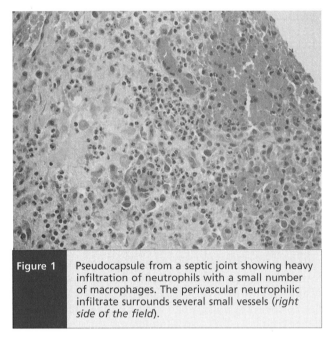

Figure 1 Pseudocapsule from a septic joint showing heavy infiltration of neutrophils with a small number of macrophages. The perivascular neutrophilic infiltrate surrounds several small vessels (*right side of the field*).

samples of the same cross-contaminated specimen, statistical criteria can be applied. If three of five (rather than one of five) cultures must be positive to make the diagnosis of infection, the number of false-positive results may decrease, improving culture specificity. In contrast, multiple meticulously obtained specimens from discrete biopsies will evaluate different sites, and even one positive culture warrants careful diagnostic consideration.

Histopathologic Diagnosis of Orthopaedic Infections

Histopathology plays an important role in the diagnosis of orthopaedic infections by providing information to corroborate the clinical and microbiologic data. Acute, chronic, persistent, and quiescent infections have well-described pathologic findings with common features related to the inflammatory response, but there can be histopathologic differences related to the underlying etiology. When there is overt purulence, a positive microbiologic culture often identifies the bacteria, and the role of histology is confirmatory; when there is no overt purulence, histopathologic examination of involved tissues has a complementary role. Sophisticated microbiologic examination of an implant that would otherwise be classified as aseptically loose may identify surface biofilm with normal skin flora such as *Staphylococcus epidermidis*. Sonication can improve the culture yield. Molecular probes and amplification methods can identify bacterial DNA and RNA, and immunofluorescence microscopy can detect fluorescent antibodies that establish the presence of bacteria. Unfortunately, the histopathologic appearance depends on the host response, which may not produce a significant inflammatory cell infiltrate in culture-negative infections without purulence.

Implant Infections

Frozen Sections

Intraoperative frozen sections are thought to be reliable for detecting infection. However, determination of the presence of infection based on a frozen section requires a skilled, highly dedicated team with an experienced pathologist. It is extremely important that the surgeon and the pathologist discuss before the procedure exactly what specimens will be obtained and how the pathologist will report the findings to the surgeon. Biopsies for frozen sections should be obtained from high-probability sites, including areas of granulation tissue, joint pseudocapsule, pseudomembrane, or periprosthetic tissue.[26] Tissue from at least two sites should be submitted for evaluation, and correlative samples from these sites should be sent to the microbiology laboratory for culture. Correlation of the histopathologic and microbiologic findings is essential. To ensure correlative data, it is a good practice for the pathologist to submit a piece of the tissue for culture from the specimen that is processed for frozen section; however, extreme care must be taken to not contaminate the piece of tissue sent for culture from the pathology laboratory. A frozen section is considered positive if 10 or more neutrophils are found per high-power field (400× magnification) in the five most cellular fields examined.

Frozen sections can be used to determine the presence or persistence of infection during revision or reimplantation arthroplasty of the knee or hip.[26-32] If the frozen section is positive for infection, implantation of a permanent prosthesis is aborted. The frozen section material must be processed for further evaluation on permanent section because the findings attributed to acute neutrophilic infiltration on frozen section may be interpreted differently on permanent section. The true value of a frozen section is in a negative finding. Frozen sections were found to have a specificity of approximately 98% to 99% and a negative predictive value of 95% to 98% for infection during revision joint arthroplasty; however, sensitivity is poor at 25% to 84%.[28,31] A finding of less than one neutrophil per high-power field is strong exclusionary evidence for infection.

Acute Implant Infection

Several studies have found that histopathology is useful in diagnosing infection of an implant.[26-30,32,33] The most reliable indicator is infiltration of the tissues surrounding the implant by inflammatory cells, especially neutrophils, including perivascular neutrophil infiltrates (**Figure 1**). Joint pseudocapsule, synovium, and pseudomembranes surrounding the implant can be involved. The presence of neutrophils is the hallmark of acute infection, whereas the presence of other inflammatory cells, including lymphocytes, plasma cells, eosinophils, and macrophages, varies significantly. Macrophages (histiocytes) and multinucleated giant cells

Table 1

Inflammatory Cell Counts Required for the Diagnosis of Orthopaedic Infections

Cell Type	Diagnosis		
	Acute Infection	Chronic Infection	Aseptic Particulate Wear
Neutrophils	Frozen section: > 10 in each of five HPFs (for two or more specimens) Permanent section: > 5 per HPF, perivascular infiltration	0 to 3 per HPF	< 1 per 10 HPFs for two or more specimens
Macrophages	Unreliable	Present	Common
Lymphocytes	Not predictive; PMNs also may be present	Present	Perivascular infiltration associated with delayed hypersensitivity from metal particulate wear
Plasma cells	> 5 per HPF	Present	Occasional
Giant cells	Rarely present	Present	Common

HPF = high-power field (400× magnification), PMN = polymorphonuclear white cells.

usually are a response to wear particles, and macrophage or giant cell infiltration therefore is not a reliable indicator of infection. The presence of more than five neutrophils per high-power field was found to be highly sensitive and specific for infection;[32] some infections were also associated with infiltration of a large number of lymphocytes and a more variable number of plasma cells.[32] The presence of more than five neutrophils per high-power field is a relatively specific marker for infection, although approximately 45% of patients have no plasma cells. A heavy lymphocytic infiltrate is not specific or sensitive for infection despite its association with a significant neutrophilic infiltrate.[32] As a result, adjacent tissues should be carefully searched for acute inflammatory cells when lymphocytic infiltrates are present. Eosinophils occasionally are seen.

The extent of inflammatory cell infiltration was found to vary greatly among the biopsy sites of an infected joint and even within a single histologic section.[32] This observation indicates the need to sample multiple sites for histopathologic and microbiologic examination and suggests that all submitted tissue should be examined by permanent section. Gram staining of tissue sections was positive only in 21.5% of patients with confirmed infection; this finding indicates that, despite its high specificity, Gram staining is unreliable for detecting infection.[28] It is imperative to correlate pathology findings with culture results, and the culture results, when available, should be reflected in the surgical pathology report (Table 1).

Aseptic Loosening

The advent of technological means of detecting biofilm on an implant surface may allow detection of quiescent infection in many cases that would otherwise be diagnosed as aseptic loosening.[24,33] The histopathology from culture-negative cases varies significantly from the

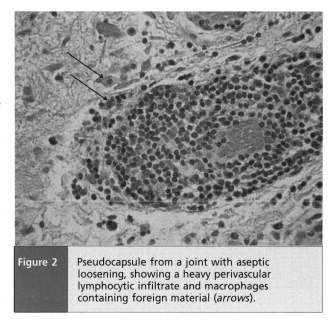

Figure 2 Pseudocapsule from a joint with aseptic loosening, showing a heavy perivascular lymphocytic infiltrate and macrophages containing foreign material (*arrows*).

histopathology of culture-positive cases. A so-called aseptic arthroplasty is more likely to have a chronic inflammatory cell infiltrate in the form of lymphocytes and macrophages (**Figure 2**). Neutrophils are far less likely to be seen; when they are present, the infiltrate usually is fewer than one cell per 10 high-power fields. A variable lymphocytic infiltrate appears to be the most common type of inflammation associated with aseptic loosening; it is present approximately 80% of the time and is commonly less than five cells per high-power field.[32] A heavy perivascular lymphocytic infiltration in the periarticular tissue of a metal-on-metal implant may indicate a delayed hypersensitivity reaction leading to formation of an aseptic lymphocytic vasculitis-associated lesion.[34,35] Plasma cells and eosinophils are

2: Diagnostic Modalities

seen only occasionally. Wear-type macrophages and giant cells are extremely common. Other findings may include fibrosis, small bone fragments, collections of hemosiderin, and fibrocartilaginous metaplasia. These changes are collectively called a fibrohistiocytic response.

The most common type of inflammatory response to biofilm is one of macrophages (histiocytes).[4] Neutrophils appear only when bacteria are shed from the surface of the biofilm. The innate self-protection strategies of the biofilm often blunt the inflammatory macrophage response, but the macrophages that are present still can release phagocytic enzymes that damage the surrounding tissues and ultimately cause bone lysis.[4] The exact role of histopathology in detecting this process has not been determined. It may be necessary to reevaluate the meaning of macrophage infiltration in periarticular structures affected by a fibrohistiocytic process if PCR molecular amplification and fluorescent in situ hybridization studies detect biofilm-related organisms on the surface of the implant. These techniques for detecting organisms are beyond the scope of many hospital laboratories, but as the use of PCR becomes more widespread, it will be possible to identify the presence of bacterial DNA and RNA from the surface of implants.[36] Precise identification of an organism requires specific probes that often are available only through a research laboratory. Discriminating between macrophages responding to biofilm and those responding to wear particles and debris may be histologically impossible, but this area needs further investigation.

Osteomyelitis

The bacterial classification of osteomyelitis as acute, subacute, or chronic is related to the duration of the disease rather than to specific pathologic findings.[37] The histopathologic findings vary significantly and depend on patient age, the specific bone involved, the blood supply to the infected area, the host immune status, and the organism. The underlying cause of the osteomyelitis also can affect the histopathologic findings; this is especially true in osteomyelitis following fracture because the pathologic changes of fracture healing also are present.[37] The classic pathology of osteomyelitis in the metaphysis of a long bone involves a fragment of dead bone (sequestrum) surrounded by new bone (involucrum). The involucrum is surrounded by a variable inflammatory cell response including neutrophils, macrophages, lymphocytes, and plasma cells, as well as a variable fibroblastic and vascular response. Neutrophils predominate in the inflammatory response to acute suppurative osteomyelitis, with a variable number of macrophages. Chronic inflammatory cells such as lymphocytes, macrophages, and plasma cells are the predominant response in subacute and chronic osteomyelitis, but neutrophils also are commonly identified in tissue samples from sites of chronic osteomyelitis.[37] The neutrophilic response probably is related to the shedding of organisms from biofilm on the surface of dead

bone fragments.[20] This factor may explain why neutrophils are readily identified in osteomyelitis that has been present for many years and may account for a recurrence of infection within the scars of treated osteomyelitis. In the future, the diagnosis of persistent infection may rely on identifying bacterial DNA and RNA using fluorescent in situ hybridization and PCR, supported by histopathology.

Fracture-Associated Infections

Histopathology can contribute to the diagnosis of infections associated with fractures, but the findings can be extremely variable and must be interpreted in light of fracture healing, the presence of internal fixation devices, and mechanical stability at the fracture site.[37] In fractures without internal fixation, the pathology is essentially identical to that of osteomyelitis. In fractures with internal fixation, the device used to immobilize the fracture eventually may become completely isolated from the surrounding bone; fibrous tissue that is continuous with the periosteum separates the implant from bone and separates an intramedullary nail from the medullary cavity.[37] A layer of compact bone forms adjacent to the fibrous tissue and ultimately becomes continuous with the original bone cortex. The pathology of infection around the fixation device is similar to that of a joint implant, although usually there is no significant macrophage or giant cell response to the fixation device within the medullary cavity, as occurs from wear debris.[37] Neutrophils predominate in an acute suppurative infection. Lymphocytes, macrophages, and plasma cells are more commonly identified in a chronic infection, but neutrophils also can be seen and are related to the shedding of bacteria from biofilm populating the surface of the fixation device. Macrophages containing hemosiderin pigment as the result of the original fracture can persist for months following the original injury.[37]

An infected nonunion can present a histopathologic challenge. Nonunion may be associated with exuberant callus formation as well as fibroblastic proliferation, woven bone formation, and cartilage deposition. Movement at the nonunion site can lead to further fibroblastic proliferation, vascular proliferation, and hemorrhage.[37] An acute suppurative infection can be readily identified by the presence of significant numbers of neutrophils. A chronic infection of a nonunion can be extremely difficult to identify because of the variable extent of chronic inflammation, which also can be a response to movement. Pathology can suggest the possibility of chronic infection, but other diagnostic modalities, especially microbiology, are more important in the diagnosis.

Summary

Specimen acquisition, processing, and analysis, in the context of a patient's clinical presentation, are the foundation for determining the appropriate antimicrobial

---

Table 2

Summary Points for Microbiologic and Histopathologic Diagnosis of Orthopaedic Infections

1. The laboratory must be informed of the clinical presentation associated with the culture and biopsy specimens.

2. Meticulous technique must be used to obtain specimens for culture to avoid contamination.

3. The culture yield may be affected by antimicrobial exposure, and antimicrobial agents therefore should ideally be withheld for 2 weeks before culture specimens are obtained for evaluation of an established orthopaedic infection.

4. Sophisticated technology not widely available in clinical laboratories is required for identifying bacteria in a culture-negative infection.

5. Antimicrobial susceptibility data should only be used to confirm the choice of clinically appropriate antimicrobial agents.

6. Accurate interpretation of culture results requires detailed knowledge of the patient's clinical presentation, accurate identification of the specimen and how it was obtained, reliable processing, and, frequently, histopathologic correlation.

7. Acute infection is associated with a neutrophilic infiltrate; chronic infection is associated with a macrophage or lymphocytic infiltrate. Neutrophils in a chronic infection probably are a response to bacteria released from biofilm.

8. The most reliable role for frozen section during an implantation procedure is in determining the absence of infection. To predict infection, large numbers of neutrophils must be seen at two or more sites. The surgeon and the pathologist should discuss the plan before obtaining frozen sections.

9. The histopathology of septic loosening and acute suppurative osteomyelitis is well established. Positive cultures and neutrophilic infiltration of tissues are well correlated.

10. The pathology of aseptic loosening of joint implants, chronic osteomyelitis, and infections around internal fixation devices should be reinterpreted in the light of the current understanding of biofilm infection.

---

regimen. Identification of the causative organisms and recognition of the pathologic response to these organisms are reliable technical tasks. Important considerations in the microbiologic and histopathologic diagnosis of orthopaedic infections are summarized in Table 2. Increased sophistication in the understanding of the biology of biofilms and the host response, as well as advances in technology, are expected to significantly improve diagnostic capabilities within the foreseeable future.

Annotated References

1. Williams REO: Epidemiology of airborne staphylococcal infection. *Bacteriol Rev* 1966;30:660-672.

2. Sherertz RJ, Bassetti S, Bassetti-Wyss B: "Cloud" health-care workers. *Emerg Infect Dis* 2001;7:241-243.

3. Donlan RM, Costerton JW: Biofilms: Survival mechanisms of clinically relevant microorganisms. *Clin Microbiol Rev* 2002;15:167-193.

4. Costerton JW: *The Biofilm Primer*. New York, NY, Springer, 2007.
   This text covers the current state of knowledge about biofilms.

5. Trampuz A, Piper KE, Jacobson MJ, et al: Sonication of removed hip and knee prostheses for diagnosis of infection. *N Engl J Med* 2007;357:654-663.
   Results of cultures of specimens collected by sonication of a removed prosthesis were compared with those of conventional cultures of periprosthetic tissue. The sonication fluid cultures were more sensitive and specific. Differences in sensitivity were especially pronounced in specimens from patients who received antibiotics within 14 days of surgery.

6. Isenberg HD (ed): *Clinical Microbiology Procedures Handbook*, ed 2. Washington, DC, ASM Press, 2004.
   The updated procedure guidelines reflect recent data on specimen collection, transport, and acceptability. Methodologies for aerobic and anaerobic bacteriology, mycobacteriology, mycology, and in vitro susceptibility testing, with analysis of bench-level microbiology work-up, also are presented.

7. Garcia LS: *Updates to the Clinical Microbiology Procedures Handbook*. Washington, DC, ASM Press, 2007.

8. Murray RP, Baron EJ, Jorgensen JH, Landry ML, Pfaller MA (eds): *Manual of Clinical Microbiology*, ed 9. Washington, DC, ASM Press, 2007.
   This desk reference includes the gold standards for clinical and laboratory microbiology, with a discussion of specimen collection, transport, methods of identifying microorganisms, and susceptibility testing. Traditional and newer molecular methodologies and applications are reviewed based on peer-reviewed publications.

9. Lee J: Efficacy of cultures in the management of open fractures. *Clin Orthop Relat Res* 1997;339:71-75.

10. Mikkelsen DB, Pedersen C, Hojbjerg T, Schonheyder HC: Culture of multiple perioperative biopsies and diagnosis of infected knee arthroplasties. *APMIS* 2006;114:449-452.
    The diagnostic criteria for infected total knee arthroplasty are determined using the number of positive surgical cultures.

2: Diagnostic Modalities

11. Calhoun JH, Manring MM: Adult osteomyelitis. *Infect Dis Clin North Am* 2005;19:765-786.

    The pathophysiology, diagnosis, treatment, and prognosis of adult osteomyelitis are discussed.

12. Trampuz A, Hanssen AD, Osmon DR, Mandrekar J, Steckelberg J, Patel R: Synovial fluid leukocyte count and differential for the diagnosis of prosthetic knee infection. *Am J Med* 2004;117:556-562.

    A prospective evaluation of white blood cell count and differential in the diagnosis of prosthetic joint infection found that the presence of more than 1,700 white blood cells per microliter and more than 65% neutrophils distinguished septic from aseptic loosening.

13. Spanghel MJ, Masri BA, O'Connell JX, Duncan CP: Prospective analysis of preoperative and intraoperative investigations for the diagnosis of infection at the sites of two hundred and two revision total hip arthroplasties. *J Bone Joint Surg Am* 1999;81:672-683.

14. Yagupsky P: Use of blood culture vials and nucleic acid amplification for the diagnosis of pediatric septic arthritis [letter]. *Clin Infect Dis* 2008;46:1631-1632.

    A letter to the editor discusses the use of blood culture vials to culture specimens from septic arthritis in young children, considering that *Kingella* is a significant pathogen in children younger than 3 years.

15. Wilson ML, Winn W: Laboratory diagnosis of bone, joint, soft-tissue, and skin infections. *Clin Infect Dis* 2008;46:453-457.

    This is an expert opinion on specimen collection and laboratory methods for the diagnosis of bone, joint, soft-tissue, and skin infections.

16. Atkins BL, Athanasou N, Deeks JJ, et al: Prospective evaluation of criteria for microbiological diagnosis of prosthetic-joint infection at revision arthroplasty: The OSIRIS Collaborative Study Group. *J Clin Microbiol* 1998;36:2932-2939.

17. Davis N, Curry A, Gambhir AK, et al: Intra-operative bacterial contamination in operations for joint replacement. *J Bone Joint Surg Br* 1999;81:886-889.

18. Patel R, Osmon DR, Hanssen AD: The diagnosis of prosthetic joint infection. *Clin Orthop Relat Res* 2005;437:55-58.

    The diagnostic considerations for prosthetic joint infections are reviewed.

19. Zimmerli W, Trampuz A, Ochsner PE: Prosthetic joint infections. *N Engl J Med* 2004;351:1645-1654.

    This review of prosthetic joint infections includes pathophysiology, histopathology, microbiology, diagnosis, and treatment.

20. Costerton JW: Biofilm theory can guide the treatment of device-related orthopedic infections. *Clin Orthop Relat Res* 2005;437:7-11.

    The biology of biofilm is reviewed, with a discussion of how it determines the diagnosis and treatment of orthopaedic infections.

21. Cunha BA: Osteomyelitis in elderly patients. *Clin Infect Dis* 2002;35:287-293.

22. Senneville E, Melliez H, Beltrand E, et al: Culture of percutaneous bone biopsy specimens for diagnosis of diabetic foot osteomyelitis: Concordance with ulcer swab cultures. *Clin Infect Dis* 2006;42:57-62.

    This retrospective review of bone biopsy and ulcer swabs in diabetic foot infections finds unreliable culture results for swabs of the ulcer.

23. Moojen DJ, Spijkers SN, Schot CS, et al: Identification of orthopaedic infections using broad-range polymerase chain reaction and reverse line blot hybridization. *J Bone Joint Surg Am* 2007;89:1298-1305.

    Broad-range 16S rRNA PCR and reverse line blot hybridization used 28 group-, genus-, and species-specific oligonucleotide probes to detect musculoskeletal infections. PCR was 97% sensitive, and culture was 81% sensitive. PCR can be important in detecting chronic infections in the musculoskeletal system. Level of evidence: III.

24. Nelson CL, McLaren AC, McLaren SG, Johnson JW, Smeltzer MS: Is aseptic loosening truly aseptic? *Clin Orthop Relat Res* 2005;437:25-30.

    This discussion of culture-negative loose arthroplasties considers the possibility that some may be infected.

25. Kamme C, Lindberg L: Aerobic and anaerobic bacteria in deep infections after total hip arthroplasty: Differential diagnosis between infectious and non-infectious loosening. *Clin Orthop Relat Res* 1981;154:201-207.

26. Lester SC: *Manual of Surgical Pathology*, ed 2. Philadelphia, PA, Elsevier Health, 2005.

    This reference text covers gross and microscopic surgical pathologic anatomy.

27. Athanasou NA, Pandey R, De Steiger R, Crook D, Smith PM: Diagnosis of infection by frozen section during revision arthroplasty. *J Bone Joint Surg Br* 1995;77:28-33.

28. Della Valle CJ, Bogner E, Desai P, et al: The analysis of frozen sections of intraoperative specimens obtained at the time of reoperation after hip or knee resection arthroplasty for the treatment of infection. *J Bone Joint Surg Am* 1999;81:684-689.

29. Fehring TK, McAllister JA Jr: Frozen histologic section as a guide to sepsis in revision joint arthroplasty. *Clin Orthop Relat Res* 1994;304:229-237.

30. Feldman DS, Lonner JH, Desai P, Zuckerman JD: The role of intraoperative frozen sections in revision total joint arthroplasty. *J Bone Joint Surg Am* 1995;77:1807-1813.

31. Lonner JH, Desai P, Decesare PE, Steiner G, Zuckerman JD: The reliability of analysis of intraoperative frozen sections for identifying active infection during revision hip or knee arthroplasty. *J Bone Joint Surg Am* 1999;78:1553-1558.

32. Pandey R, Drakoulakis E, Athanasou NA: An assessment of the histological criteria used to diagnose infection in hip revision arthroplasty tissues. *J Clin Pathol* 1999;52:118-123.

33. Savarino L, Baldini N, Tarbusi C, Pellacani A, Giunti A: Diagnosis of infection after total hip replacement. *J Biomed Mater Res B Appl Biomater* 2004;70: 139-145.

    An investigation of revision hip replacements for loose or infected implants found unexpected positive cultures in 52% of so-called aseptic loose implants. Primary hip replacements having no indication or risk for infection served as a control group,

34. Davies AP, Willert HG, Campbell PA, Learmonth ID, Case CP: An unusual lymphocytic perivascular infiltration in tissues around contemporary metal-on-metal joint replacements case. *J Bone Joint Surg Am* 2005;87: 18-27.

    Histopathologic analysis of 25 retrieved metal-on-metal hip implants found lymphocytic perivascular infiltrates.

35. Willert H, Buchorn G, Fayaayazi A, Lohmann C: Histopathological changes around metal/metal joints indicate delayed type hypersensitivity: Preliminary results of 14 cases. *Osteologie* 2000;9:2-16.

36. Dempsey KE, Riggio MP, Lennon A, et al: Identification of bacteria on the surface of clinically infected and non-infected prosthetic hip joints removed during revision arthroplasties by 16S rRNA gene sequencing and by microbiological culture. *Arthritis Res Ther* 2007;9:R46.

    Culturing and PCR evaluation of 10 implants revealed bacteria on all implants, with more diverse microflora detected by PCR.

37. Rosai J: *Rosai and Ackerman's Surgical Pathology*, ed 9. St. Louis, MO, Mosby, 2004.

    This is a reference text for surgical pathology.

2: Diagnostic Modalities

Approach to Treatment

SECTION EDITOR:

GEORGE CIERNY III, MD

Chapter 8

Surgical Débridement and Lavage

*Kevin Tetsworth, MD, FRACS

Introduction

The importance of débridement and lavage in treating orthopaedic infections, open fractures, and battlefield injuries has been recognized for many years. For effective control of infection, débridement must include the complete removal of all necrotic bone, foreign material, and tissue with compromised viability. However, the sole use of the original principle of surgical débridement resulted in recurrent sepsis in 30% of chronic osteomyelitis wounds.[1] Improvements in microsurgical techniques, methods of soft-tissue transfer, and graft augmentation have led to reconstructions that support more complete débridement and an improved outcome.[2]

The goals of treatment include both eradication of infection and reconstruction of form and function in the affected limb. The development of sophisticated implants and external fixation devices during the past 20 years has expanded the options for reconstruction. The standard of care now includes local antibiotic delivery using polymethylmethacrylate (PMMA) beads and other methods of dead space treatment, which have allowed the implementation of staged reconstruction protocols. External fixation for gradual, controlled mechanical distraction has been effective for both skeletal and soft-tissue reconstruction.[3,4] The addition of newer methods and devices to the surgical armamentarium has yielded a dramatic improvement in results; clinical success in arresting infection has repeatedly been reported in more than 90% of patients.[1,5,6]

Débridement

The most critical factor in the successful treatment of an acute or chronic orthopaedic infection remains the quality of the surgical débridement. In a prospective, randomized study, all patients who received aggressive débridement with a wide resection margin (at least 5 mm) had virtually complete eradication of infection lasting at least 1 year.[7] In contrast, intralesional biopsy and curettage was uniformly unsuccessful.

The goal of débridement is to achieve a clean, viable wound through an atraumatic exposure. The wound is cleansed of any potentially infectious agent or contaminated material, including foreign objects, necrotic bone, and devitalized tissue. Any residual contaminated material can harbor microorganisms within adherent biofilms and thereby lead to treatment failure.[8]

For an acute infection, the simplest form of débridement is incision and drainage. Coupled with lavage, this procedure often is adequate to treat a simple abscess or acute joint sepsis. The local tissue usually is viable, and the release of purulent fluids can reduce the bacterial load sufficiently to allow host defenses and antibiotics to resolve the infection.

In a chronic infection, simple incision and drainage usually is unsuccessful because of the presence of tissue and host compromise, foreign bodies, and adherent biofilms.[5,9,10] Even when a complete, thorough débridement seems impossible, the likelihood of success can be enhanced by a systematic approach, attention to detail, and gentle handling of soft tissues.[10]

Presurgical Considerations

A careful physical examination and assessment of radiographic studies are useful in estimating the required extent of débridement and determining the likelihood of success. However, the extent of the débridement ultimately is determined by intrasurgical findings. Planning is required before treating anticipated soft-tissue and bone defects as well as any dead space that is created. If the affected limb has undergone an earlier reconstruction using a microvascular free tissue transfer, the anasto mosis should be located and then protected during débridement. Due to atrophy, the flap often is stiff and fibrotic, with diminished compliance and limited potential for further transposition.

High-quality plain radiographs can reveal a dense intramedullary cortical sequestrum, endosteal scalloping, or an involucrum.[5,10] More sophisticated studies are necessary if routine radiographs do not provide information adequate for determining the extent of the pathology and the potential resection margins.[11] CT often is the best method of evaluating a bony infection and selecting the optimal approach for débridement or biopsy in a united fracture.[10] MRI is the best means of detecting extension of a superficial infection into the medullary canal or the presence of skip lesions above or below the primary site of infection. MRI and nuclear studies can define the zone of inflammation and indicate the resection margins.[11]

*Kevin Tetsworth, MD, FRACS or the department with which he is affiliated has received research or institutional support from Smith & Nephew.

3: Approach to Treatment

Soft-Tissue Débridement

Complex soft-tissue considerations usually dictate the optimal surgical approach. Soft-tissue injury related to the original trauma may have led to extensive scarring that obscures most normal anatomic planes. The difficulty associated with dissection through dense scar and distorted anatomy may be compounded by the consequences of earlier surgery, as local tissues are often transposed during efforts to obtain soft-tissue coverage. The viability of local soft tissue must be preserved by gentle handling and by following the planes of earlier surgical and traumatic dissection. If possible, earlier incisions and approaches should be followed, although doing so can be difficult in a traumatized limb. If a linear scar is encountered and is not to be incorporated in the approach, the new incision should cross the scar at an angle as close as possible to 90° so that the risk of margin necrosis and wound breakdown is minimized.[10]

The character and quality of the soft tissue should be critically examined to determine its healing potential. Palpation and manipulation are useful in determining local soft-tissue compliance, and the presence or absence of peripheral pulses can help determine whether vascular studies and transcutaneous oxygen pressures should be obtained.[10] Insufficient tissue vascularity may impede wound revascularization and healing.

An expansile exposure is used for débridement,[5,10] with preparation for a more extensile approach as needed. The procedure may evolve based on the intrasurgical findings. Overlying scar can obscure anatomic landmarks and conceal the precise location of a focus of infection. The most likely area of involvement is initially exposed, and the wound is extended as necessary. Elevation of soft tissue from the bone is avoided outside the region of interest because subperiosteal exposure strips the cortex of an important source of vascularity. The exposure is otherwise in the extraperiosteal plane.[10]

An incision made through an earlier exposure can be prepared for closure by excising the original scar, with a margin of several millimeters on either side. The pathologic tissue often extends from the surface through soft tissue and into bone.[5,10] A sinus tract often is included, if present. Sinus tracts distant from the intended course of the exposure are not routinely excised because they close spontaneously after the source of infection (and drainage) has been eliminated.[10] A thorough surgical débridement may be unsuccessful, however, if viable soft tissue is not available to cover and protect the wound. Soft-tissue transposition and transfer should be considered whenever primary soft-tissue closure cannot be achieved.

Bone Débridement

Necrotic bone must be sought and removed. Stabilization of the limb segment should be considered if the débridement defect will lead to skeletal instability or leave the bone at risk for subsequent fracture. Wide resection margins are advantageous, even though some normal bone will be lost.[7] Close histologic examination of intralesional margins often reveals osteoblasts containing intracellular organisms that are insensitive to antibiotics.[12,13] Such findings have implications for antibiotic resistance. In theory, intracellular organisms can remain dormant for decades, biologically inert and clinically quiescent, and in this state be impervious to antibiotics that interfere with bacterial replication or block the production of critical proteins. Their subsequent reactivation could be responsible for a late recurrence of chronic osteomyelitis.

Healthy, viable bone is a valuable resource, and its vascular supply must be preserved. If the overlying periosteum was removed during exposure, débridement of the adjacent medullary canal devitalizes the cortex and creates a significant risk that a new sequestrum will develop. A long segment of diaphyseal bone can be devitalized if intramedullary rod placement is done during the same procedure as plate and screw removal. The risk should be minimized, if possible, by performing the exchange in two stages and allowing at least 6 weeks between procedures so that the medullary canal can recover adequately.[10]

Although sequestered bone must be identified and removed, reactive new bone forming an involucrum around an area of chronic infection may have substantial volume and structural integrity. By definition, the reactive bone is living, does not require débridement, and can be relied on to revascularize cancellous grafts after reconstruction.

Sharp, precise, rapid débridement of bone is best done using high-speed burrs and cooled by continuous saline irrigation to limit thermal necrosis.[10] The use of fresh burrs maximizes cutting efficiency and limits the risk of injury. Osteotomes and curets are inefficient and can cause stress risers, which can increase the risk of a stress fracture.

During débridement, the surface of the bone is carefully assessed and constantly monitored to detect the scattered pinpoints of bony bleeding that indicate adequate vascularity. This uniform punctate haversian bleeding, called the paprika sign, is characteristic of living bone and is useful in establishing the limits of débridement.[5,10] Dense cortical bone generally is less vascular than other bone, with characteristic anatomy-specific variations. The laser Doppler probe may provide an objective means of measuring bone viability,[5,10,14-17] but it is not a substitute for surgical experience.

Reaming may be adequate for débriding infection restricted to the medullary canal. To limit the thermal effects of reaming, a slow pace and sharp reamer tips are used. A saline-soaked cotton gauze pad can be draped to cool a subcutaneous bone such as the tibia. A standard nasogastric tube is used to irrigate debris from the canal by washing distal to proximal, creating a constant outward flow. The limb should be positioned to promote fluid and debris removal. A nasogastric tube is useful for distal-to-proximal suction directly from the

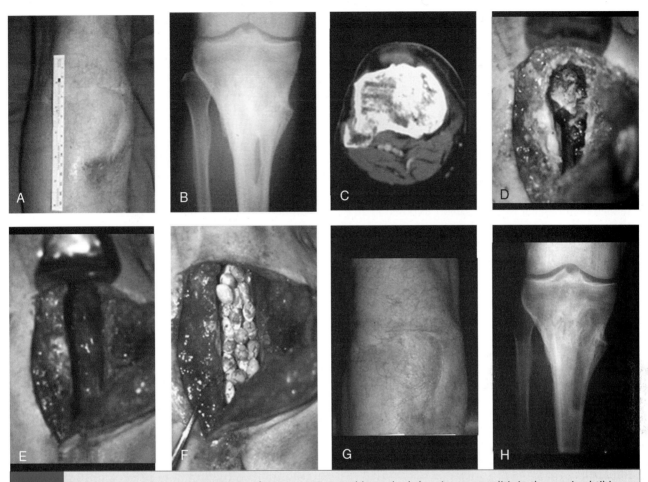

Figure 1 Twelve years after sustaining an open fracture, a 53-year-old man had chronic osteomyelitis in the proximal tibia, caused by methicillin-resistant *Staphylococcus aureus*. He had undergone unsuccessful treatment, including débridement with a cortical trough and a medial gastrocnemius rotational myoplasty. **A,** Area of persistent drainage slightly distal to an earlier trough at the inferior margin of the muscle flap. **B,** Presurgical AP radiograph of the region, showing remnants of trough too far distal to persistent sclerotic metaphyseal bone. **C,** CT scan through persistent sclerotic metaphyseal bone, which was the apparent nidus of infection. **D,** Intrasurgical view through the oval cortical biopsy window, showing sequestrum of bone as seen on presurgical studies. **E,** Débridement defect in the proximal tibial metaphysis after removal of sequestrum. **F,** PMMA beads used to obliterate dead space and deliver high concentrations of local antibiotic. A clinical photograph **(G)** and an AP radiograph **(H)** taken 18 months after surgery show successful control of infection.

canal; the characteristic sound can be helpful in determining whether irrigation and débridement of the medullary canal are complete.[5,10]

Reaming alone is inadequate if the infection involves an area proximal or distal to the isthmus of the bone because the canal's internal width is greater in these areas.[10] Reaming also is inadequate in the presence of endosteal scalloping, as seen on presurgical radiographs. To obtain access to the medullary canal, sometimes it is necessary to perform a longitudinal osteotomy of the involved region. After open débridement, the osteotomized fragment can be replaced and secured with cerclage wires, taking care to preserve bone viability. Alternatively, a longitudinal trough can be created, with the canal débrided directly (**Figure 1**). This elongated oval cortical window provides access to the medullary canal and its contents. Biomechanical studies show that the ideal biopsy portal is oval, with circular ends. The

trough thus created has limited width and smooth margins that can be extended a substantial longitudinal distance, with only slight diminution of torsional strength.[5,10] The region of interest is first exposed in an extraperiosteal fashion, and the periosteum is gently lifted from the underlying cortex. A longitudinal trough parallel to the long axis of the bone is created using a high-speed burr under continuous cool-saline irrigation. The width and length of the trough should be no greater than is necessary to view and débride the endosteal nidus.

If 70% or more of the original cortical circumference is intact at the level of débridement, the risk of stress fracture is low, and stabilization usually is unnecessary.[10] For a larger débridement defect, external fixation is generally the preferred method of stabilizing the at-risk bone while preserving local vascularity. The need for stabilization can be difficult to determine

3: Approach to Treatment

during surgery, and occasionally a simple external fixator must be provisionally applied to an intact limb segment.[10,18] The external fixator is removed if residual bone volume is found to be adequate on postsurgical radiographic studies.

Wide bone resection is an excellent method of treating refractory infection in a nonunited fracture, provided the resulting defect is amenable to a functional reconstruction.[1,3,4] In some patients, the limb is stabilized with an external fixator before débridement. Blood loss can thereby be minimized, and the fixator may be technically easier to apply to an intact limb segment. Immediately before stabilization, the region of intended débridement is provisionally exposed in an extraperiosteal fashion under tourniquet control. The tourniquet is released, hemostasis is obtained, and the wound is loosely closed to restore skin alignment before fixator placement. The fixator components can be used as alignment guides during the reconstruction.[10]

The exposure during a segmental resection must be adequate to allow retractors to be placed for protection of surrounding soft tissues and neurovascular structures. An oscillating saw is used for osteotomies, with continuous cool saline irrigation to limit the risk of thermal necrosis at the resection margins. Each osteotomy can be completed using an osteotome to avoid inadvertent injury to vital structures. After segmental resection, the medullary canal and cortical bone of the cut surfaces are inspected to ensure viability and satisfactory resection margins. The margins can be extended if necessary.[10] If the surrounding periosteum is fibrotic or partially ossified, débridement may be required.

Lavage

Lavage is vital after thorough débridement of an infected wound and physical removal of macroscopic debris. Copious irrigation facilitates the mechanical removal of residual adherent bacteria and microscopic pathologic remnants.[19] The efficacy of lavage depends on the volume of irrigation, the type of bacteria, and the nature of the surface to which the bacteria are adhering.[20] A direct relationship has consistently been found between increasing volume of irrigation and greater reduction in bacterial load; 3 to 9 L of irrigation fluid typically are used.[21] The addition of antibiotics to the saline irrigation fluid appears to offer little advantage.[20] In one study, antibiotic irrigation after débridement of open fractures led to an unexpected increase in the risk of subsequent wound complications.[22]

A mild soap added to the irrigation fluid acts as a surfactant, disrupting the chemical bond holding an organism to a surface and thus facilitating the removal of some bacterial contaminants. In particular, mild soap is effective in removing *Staphylococcus epidermidis* from metal implants.[20] Studies of metal implants, fractured bones, and damaged soft tissues demonstrated that a surfactant irrigation fluid is superior to saline or antibiotic fluid.[20,22]

Low-pressure pulsed lavage with a mild soap solution appears to be most effective in removing the bacteria adhering to bone while preserving bone viability.[23] Low-pressure pulsed lavage is more efficient than use of a bulb syringe in reducing the bacterial load in a contaminated wound.[21] High-pressure pulsed lavage can damage bone and soft tissues.

Dead Space Management

The bone and soft-tissue defect created by débridement can become a dead space filled with a hematoma susceptible to recurrent infection. Active treatment is necessary.[5,10] Obliteration of a possible dead space can be achieved by biologic and nonbiologic techniques, including local myoplasty, free tissue transfer, bone grafting, and an antibiotic-impregnated depot. PMMA beads are most commonly used for a local antibiotic depot, and their use is fundamental to staged reconstruction protocols for musculoskeletal sepsis.[24]

Staged procedures have become key to successful treatment of chronic osteomyelitis.[5,10,25] As the initial procedure is completed, an antibiotic depot is used to deliver a high local concentration of antibiotic and simultaneously obliterate possible dead space. Fortuitously, the depot preserves dead space for the subsequent reconstruction.[10] Antibiotic-loaded PMMA beads generally are removed after the soft tissues have had 3 to 6 weeks to recover from the trauma of surgery.

A free flap used for soft-tissue coverage usually cannot safely be reelevated until its margins or the associated split-thickness skin graft has matured, generally after 6 to 8 weeks. Therefore, when a free flap has been placed over antibiotic beads, the second stage of bead removal and exchange for bone graft must be delayed at least 6 to 8 weeks. Beads placed within the medullary canal must be removed within 10 to 14 days because the formation of granulation tissue makes later removal difficult.[10] Alternatively, antibiotic PMMA cylinders can be placed and easily removed after prolonged use.

The second stage consists of bead removal, repeat irrigation and débridement, and possibly a bone graft[5,10,26] (**Figure 2**). Careful inspection is required to confirm the complete removal of all beads and any residual debris. Using an autogenous cancellous bone graft is preferable, although allograft cancellous chips are sometimes used to augment the graft material. The bone graft definitively obliterates residual dead space, and it can serve as a local antibiotic depot if a pathogen-specific powdered antibiotic is mixed into the graft material immediately before the defect is filled.[27]

Wound Closure

When the surgical procedure is complete, the wound must be either closed without tension or left open. Local advancement flaps are used as necessary to achieve

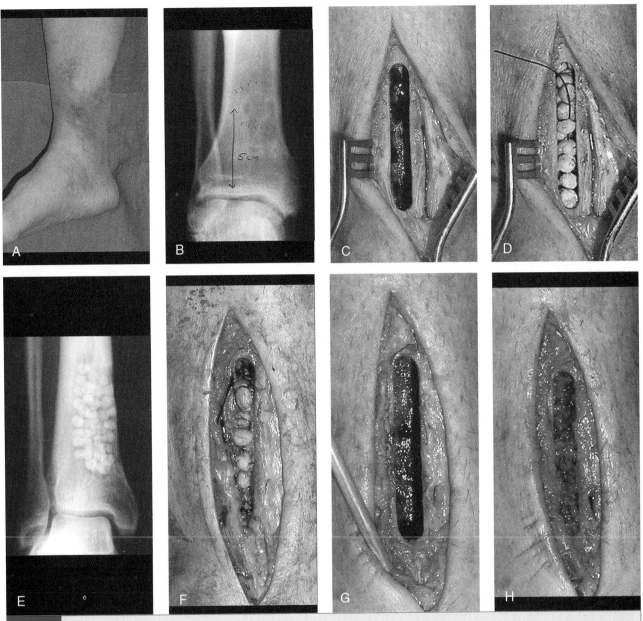

Figure 2 Four years after external fixation of an open fracture, a 37-year-old man had chronic osteomyelitis in the distal tibia, caused by methicillin-resistant *S aureus*. **A,** Area of recurrent episodic drainage corresponding to distal pin sites from the external fixation. **B,** Presurgical AP radiograph of the involved region, showing a distal tibial metaphyseal cavitary osteomyelitis lesion. **C,** Intrasurgical photograph showing the trough used for débridement of the region involved in the distal tibial metaphysis. **D,** PMMA beads used to obliterate dead space and deliver high concentrations of local antibiotic. **E,** Postsurgical AP radiograph showing antibiotic beads in the distal tibial metaphysis. **F,** Initial appearance of the antibiotic beads when exposed 8 weeks later during the second-stage procedure. **G,** The débridement defect after bead removal. **H,** The beads were exchanged for autogenous cancellous bone graft.

a watertight closure. Optimal soft-tissue treatment requires eversion of wound margins, even after activation of suction drains; excision or mobilization of adjacent scar tissue limits the possibility of inversion of the wound margins after closure. Judicious drain placement can be done at the time of wound closure.

Both braided and absorbable sutures can contribute to wound complications and treatment failure. Microorganisms harbored in the complex geometric structure

of braided suture may become a source of recurrent sepsis. Absorbable suture by design stimulates an inflammatory response, which generally is undesirable. Nylon and stainless steel are preferred as the least reactive suture materials, and nylon is far more convenient for clinical use. Monofilament nylon suture used in a vertical or horizontal mattress fashion is preferred for achieving a tension-free, watertight wound closure.[10] Animal studies suggest that antimicrobial-impregnated

3: Approach to Treatment

suture materials are beneficial in preventing surgical site infection in a critically contaminated wound.[27]

Negative Pressure Wound Therapy

Negative pressure wound therapy (NPWT) or vacuum dressing has been studied for wound care during the past decade.[28-30] NPWT involves the indirect application of suction or a vacuum force to the exposed surface of an open wound. Usually a suction tube is placed into a sterile, semicollapsible foam sponge conforming to the dimensions of the wound. An impermeable plastic adhesive film is draped over the sponge and suction tube to create an isolated space, and subatmospheric pressure is continuously or intermittently applied through the suction tube. It is possible to vary the amount of negative pressure, but a small animal study concluded that a minimum suction force of 50 mm Hg is required for efficacy.[31] The dressing is left in place for 48 to 72 hours, with regular dressing changes thereafter on a similar schedule extending indefinitely. During the next several weeks, the wound gradually contracts in size, and healthy granulation tissue forms.

The use of NPWT has dramatically changed the clinical care of open fractures and challenging wounds, although a meta-analysis found insufficient evidence to prove clinical benefit.[32] In some large medical centers, NPWT is used for almost half of all open fracture wounds.[33] The proposed clinical mechanisms of action responsible for the possible benefits of NPWT include enhanced angiogenesis, increased blood flow, improved drainage, and decreased interstitial fluid.[34] The dressing material used in NPWT appears to be influential. When negative pressure is applied through cotton gauze rather than a sponge dressing, the rate of cell death is greater, and the stimulation of cell migration and cell proliferation is less. Cell apoptosis in gauze-covered tissues is significantly higher under suction than not under suction.[34] The possible benefits of NPWT may be related to the ability of a treated wound to support cell growth and stimulate chemotaxis, thus promoting cellular proliferation without increasing apoptosis.[34]

NPWT primarily should be considered for difficult wounds, particularly diabetic foot wounds and high-energy open traumatic wounds. For a diabetic foot wound, NPWT can be used for adjunctive care or as a definitive alternative to other nonsurgical methods such as total contact casting. In a retrospective study of 15 patients with 18 foot or ankle wounds treated using NPWT, 13 wounds healed at an average 2.5 months. The use of NPWT appeared to hasten the closure of these difficult wounds and obviated the need for further surgery in many patients.[28]

For wounds related to high-energy trauma or open fracture, NPWT can be used to postpone definitive wound coverage until conditions are more favorable. NPWT requires less frequent dressing changes than many other forms of wound care and thereby dimin-ishes the risk of nosocomial contamination and significantly reduces the nursing resources required. Contracture of the wound margins and robust induction of granulation tissue after NPWT may allow a less elaborate soft-tissue reconstruction.[29,30] However, a retrospective review of 38 type IIIB open fractures found that a delay of 7 or more days from initial NPWT to definitive soft-tissue coverage increased the rate of deep infection from 12.5% to 57%.[35]

Summary

The single most important aspect in the management of orthopaedic infections remains the quality of the surgical débridement. Eradication of chronic infection is significantly more likely when a wide resection margin is achieved. Meticulous surgical technique, with preservation of local soft tissue vascularity, is another important consideration. The standard of care now involves staged management, often including local antibiotic delivery using PMMA beads. After débridement, copious lavage with a mild detergent solution is an effective method of removing residual adherent bacteria and microscopic pathologic remnants. NPWT has become popular for managing difficult wounds.

Annotated References

1. Cierny G III: Infected tibial non-unions (1981-1995): The evolution of change. *Clin Orthop Relat Res* 1999; 360:97-105.

2. Gonzalez MH, Weinzweig N: Muscle flaps in the treatment of osteomyelitis of the lower extremity. *J Trauma* 2005;58:1019-1023.

   A retrospective review of 31 consecutive patients with tibial osteomyelitis found that the success rate after coverage of soft-tissue defects by muscle flaps was higher than 80% at an average 34-month follow-up.

3. Cierny G III, Zorn KE: Segmental tibial defects: Comparing conventional and Ilizarov methodologies. *Clin Orthop Relat Res* 1994;301:118-123.

4. Watson JT, Anders M, Moed BR: Management strategies for bone loss in tibial shaft fractures. *Clin Orthop Relat Res* 1995;315:138-152.

5. Heitmann C, Patzakis MJ, Tetsworth KD, Levin LS: Musculoskeletal sepsis: Principles of treatment. *Instr Course Lect* 2003;52:733-744.

   This review article provides detailed strategies and protocols for treatment of orthopaedic infections, including débridement techniques, dead space treatment, local antibiotic delivery, and antibiotic selection.

6. Beals RK, Bryant RE: The treatment of chronic open osteomyelitis of the tibia in adults. *Clin Orthop Relat Res* 2005;433:212-217.

In a case-control study of 30 consecutive adult patients with chronic osteomyelitis of the tibia, a variety of techniques specific to each patient achieved a 90% success rate. Débridement, bone graft, and soft-tissue coverage were used for most patients, augmented by distraction osteogenesis techniques in 14 patients.

7. Simpson AH, Deakin M, Latham JM: Chronic osteomyelitis: The effect of the extent of surgical resection on infection-free survival. *J Bone Joint Surg Br* 2001;83: 403-407.

8. Costerton JW: Biofilm theory can guide the treatment of device-related orthopaedic infections. *Clin Orthop Relat Res* 2005;437:7-11.

Important considerations in bacterial biofilm formation, bacterial adhesion to implants, and the persistence of chronic infection are comprehensively discussed. Bacterial colonies within biofilms are protected from host defenses and antibiotics and must be physically removed from the wound before the infection can be resolved.

9. Brady RA, Leid JG, Calhoun JH, Costerton JW, Shirtliff ME: Osteomyelitis and the role of biofilms in chronic infection. *FEMS Immunol Med Microbiol* 2008; 52: 13-22.

The nature of biofilms and their critical role in persistent infection are discussed, with exploration of the nature of molecular interactions between bacteria as well as between bacteria and the local environment, including the host.

10. Tetsworth K, Cierny GC: Osteomyelitis debridement techniques. *Clin Orthop Relat Res* 1999;360:87-96.

11. Gross T, Kaim AH, Regazzoni P, Widmer AF: Current concepts in post-traumatic osteomyelitis: A diagnostic challenge with new imaging options. *J Trauma* 2002;52: 1210-1219.

12. Webb LX, Wagner W, Carroll D, Tyler H, Coldren F, Martin E: MCSIR: Osteomyelitis and intraosteoblastic Staphylococcus aureus. *J Surg Orthop Adv* 2007;16: 73-78.

A successful osteoblast cell culture revealed the intraosteoblastic location of a human osteomyelitis *S aureus* isolate. A possible mechanism is suggested for the periodic protracted quiescence typical of chronic osteomyelitis, with implications for the required width of margins during débridement.

13. Ellington JK, Harris M, Hudson MC, Vishin S, Webb LX, Sherertz R: Intracellular Staphylococcus aureus and antibiotic resistance: Implications for treatment of staphylococcal osteomyelitis. *J Orthop Res* 2006;24:87-93.

In a laboratory study using cultured mouse and human osteoblast cells, cell cultures were infected with *S aureus,* and the bacteria were allowed to invade the osteoblasts. Intracellular bacteria were found to be less sensitive to antibiotics capable of eukaryotic cell penetration.

14. Duwelius PJ, Schmidt AH: Assessment of bone viability in patients with osteomyelitis: Preliminary clinical experience with laser Doppler flowmetry. *J Orthop Trauma* 1992;6:327-332.

15. Swiontkowski MF: Surgical approaches in osteomyelitis: Use of laser Doppler flowmetry to determine nonviable bone. *Infect Dis Clin North Am* 1990;4:501-512.

16. Swiontkowski MF: Criteria for bone débridement in massive lower limb trauma. *Clin Orthop Relat Res* 1989;243:41-47.

17. Swiontkowski MF, Hagan K, Shack RB: Adjunctive use of laser Doppler flowmetry for débridement of osteomyelitis. *J Orthop Trauma* 1989;3:1-5.

18. Fodor L, Ullmann Y, Soudry M, Calif E, Lerner A: Prophylactic external fixation and extensive bone debridement for chronic osteomyelitis. *Acta Orthop Belg* 2006; 72:448-453.

In a small study, patients with chronic osteomyelitis were treated with aggressive débridement, dead space management, and antibiotics, as well as prophylactic external fixation to stabilize the limb. No recurrences were found within the follow-up period.

19. Bahrs C, Schnabel M, Frank T, Zapf C, Mutters R, von Garrel T: Lavage of contaminated surfaces: An in vitro evaluation of the effectiveness of different systems. *J Surg Res* 2003;112:26-30.

An in vitro comparison of three different lavage techniques on four different surfaces found that bacterial reduction was effective on all four surfaces using all three lavage techniques. A continuous manual pump irrigator was found to be practical, economical, and effective.

20. Anglen J, Apostoles PS, Christensen G, Gainor B, Lane J: Removal of surface bacteria by irrigation. *J Orthop Res* 1996;14:251-254.

21. Svoboda SJ, Bice TG, Gooden MA, Brooks DE, Thomas DB, Wenke JC: Comparison of bulb syringe and pulsed lavage irrigation with use of a bioluminescent musculoskeletal wound model. *J Bone Joint Surg Am* 2006;88:2167-2174.

Bioluminescent bacteria were used in an animal model to quantify the efficacy of pulsed lavage compared with lavage using a bulb syringe. Both device and volume effects were found, and pulsed lavage proved significantly more effective than a bulb syringe.

22. Anglen JO: Comparison of soap and antibiotic solutions for irrigation of lower-limb open fracture wounds: A prospective, randomized study. *J Bone Joint Surg Am* 2005;87:1415-1422.

In a prospective, randomized study of 458 open fracture wounds treated using antibiotic irrigation or a mild detergent, the infection rate was 18% in wounds treated with antibiotic irrigation and 13% in those treated with detergent. This difference was not significant. Antibiotic irrigation was associated with a minor, not-significant increase in wound complications.

3: Approach to Treatment

23. Bhandari M, Adili A, Schemitsch EH: The efficacy of low-pressure lavage with different irrigating solutions to remove adherent bacteria from bone. *J Bone Joint Surg Am* 2001;83:412-419.

24. Zalavras CG, Patzakis MJ, Holtom P: Local antibiotic therapy in the treatment of open fractures and osteomyelitis. *Clin Orthop Relat Res* 2004;427:86-93.

    This comprehensive discussion of local antibiotic delivery, including antibiotic polymethylmethacrylate beads and bioabsorbable alternatives, concludes that local antibiotic therapy is safe and results in a high local concentration of antibiotics with a minimal systemic level.

25. Tulner SA, Schaap GR, Strackee SD, Besselaar PP, Luitse JS, Marti RK: Long-term results of multiple-stage treatment for posttraumatic osteomyelitis of the tibia. *J Trauma* 2004;56:633-642.

    Retrospective review of 47 patients with chronic osteomyelitis who were treated using a standard staged protocol found that 91% had infection control at an average 94-month follow-up.

26. Chen CE, Ko JY, Pan CC: Results of vancomycin-impregnated cancellous bone grafting for infected tibial nonunion. *Arch Orthop Trauma Surg* 2005;125: 369-375.

    No recurrent infection was found in a retrospective review of 18 patients with tibial osteomyelitis who were treated using vancomycin-impregnated cancellous bone grafts for final osseous reconstruction.

27. Marco F, Vallez R, Gonzalez P, Ortega L, de la Lama J, Lopez-Duran L: Study of the efficacy of coated Vicryl plus antibacterial suture in an animal model of orthopaedic surgery. *Surg Infect (Larchmt)* 2007;8:359-365.

    S epidermidis was used to contaminate surgical steel suture in the deep zone of surgical wounds closed with Vicryl Plus suture (Vicryl impregnated with triclosan) or untreated Vicryl suture. The incidence of positive cultures in specimens retrieved after 16 days was higher in wounds closed with untreated Vicryl ($P = 0.005$).

28. Mendonca DA, Cosker T, Makwana NK: Vacuum-assisted closure to aid wound healing in foot and ankle surgery. *Foot Ankle Int* 2005;26:761-766.

    Retrospective review of 18 difficult foot or ankle wounds treated with NPWT found that satisfactory healing was achieved in 13 at an average of 2.5 months, leading to more rapid wound closure and avoiding the need for further surgery.

29. Herscovici D Jr, Sanders RW, Scaduto JM, Infante A, DiPasquale T: Vacuum-assisted wound closure (VAC therapy) for the management of patients with high-energy soft tissue injuries. *J Orthop Trauma* 2003;17: 683-688.

    In a consecutive, nonrandomized study of 21 patients with a high-energy soft-tissue wound who were initially treated using NPWT for an average of 19.3 days, 57% required no further treatment or a split-thickness skin graft. Only 43% required a free tissue transfer.

30. Dedmond BT, Kortesis B, Punger K, et al: The use of negative-pressure wound therapy (NPWT) in the temporary treatment of soft-tissue injuries associated with high-energy open tibial shaft fractures. *J Orthop Trauma* 2007;21:11-17.

    In a retrospective study of 50 consecutive grade III open tibial shaft fractures initially treated with NPWT, the overall infection rate was relatively high (30%). NPWT appeared to decrease the need for free tissue transfer or rotational myoplasty.

31. Isago T, Nozaki M, Kikuchi Y, Honda T, Nakazawa H: Effects of different negative pressures on reduction of wounds in negative pressure dressings. *J Dermatol* 2003;30:596-601.

    A laboratory study used rats to investigate the optimal pressure level for NPWT. Reduction in wound area was satisfactory at 50 mm Hg and all higher pressure levels. Pressure below 50 mm Hg did not improve the response, and reduction in wound area was suboptimal at 25 mm Hg.

32. Gregor S, Maegele M, Sauerland S, Krahn JF, Peinemann F, Lange S: Negative pressure wound therapy: A vacuum of evidence? *Arch Surg* 2008;143:189-196.

    This meta-analysis found 255 published articles on NPWT, but only 17 satisfied the inclusion criteria. The available evidence was insufficient to prove an added clinical benefit to NPWT. The large number of terminated or unpublished studies concerned the authors.

33. Parrett BM, Matros E, Pribaz JJ, Orgill DP: Lower extremity trauma: Trends in the management of soft-tissue reconstruction of open tibia-fibula fractures. *Plast Reconstr Surg* 2006;117:1315-1322.

    This retrospective review of 290 consecutive open tibial fractures discusses changes in treatment over a 12-year period. NPWT now is used to treat almost half of all open fracture wounds, and there is a trend toward less elaborate soft-tissue reconstruction.

34. McNulty AK, Schmidt M, Feeley T, Kieswetter K: Effects of negative pressure wound therapy on fibroblast viability, chemotactic signaling, and proliferation in a provisional wound (fibrin) matrix. *Wound Repair Regen* 2007;15:838-846.

    This industry-supported study investigated cellular mechanisms responsible for the possible benefits of NPWT. Fibroblasts grown in a three-dimensional matrix were treated with or without suction and using different dressings. The ability of NPWT to support cell growth, stimulate chemotaxis, and support cell proliferation may be partly responsible for clinically observed results.

35. Bhattacharyya T, Mehta P, Smith M, Pomahac B: Routine use of wound vacuum-assisted closure does not allow coverage delay for open tibia fractures. *Plast Reconstr Surg* 2008;121:1263-1266.

    In a retrospective review of 38 grade IIIB open tibial fractures initially treated using NPWT, the infection rate in wounds definitively covered before 7 days was 12.5%, compared with a 57% infection rate in those covered at 7 days or later.

Chapter 9
Local Antimicrobial Treatment

Alex C. McLaren, MD   Felipe N. Gutierrez, MD, MPH   Mary Martin, PharmD   Ryan McLemore, PhD

Introduction

The local delivery of antimicrobial agents to the site of orthopaedic infections is based on the need for high concentrations of these drugs to kill planktonic and biofilm-based bacteria. Although the mainstay of treatment remains surgical resection, most resections are intralesional and leave the resection surfaces exposed to contaminating bacteria. The debris that remains in the wound, even following a thorough low-pressure pulse lavage, almost certainly includes clumps of biofilm that contain the causative organisms. Even small biofilm fragments with a few organisms are unresponsive to antimicrobial agents in the usually effective concentrations. Systemic toxicity usually precludes parenteral dosing at those levels. Pharmacokinetic factors, including alterations in local tissue perfusion, make local delivery the best method of achieving an extremely high antimicrobial level.

History

Local delivery of antimicrobial agents to infected wounds has been used throughout history. As early as 1600 BC in Greece and 1500 BC in Egypt, mold was placed into wounds to prevent and treat bacterial infections.[1] The Romans used silver nitrate in open fractures, and this modality was again promoted in the late 1800s.[2] Silver-coated fabrics were used in the 1970s to treat osteomyelitis.[3] The use of bone cement impregnated with antimicrobial agents to prevent infection in total hip arthroplasties was first reported in 1970.[4] Antimicrobial-loaded bone cement (ALBC) has since been used in the treatment of soft-tissue infections, open fractures, long bone osteomyelitis, and arthroplasty infections.[5-10] Fixation of prosthetic components has been performed using ALBC for prophylaxis in primary procedures. The pharmacokinetics of antimicrobial delivery from ALBC have been studied extensively in vitro and in vivo. Alternative materials have been suggested to address concerns about incomplete antimicrobial release, leading to prolonged subtherapeutic antimicrobial levels, and potential surface colonization of ALBC by resistant organisms.[11]

General Considerations

The Zone of Local Antimicrobial Activity

It is important to coordinate the local and systemic administration of antimicrobial agents.[12] During resection, bacteria are shed from the infected site, and these planktonic bacteria have the potential to seed and survive in sites remote from the local antimicrobial depot. The antimicrobial level required to kill bacteria in biofilm often is more than 100 times higher than the level required to kill the same bacteria in planktonic form.[13,14] The extreme antimicrobial concentration achieved from high-dose ALBC is limited to penetration of the wound hematoma and approximately 1 cm of bone and a few centimeters of soft tissue immediately adjacent to the delivery depot.[9,15] The concentrations fall to a subtherapeutic level over a short distance, and systemic antimicrobial agents are required to control planktonic bacteria in tissue beyond the therapeutic range of the local depot.

Delivery Mechanisms: Surface Bonded or Local Release

Local delivery of antimicrobial agents falls under two main concepts: surface bonded and local release. The distinction between these two concepts is the target of intended activity. Antimicrobial agents bound to the implant surface are intended to protect the surface of the implant, not to release into the surrounding fluid and adjacent tissues.[16] Examples of surface activity include antiseptic- or antimicrobial-impregnated materials used for indwelling catheters,[17] antimicrobial sutures,[18] antimicrobial vascular grafts,[19] vancomycin-polyethylene glycol-acrylate polymerized to orthopaedic implant materials,[20] and vancomycin covalently bonded to titanium[21] and bone.[22] Surface protection is durable and effective in vitro. Surface-active indwelling catheters and antimicrobial sutures are in clinical use. The use of antimicrobial agents covalently bonded to implant or bone surfaces is still under investigation. The commercial development of an implant with antimicrobially active surfaces is a complex process, and the technologies currently under study may not be available as clinically usable devices for several years. One possible method currently available for delivering antimicrobial activity to an implant surface is to fill the interstices of a porous implant material with a

3: Approach to Treatment

resorbable antimicrobial depot. The goal is to provide antimicrobial activity at the surface of implants where ALBC will not be used. This technique is under investigation.

For materials that are intended to release the antimicrobial agent, the target of activity is the adjacent fluid, soft tissue, and bone in postresection surgical wounds. The antimicrobial levels delivered to the target tissues depend on fluid dynamics in the local wound and release characteristics of the depot. The release performance of a delivery material depends on the penetration of fluid into the depths of the material, dissolution of the contained antimicrobial agent, and diffusion of the antimicrobial agent from the depot. Surface protection of the depot material is assumed, although it may not be absolute. There is concern that bacteria could populate the surface of the delivery material as the concentration of the released antimicrobial agent falls below therapeutic levels. Although there have been reports of bacteria growing on ALBC surfaces,[23] secondary infections have not been a clinical problem. More important is that any bacteria present are probably resistant to the antimicrobial agent in the cement, and this factor should be considered if an infection does occur in the presence of ALBC.[24]

Pharmacokinetics and Pharmacodynamics

Local antimicrobial concentration and duration of delivery are key determinants of clinical success. The goal of achieving antimicrobial levels that are sufficiently high and sufficiently long lasting to eradicate all living microbes is balanced against the risk of drug toxicity and premature antimicrobial depletion. Both pharmacokinetics (the absorption, distribution, metabolism, and elimination of the antimicrobial agent) and pharmacodynamics (the action of the antimicrobial agent on the microbes) are important. The pharmacokinetics associated with a specific delivery vehicle are highly specific to that vehicle and are dependent on the material and preparation methods used to make the delivery vehicle, the anatomic site to which it is delivered, and site-specific pathophysiology. The performance of one vehicle cannot be assumed to apply to another vehicle, even if there is only a minor change in preparation methods using the same material.

Killing Time: Time-Dependent Versus Concentration-Dependent Agents

The optimal length of time for local delivery systems to release antimicrobial agents is undetermined. A 6-week period has been suggested, based on the traditional parenteral regimen for osteomyelitis. This regimen is largely empirical and is based on the clinical response of patients who have not undergone resection; in these patients, antimicrobial distribution often is hindered by areas of poor penetration. The 6-week regimen may not be necessary if the antimicrobial agents are locally delivered to a completely resected site in very high concentrations.

Many factors can affect the killing time for a specific antimicrobial agent to kill a specific pathogen, including bacterial load, bacterial replication rate, the presence of resistant subpopulations, and the host immune response. Sophisticated pharmacokinetic-pharmacodynamic models have been developed to realistically simulate the in vivo environment.[25,26] By exposing pathogens in vitro to antimicrobial agents in fluctuating concentrations, time-kill curves can be generated to determine the time and concentration conditions that effect bacterial killing for specific drug-bacterium pairs. Time-kill data pertain to planktonic bacteria. However, the principles can be used to guide release duration goals in the formulation of ALBC when the biology and pharmacodynamics data for biofilm-based bacteria are considered.[27,28]

Understanding the minimum inhibitory concentration (MIC) and static concentration is important to understanding the application of time-kill data. MIC is an in vitro measure of the lowest concentration that will inhibit bacterial growth over 18 to 24 hours of exposure to a constant concentration of the antimicrobial agent. Specific bacteria generally are considered susceptible to an antimicrobial agent when serum levels above the MIC of the agent for that bacterium can be reliably achieved using normal doses.

For each antimicrobial-bacterium pair, there is a specific antimicrobial concentration at which the number of bacteria remains static. At this static concentration, cell replication matches cell death, so that the bacterial population is neither increasing nor decreasing. However, the bacteria are still viable, and replication is continuing. Elimination of the bacteria therefore depends on host immune killing. For time-dependent antimicrobial agents such as the β-lactams, the static concentration is close to the MIC. As the concentration of the antimicrobial agent increases, the killing increases linearly until the antimicrobial concentration reaches approximately four times the MIC. Above four times the MIC, the killing rate does not increase.[26,29] More time is required to effect complete bacterial eradication. This is called time-dependent killing. For systemically administered antimicrobial agents that act by time-dependent killing, the antimicrobial concentration should typically be maintained at a level more than four to five times the MIC for a portion of the interval between doses that is agent specific (for example, penicillin 50%, cephalosporin 70%).[30] During local delivery, antimicrobial concentrations are continuously high and do not fluctuate.

For antimicrobial agents that have concentration-dependent killing, the static concentration is typically much lower than the MIC. Killing continues to increase at concentrations that are typically much higher than the concentrations at which time-dependent antimicrobial agents no longer increase their killing rate. Gentamicin is known to be concentration dependent for killing of *Pseudomonas* at concentrations 10 times the MIC and greater.[29] However, aminoglycosides may not have concentration-dependent killing of gram-positive organisms. The *Staphylococcus* kill rate does not increase with concentrations as high as 80 times the MIC.[31] At the concentrations delivered by ALBC, aminoglycosides exhibit concentration-dependent killing of gram-negative organisms but time-dependent killing of gram-positive organisms.[29] The data for vancomycin suggest a combination; clinical efficacy is reported to depend on the time of exposure to more than four to five times the MIC, but in vitro data show that bacterial eradication depends on the area under the time-kill curve, increasing with both concentration and time.

The application of in vitro time-kill data to clinical infections is an imprecise process because the bacterial burden in clinical infections is unknown, antimicrobial penetration at the infection site may be inconsistent, resistant bacterial subpopulations may be present, and the host's local and systemic immune response can vary widely. The biologic diversity of the bacteria in biofilm magnifies the challenge in orthopaedic infections. An otherwise intact immune system may not detect or respond to bacteria in biofilm, and bacteria in biofilm have decreased susceptibility to antimicrobial agents. Nonetheless, the concepts should be considered when formulating ALBC.

Time-kill data show a 99.9% reduction of a 10^7 *Staphylococcus* load within less than 2 hours for gentamicin and less than 16 hours for vancomycin, with the concentration of both drugs below 20 μg/mL.[29] Eliminating all viable bacteria requires multiple dosing cycles for systemic administration because the antimicrobial levels fall below the MIC for part of each cycle. With continuously high levels from local delivery, the time to eradication may be less than with intermittent parenteral dosing. High-dose ALBC delivery of vancomycin and gentamicin provides the necessary concentration for activity against biofilm-based bacteria, exceeding 100 times the usually expected MIC. If the killing rate in biofilm at concentrations exceeding 100 times the MIC is similar to published data for killing planktonic bacteria at the MIC, the bacterial load will be reduced by 10^9 during the initial 48 hours (three times the 16 hours required by vancomycin for a 99.9% kill). Animal and clinical data suggest that high-dose ALBC will deliver these levels for aminoglycosides and vancomycin for more than 48 hours.[5,9,10,32-44] The time required for the eradication of all viable bacteria from an orthopaedic infection site with continuous high-concentration antimicrobial exposure following resection is not known; it must be less than the time required when high concentrations are delivered by the ALBC used clinically because long-term infection control is generally achieved in at least 90% of patients.[5,7,12,33,36,42,45-50] Some susceptibility data but no time-kill data are available for biofilm-based bacteria.[27,28] Time-kill data for constant exposure of biofilm-based bacteria to the antimicrobial levels achievable by local delivery are needed to more accurately define the required duration of exposure.

Bacteriostatic and Bacteriocidal Agents

It is widely accepted that the antimicrobial agents used for local delivery should be bacteriocidal, but this may not be true if delivery is continuous at a high concentration. Bacteriocidal activity is concentration dependent, and bacteriostatic agents can be bacteriocidal above the static concentration. The distinction between bacteriostatic and bacteriocidal is hotly debated but may have practical importance only if the host's immune status is sufficiently compromised that the remaining viable bacteria cannot be eliminated at static concentrations. Biofilm may impair local immune activity so greatly that the host is not able to eliminate the remaining viable bacteria. The bacteriostatic-bacteriocidal status of an antimicrobial agent also is affected by bacterial load, local wound factors, host immune status, the length of time the antimicrobial agent is above or below therapeutic levels, and the susceptibility of the bacterium. Vancomycin, gentamicin, and β-lactams are considered to be bacteriocidal agents, but they may perform differently in vivo against biofilm-based bacteria, even when they are delivered in extreme concentrations.

Antimicrobial Agents Commonly Used in ALBC

Gentamicin, tobramycin, vancomycin, and cefazolin are the antimicrobial agents most commonly used in ALBC. These drugs have been investigated in elution and clinical studies. Pilot data are available for many other antimicrobial agents, but most antimicrobial agents lack comprehensive in vitro and in vivo performance data. There are no widely accepted guidelines for using a drug that lacks elution and clinical data to define its performance. A prudent approach might be to add the equivalent of a 24-hour systemic dose to an ALBC formulation having the optimal amount of poragen (10 g for high-dose ALBC). Poragens are materials that are used to create pores. In ALBC, the antibiotic powder or soluble particulate filler dissolves and diffuses into the surrounding fluid, leaving pores. A poragen is not needed in the formulation of a soluble or highly porous alternative material. Elution data and animal studies suggest that release of the entire dose is not expected within the first 24 hours, even with highly porous polymethylmethacrylate (PMMA) or an alternative material.[34] Although general clinical experience suggests that little or no systemic exposure should be expected, the clinical need must be weighed against an undefined risk of toxicity.

Antimicrobial Agents for Anaerobic Bacteria and Fungi

Antimicrobial agents can be mixed with bone cement to treat infections caused by anaerobes and fungi. For anaerobic coverage, second-generation cephalosporins and penicillin elute well from ALBC, but metronidazole and clindamycin are not available as powder. The

3: Approach to Treatment

in vitro elution data on antifungal agents in ALBC are limited, and there are few reports on their clinical use.[51-53] Antifungal agents present specific challenges. Fluconazole is available only in nonsterile tablets that must be crushed and sterilized. Amphotericin deoxycholate chemically binds with PMMA, preventing its release.[52] However, amphotericin deoxycholate will elute if 50 mg are added to 10 g of poragen (typically an antimicrobial powder) in ALBC.

Liquid Antimicrobial Agents in ALBC

Antimicrobial agents are used in powder form in ALBC because water and methacrylate monomer are not miscible. Most of the liquid separates from the PMMA during the polymerization process if more than a few milliliters of water are used. It is not possible to carry enough drug in the few milliliters of solution that will stay in the PMMA to achieve an adequate antimicrobial load. Low-dose liquid gentamicin (6 mL of concentration 40 mg/mL) is reported to cause a 49% degradation in compressive strength of the ALBC and inadequate elution (average, 26.4 µg/mL over 24 hours).[54] Marginally higher elution of the antimicrobial agent may occur when a similar dose of liquid gentamicin is used in addition to 4 g of vancomycin, but there is still a 37% to 45% loss of compressive strength.[55] The powder form of the antimicrobial agent should be used in hand-mixed ALBC formulations until a satisfactory procedure is established for mixing a liquid antimicrobial agent into PMMA.

Adverse Reactions, Allergy, and Desensitization

Adverse reactions to antimicrobial agents in ALBC are extremely rare. With the exception of reports of isolated renal toxicity to aminoglycosides,[42,44,56,57] anecdotal experience suggests that patients who have had an adverse reaction to a specific antimicrobial agent (including a severe type 1 hypersensitivity reaction) do not react when the agent is locally delivered in ALBC. The explanation may be inherent in the kinetics of local delivery. For example, many of the adverse reactions to early generic formulations of vancomycin were caused by impurities; however, such reactions were not found with local delivery in ALBC. It is reasonable to assume that systemic exposure to the impurities, like the systemic exposure to vancomycin, was at subthreshold levels.

The risk of red man syndrome, an anaphylactoid reaction, also is avoided when vancomycin is delivered in ALBC. Red man syndrome is characterized by the release of histamine from mast cells; the extent of histamine release is predominantly related to the rate of vancomycin infusion and may be attenuated by reducing the rate of administration. The systemic exposure from ALBC is limited, with very low serum levels that require 12 hours or longer to reach their maximum.

Classic anaphylaxis is the result of an IgE-mediated immediate type 1 allergic reaction. Type 1 hypersensitivity reactions can be life threatening but are amenable to desensitization. Rapid desensitization is a highly effective process in which a sensitized patient receives a slowly increasing dose over several hours to avoid mast cell degranulation and allow T-suppressor cell induction. Desensitization starts with an extremely small exposure, typically an infusion of 10^{-5} times the therapeutic dose. The exposure is incrementally increased at 15- to 20-minute intervals over 4 to 6 hours to the full dose. It is essential that no desensitization or therapeutic dose is missed; if therapy is interrupted, it is necessary to repeat the desensitization process.[58,59] Serendipitously, local delivery produces precisely these kinetics. Desensitization by local delivery occurs as the drug is released; the required gradual rise in serum concentration occurs over 4 to 6 hours. The rise in antimicrobial concentration continues to a peak at 12 to 24 hours and then decreases to nonmeasurable levels within 72 to 96 hours. There is no interruption in exposure to the drug, and the process occurs in the operating and recovery rooms under maximal medical surveillance. The tolerance resulting from this pattern of exposure is associated with a mild and usually undetectable response.

Delayed hypersensitivity to the antimicrobial agents delivered in ALBC has not been an issue, although in a German case study a delayed hypersensitivity reaction to PMMA was reported to require exchange to an implant with a different fixation.[60]

Local Tissue Toxicity

Local delivery of antimicrobial agents leads to an extremely high antimicrobial concentration that can reach thousands of micrograms per milliliter. Drain fluid levels have been measured in excess of 2,000 µg/mL. Antimicrobial agents at these levels are directly in contact with the healing surgical wound, which often is the site of bone defect reconstruction. There is concern about possible toxicity to the local biology, downregulation of immune activity, or cellular toxicity and death. The effect on local immune response and wound healing has not been studied directly, but fibroblast and osteoblast cell response has been studied. Fibroblast growth is not inhibited by high levels of gentamicin in cell culture.[10] Osteoblast cell culture studies found a progressive effect with increasing levels. A decrease in metabolic activity (indicated by a decreased alkaline phosphatase level) occurs with exposure to more than 100 µg/mL of gentamicin. Cellular replication decreases in response to more than 200 µg/mL of cefazolin or more than 400 µg/mL of tobramycin. Cell death is seen with exposure to more than 10,000 µg/mL of tobramycin, vancomycin, or cefazolin.[61-63] Although impaired wound healing and bone graft incorporation have not been clinically associated with local delivery of antimicrobial agents, these cell culture studies clearly show deleterious effects on local cellular biology. Further study of molecular and cellular responses is needed, as is greater knowledge of the antimicrobial levels that occur in clinical application.

In clinical use, high-dose porous ALBC is very tissue compatible. The tissue directly apposed to ALBC generally is a thin, fibrous layer that is adherent to the surfaces, and this factor should be considered when attempting to aspirate fluid adjacent to ALBC for evaluation before delayed reconstruction. There is no free fluid adjacent to high-dose ALBC, in contrast to low-dose ALBC. Host tissue does not grow onto the surface of nonporous low-dose ALBC. Small amounts of fluid may be present in the joint space of articulating spacers. The amount of fluid in uncontrolled infection varies, and aspiration therefore should be planned on a case-by-case basis. Multiple failed attempts and injection of fluid to retrieve a specimen should not be performed for dry taps adjacent to high-dose ALBC.

Bacterial Resistance

Induction or selection of resistant organisms is a prevailing concern with the use of ALBC and local depots using other materials. Local delivery always progresses to a low-level delivery that can persist for months or years. The declining antimicrobial levels do not prevent subpopulations with low susceptibility from establishing a biofilm on the surface of the depot, even if only temporarily, as can happen before resorbable materials disappear. Microbial organisms do not have the ability to correct errors in genetic translation; errors can occur whenever an organism is reproducing, even with the slow replication that occurs in biofilm. A locally impaired immune response and subtherapeutic antimicrobial levels provide a selective advantage for mutations that have decreased susceptibility. In addition, genetic transfer by plasmid or other means can introduce resistance in any bacteria occupying the surface.

Clinical and in vitro data irrefutably confirmed that gentamicin-resistant organisms grow on the surface of gentamicin-loaded bone cement and that the incidence may increase with time.[23,24] The incidence of clinical progression to infection and hardware failure is low, however. Perhaps the most concerning possible explanation of the low incidence of clinical manifestations of bacteria growing on the surface of PMMA is that organisms are indeed growing on ALBC or other PMMA surfaces but are not inciting a purulent or symptomatic response. Instead, they may be slowly inciting a fibrohistiocytic response and eventual mechanical looseness. There is considerable evidence that this may be the case in many so-called aseptic arthroplasty failures, which may be truly infectious despite the lack of a classic clinical infection or the ability to isolate the microbes.[64] Although the prevalence and morbidity of these subclinical infections are impossible to determine, the possible presence of resistant organisms must be considered whenever revision surgery is performed after ALBC use. Any bacteria present when the revision is performed probably are resistant to the antimicrobial agent used in the original ALBC, and therefore it may be prudent to use an alternative or additional antimicrobial agent in the ALBC used at revision surgery.

The development of secondary infection does not appear to be an important concern when high-dose ALBC spacers are used. Radiographs show an absence of radiolucent zones surrounding high-dose ALBC spacers, and more than 90% of patients remain symptom free and have no evidence of infection on laboratory tests.[5,6,12,32,36,47,48,50,65-68] Thus, it can be concluded that high-dose ALBC spacers do not carry a short-term risk of subclinical infection, any more than non–antimicrobial-loaded PMMA does.

When local delivery is used to treat established infections caused by resistant organisms, it is important to consider how susceptibility is designated. For some antimicrobial agents, notably those associated with concentration-dependent killing, the concentration that determines susceptibility may be far below the levels achieved in a wound treated with local delivery. Many of these organisms are not resistant at the levels delivered by high-dose ALBC.

Methicillin-resistant *Staphylococcus aureus* (MRSA) and methicillin-resistant *Staphylococcus epidermidis* are becoming increasingly important as primary pathogens in implant infections and osteomyelitis, and there is considerable pressure to use vancomycin. However, unconstrained use of vancomycin carries an unacceptable risk for developing vancomycin-resistant organisms. Local delivery of vancomycin is not associated with as high a risk of developing resistance as systemic use. Locally delivered high-dose tobramycin is good prophylaxis for the common commensal organisms, including resistant strains, so there is less pressure to indiscriminately use vancomycin in ALBC. Vancomycin in ALBC is appropriate for a patient who has a history of MRSA infection, is an MRSA carrier, or is in an institution where MRSA is prevalent.

Materials for Local Delivery of Antimicrobial Agents

The gold standard for delivery materials is bone cement. Although there is an extensive literature with a positive consensus, few level I studies have been published. The US Food and Drug Administration (FDA) has approved only low-dose ALBC (0.5 or 1 g of antibiotic per batch of cement). High-dose ALBC (at least 10 g of antibiotic powder per batch of cement) for treating orthopaedic infections is considered an off-label application of PMMA. A thorough understanding of the factors affecting the performance of local delivery materials therefore is essential.

Concern about bacterial growth on the surface of retained ALBC has led to a belief that all ALBC should be removed unless needed for implant fixation. This concern prevails despite the knowledge that there is long-term retention of ALBC in millions of arthroplasties that are not clinically infected. Although bacteria on the surface of PMMA used for implant fixation may lead to so-called aseptic loosening, infection of retained

3: Approach to Treatment

Table 1

Non-PMMA Materials Used for Local Delivery of Antimicrobial Agents

Protein
Albumin
Autologous blood clot
Elastin-like polypeptides
Gelatin
Human fibrinogen and thrombin (fibrin clots)
Lyophilized collagen sponge
Microfibrillar type-I collagen (bovine or porcine)

Bone Graft and Substitutes
Bioactive glass
Calcium sulfate
Hydroxyapatite
Morcellized cancellous bone (autograft or allograft)
Tricalcium phosphate

Polymers
Polyanhydride P
Polycaprolactone microspheres
Poly-DL-lactide-co-glycolide microspheres
Polyglycolide
Polyhydroxyalkanoate
Polyhydroxybutyrate-co-hydroxyvalerate
Polylactide and poly-DL-lactide microspheres
Polypropylene fumarate-methylmethacrylate
Polysaccharide (D-glucosamine, N-acetyl-D-glucosamine)

ALBC has not become a clinical problem. In some patients, removal is warranted for mechanical reasons when a secondary reconstruction procedure is not otherwise necessary. A resorbable delivery material that does not require removal is therefore desirable.

Non-PMMA Delivery Materials

Numerous alternative materials have been investigated, and limited clinical data are available for some [11,69] (Table 1). These materials can be divided into three groups: protein and peptide based, bone graft and substitutes, and synthetic polymers. The alternative materials are resorbable, with the exception of β-tricalcium phosphate, hydroxyapatite, and bioactive glass. Several are intended to directly promote bone regeneration in the defect; they include morcellized cancellous bone (MCB), calcium sulfate, β-tricalcium phosphate, and hydroxyapatite. In vitro, most of the contained antimicrobial agent is dumped within the first 24 to 48 hours. In vivo performance varies widely; in the low-flow en-

vironment of an intramedullary canal, high local levels may be sustained for several weeks. With the exception of MCB and possibly calcium sulfate, the in vivo pharmacokinetic and clinical data are insufficient to establish a clinical role for any of these materials. None of the materials are FDA approved for use in the local delivery of antimicrobial agents. Only anecdotal clinical information and small case studies are available, and they are largely uncorroborated. Data correlating in vitro, in vivo, and clinical performance are limited or nonexistent. Some materials have local effects that may not be predictable; for example, calcium sulfate can cause draining wound seromas, and polyanhydride remains as a gelatinous mass long after the antimicrobial agent is gone.[11,15,70]

Antimicrobial-Loaded Bone Graft

In vitro, in vivo, and clinical data are available to support the use of two alternative materials, MCB and calcium sulfate α-hemihydrate, which also have an application in bone defect regeneration. Calcium sulfate is in limited use as a bone graft substitute. The loading of calcium sulfate with antimicrobial agents is an off-label application in the United States and has been associated with wound seroma and fistula formation. There are release data for tobramycin and vancomycin in calcium sulfate, and good clinical performance has been reported.[11,71]

Grafts of MCB are widely used for reconstructing nonstructural bone defects and stimulating healing. Loading MCB with antimicrobial agents is straightforward, has no important disadvantages, and increases the cost only by the price of the antimicrobial agent. High local antimicrobial levels protect the reconstruction while the graft is being incorporated. Host defenses are recruited before the antimicrobial release falls to subtherapeutic levels, and complete absence of antimicrobial agents is expected by the time the graft is fully incorporated. In vitro and in vivo data suggest a substantial margin of safety, with high local levels of tobramycin and vancomycin in the graft (remaining above the MIC for 3 weeks) and low serum levels (below 9 µg/mL, with a maximum at 4 hours).[72-75] Clinical pharmacokinetic data showed 10 to 100 times the MIC in drain fluid during the first 48 hours and serum levels below 10 µg/mL, with a maximum at 12 hours.[74,75] No complications were attributable to the loading of antimicrobial agents in bone graft. The formulation of antimicrobial-loaded MCB during the 1980s involved simply stirring the antimicrobial powder into a variable amount of MCB at the time of surgery; generally 1 g of vancomycin and 1.2 g of tobramycin were used with 100 to 400 mL of morcellized bone. Excellent infection control and graft incorporation were reported when bone defect reconstruction was done as a second-stage procedure following resection of infected long bones and arthroplasties.[68,76]

Antimicrobial-loaded MCB continues to be used clinically. The opportunity to use antimicrobial-loaded

MCB is widespread, but no mechanism is available to document its use; it does not require commercial products used only for this application, has no directly related complications, and is not documented by specific procedural codes. Anecdotal reports suggest that a wide spectrum of antimicrobial agents has been used, in varying dosages, and that the concept has progressed over time. The use of reamings from allograft femoral heads has been replaced by the use of bone material that is commercially cleaned to remove all cellular marrow material and is ground into particles of specific sizes. The pharmacokinetic data from the initial studies using fresh frozen allograft bone containing all the marrow elements do not establish an appropriate dose to be used with the contemporary bone products. Pharmacokinetic studies must be completed for each new graft material because of the difficulty of predicting release characteristics from the new materials. For some newer materials, including bone particles in glycerin, data are available on the release of hand-mixed antimicrobial agents. Antimicrobial-loaded MCB also is used in impaction grafting; more than 95% control of infection was found 2 years after treatment of infected hip replacements.[56,77] Enhanced loading of gentamicin and flucloxacillin into cortical bone segments using iontophoresis was reported, with supportive serum and wound drain levels.[78] None of 12 patients undergoing second-stage reconstruction had a recurrence of infection; infection occurred in only 2 of 19 patients after a high-risk primary segmental allograft procedure.[78] Covalent bonding of vancomycin to the surface of bone is under investigation as a method of surface protection of the graft material,[22] but this method is not yet clinically available.

Antimicrobial-Loaded Bone Cement

Continuing investigations are likely to define where some of the alternative materials fit into the clinical armamentarium. In the interim, ALBC is the local delivery material of choice, and Septopal (Biomet Europe, Dordrecht, Netherlands) is the clinical standard by which ALBC is measured. Septopal is a commercial formulation of highly porous PMMA beads that release high concentrations of genamicin.[10,33,45,49,79,80] Septopal is used throughout Europe and in other countries but is not available in the United States. The elution of antimicrobial agents from ALBC hand made from different brands of PMMA differs considerably.[10] Palacos (Zimmer, Warsaw, IN) has been associated with the highest elution rates in the past; however, changes in its manufacturing may have significantly decreased elution from its current form.[81]

Low-Dose Versus High-Dose ALBC

ALBC is categorized by dose. One to two grams of antimicrobial powder per batch of bone cement (40 g of polymer powder and approximately 20 mL of monomer liquid) are considered a low dose. Ten or more grams of antimicrobial powder per batch of bone ce-

ment are considered a high dose. The distinction between a low dose and a high dose is based on the extent to which the antimicrobial powder acts as a poragen. As a soluble particulate filler, high-dose antimicrobial powder dissolves when exposed to fluid in the wound. The dissolved antimicrobial agent diffuses from the ALBC, leaving pores that provide access to deeper antimicrobial particles. At low doses, the antimicrobial particles are encased in PMMA, and the deep particles are not accessible for release.

The initial formulations of ALBC contained only 0.5 to 1 g of gentamicin per batch and released only 3% to 7% of the contained gentamicin. Gentamicin release was based primarily on the inherent microporosity of the PMMA rather than the secondary porosity that developed from dissolution of the particulate gentamicin. In a recent clinical pharmacokinetic study of Simplex P with 1 g of tobramycin per batch (Howmedica, Limerick, Ireland), 3% of the tobramycin was excreted in urine at 48 hours.[82] The release of intermediate-dose ALBC (3 to 6 g) is somewhat higher; as much as 12% of the contained antimicrobial agent is released, still primarily from near the surface of the ALBC.[5,6] When enough antimicrobial powder is added, the release behavior changes dramatically. An interconnecting, open-cell porosity develops as the antimicrobial powder elutes from the ALBC, providing a mechanism for antimicrobial agents to be released from deep in the ALBC. With 14 g of antimicrobial powder, fluid penetrates to the center of 7-mm beads within 14 days in vitro.[53,83]

The poragen load at which low-dose ALBC transitions to high dose-ALBC is not clear. Based on pilot in vitro studies and anecdotal clinical experience, the load required to achieve the secondary porosity of high-dose ALBC was estimated to be approximately 10 g of antimicrobial powder or inert particulate poragen per batch of PMMA;[84] however, clinical success using 3 to 5 g of antimicrobial agent per batch of bone cement has been reported.[5,6,36,50,65]

PMMA Permeability

The amount of antimicrobial powder clinically used in hand-mixed ALBC generally is based on the gram dose of the antimicrobial agent, without a good understanding of the determinants that control the release of the antimicrobial agent from ALBC. These determinants include the volume fraction (the percentage of the ALBC volume that is antimicrobial powder), particle shape, particle size, homogeneity of distribution in the PMMA, and drug solubility. Each antimicrobial agent has a different density; therefore, identical gram doses of an antimicrobial agent can have different volume fractions. These variables generally have not been used to determine how clinical preparations are formulated.

Fluid penetration studies confirmed that the permeability of ALBC depends on the volume fraction, and the most uniform fluid penetration occurs when particles are small (100 to 200 μm) and homogeneously distributed in the PMMA.[53] With an inert particulate

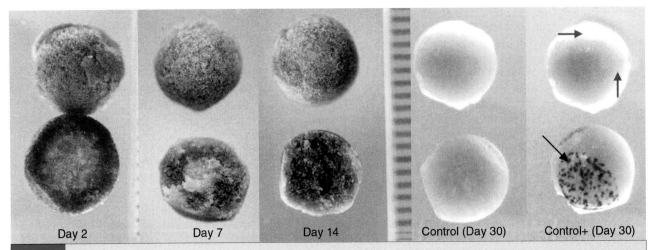

Day 2   Day 7   Day 14   Control (Day 30)   Control+ (Day 30)

Figure 1   PMMA beads (diameter, 7 mm) were loaded with 14 g of xylitol (particle size, 106 µm) as a poragen and 500 mg of phenolphthalein as an indicator. The beads were split after soaking in a sodium hydroxide solution for 2, 7, or 14 days. The external surfaces *(top row)* show porosity resulting from xylitol dissolution. The cut, interior surfaces *(bottom row)* show fluid penetration. A drop of the sodium hydroxide solution on the Control+ bead (containing phenolphthalein but no xylitol) shows that the phenolphthalein locked inside the PMMA *(single black arrow)* is not accessible to surface fluid *(between the two gray arrows)*.

filler, PMMA is minimally permeable at a weight fraction of 1.5% (950 mg per batch). The penetration of fluid is incongruous and limited to approximately 1 mm over 30 days.[83] When the weight fraction is increased to approximately 11% (7.5 g per batch), fluid penetration is more diffuse but still slow, at approximately 2 mm over 30 days. PMMA becomes highly permeable at weight fractions of 19% and 32% (14.1 and 28.5 g per batch, respectively) with penetration of 1 to 2 mm by 2 days and approximately 3 mm by 7 days[83] (Figure 1). Although depth of penetration occurred faster when particles were larger (850 µm), greater volumes of intervening PMMA between the particles were left unpenetrated by fluid.[53] Unfortunately, these data are expressed in weight fraction. To accurately compare poragens of different density and particle morphology, including antimicrobial powders, the data should be expressed in terms of volume fraction.

Further work is needed to determine the optimal particle morphology and volume fraction. Current data suggest, however, that the initial estimate of 10 g of powder to achieve an open-cell porosity is remarkably accurate. Elution studies and reports of postoperative levels in wound drains suggest it is unlikely there is a need to exceed a volume fraction of 20% if a small particle size (approximately 100 µm) is used.[10,36,67,74,80] If inert poragens are not available in the hospital pharmacy, cefazolin powder can be used as an inexpensive, low-toxicity poragen. The particle morphology of cefazolin powder appears to be effective on empiric grounds.

Elution Experiments to Compare Delivery Vehicles
Engineering for drug delivery involves terminology and concepts that are not common to orthopaedics but nonetheless are essential to understanding local antimi-

crobial delivery. Elution experiments, in which drugs are leached out of the delivery material into the surrounding fluid (eluent), are commonly used to characterize the release performance of different drug delivery systems (different drugs in different materials, combined in different ways). Consistent protocols and analyses have not been used in these experiments but would be required to allow reliable comparisons of antimicrobial release from one system to another. It must be emphasized that elution data characterize the release performance of a delivery system in highly controlled laboratory conditions; because of the broad spectrum of in vivo conditions, they do not predict tissue concentrations achieved clinically.

A protocol for an ideal elution experiment illustrates the engineering principles that apply.[85] All of the drug that can possibly be released from the depot is recovered in infinite sink conditions. M_{inf} is the mass of antimicrobial agent recovered in infinite sink conditions after an infinite time of elution (approximated by the total amount of drug recovered up to the point at which no further release can be measured). Infinite sink conditions require that release of the drug from the depot is not resisted by a high concentration of drug in the surrounding eluent. To achieve infinite sink conditions, the eluent must be of a relatively large volume and must maintain a very low concentration of the antimicrobial agent relative to the depot. The concentration gradient between the depot and the eluent is important because antimicrobial release is largely by diffusion, and diffusion is dependent on the concentration gradient (Fick's first law). As diffusion progresses, the drug mass moves from the depot into the eluent, causing a change in the concentration gradient over time (Fick's second law).

In an elution experiment, the concentration of the antimicrobial agent could quickly increase in immediate proximity to the depot (for example, beads), decreasing the concentration gradient and thereby compromising the infinite sink condition. To prevent an increasing concentration near the depot, the eluent must be well mixed, with the eluted antimicrobial agent equally distributed throughout an adequate volume of fluid. Constant agitation is used to achieve a well-mixed fluid state in the eluant. The eluent must be changed before the released drug increases the concentration sufficiently to slow diffusion of the antimicrobial agent from the depot. Well-mixed infinite sink conditions can be achieved using several milliliters of eluent for a 7-mm diameter bead; all of the eluent is removed and replaced with fresh eluent when the antimicrobial concentration in the eluate is high enough to be measured accurately. The antimicrobial concentration in the eluate is assayed, and the cumulative mass of recovered antimicrobial agent at that time (M_T) is calculated.

The mechanism of antimicrobial delivery may be by diffusion, redistribution between partitions, or convection. Delivery from PMMA is mostly by diffusion. Redistribution between partitions can be important if the solubility of the antimicrobial agent in the delivery material is close to its solubility in the eluant, as may be the case for some bioabsorbable materials. At equilibrium, a portion of the antimicrobial agent is in the delivery material partition, and a portion is in the surrounding fluid partition. The solubility of antimicrobial agents is thousands of times less in PMMA than in a fluid such as water, saline, or plasma. PMMA does not absorb or transmit antimicrobial agents well, and partition-based delivery from ALBC therefore is extremely limited. Partition delivery may be more important for alternative materials in which an antimicrobial agent is soluble or for PMMA that has been altered to increase its antimicrobial solubility by, for example, combining it with poly(N-vinyl-2-pyrrolidone).[34] Convection transport of the antimicrobial agent from the delivery material generally is not measured. Convection is bulk fluid flow in response to changes in temperature, transmission of arterial pulse, pressure changes from muscle contraction, and weight bearing. Convection may be more important in the fluid surrounding the depot than in the movement of antimicrobial agents through the pores in the delivery material.

Ultrasonography was reported to significantly enhance the release of gentamicin from Septopal beads but not from commercially prepared low-dose ALBC. This result was attributed to microstreaming through the pores of the Septopal beads, which cannot happen in comparatively nonporous low-dose ALBC.[86] The efficacy of antimicrobial agents from ALBC, however, may be enhanced by applying ultrasonography to the site of low-dose ALBC, thus improving bacterial kill rates in suspension and in biofilm.[87] This technique has not been widely adopted.

Zero-Order, Diffusion-Controlled, and Burst Release
Kinetic release order is determined by the rate at which a drug is released over time.[85,88] Antimicrobial delivery at a constant rate is referred to as zero-order kinetics; M_T is not dependent on the concentration of the antimicrobial agent. Zero-order kinetics occur when antimicrobial agents at the surface of a delivery material are dissolved directly into the surrounding fluid until the surface-exposed antimicrobial agent is depleted.

In a first-order system, the release rate is diffusion controlled; it is dependent on the concentration of the antimicrobial agent and concentration changes with time. Antimicrobial agents generally are released from bone cement following diffusion-controlled kinetics. However, to some extent the release of antimicrobial agents from many alternative materials initially follows zero-order kinetics when dissolution of the antimicrobial agent at the surface of the material occurs directly into the eluant. The zero-order release is likely to be greater for materials with higher permeability, such as collagen sponge, although these materials are still likely to approach diffusion-controlled release with time. An instantaneous release of drug upon exposure to fluid is called burst release; little or no antimicrobial release from ALBC follows initial-burst kinetics.

To reliably compare materials used for local delivery of antimicrobial agents, the elution data should be generated and analyzed following these engineering principles. Unfortunately, it is difficult to make true quantitative comparisons between local delivery systems because the data in the orthopaedic literature generally are not generated in infinite sink conditions and are not expressed in terms of M_T/M_{inf}, diffusion, and partitions.

Mechanical Properties of ALBC
Adding antimicrobial powder to PMMA affects its mechanical properties, and the mechanical properties change over time with elution of the contained antimicrobial agent.[89,90] PMMA had an unacceptable loss in strength when 4.5 g of antimicrobial powder were added; for this reason, the ALBC used for implant fixation should be formulated with less than 4.5 g of antimicrobial powder.[91,92] The volume fraction of the antimicrobial agent in the ALBC probably is the important factor, rather than the gram weight. The volume of powder per gram weight of any specific antimicrobial agent is not readily known, and the material strength of the ALBC that will lead to clinical mechanical failure also is unknown. Therefore, uncertainty exists about the amount of antimicrobial agent that can be added to PMMA without unacceptably compromising its mechanical performance.

The FDA has approved several commercially formulated low-dose ALBCs, containing doses of aminoglycoside ranging from 500 mg to 1 g of active drug. Aminoglycosides vary in potency, with the activity per gram differing as much as 100%. In commercially prepared ALBC, the weight of the aminoglycoside powder

3: Approach to Treatment

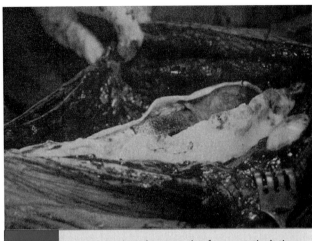

Figure 2 | Intraoperative photograph of a nonarticulating knee spacer fusion showing thin layers of ALBC in the gutters and suprapatellar pouch. (The femur is to the right in this photographic view.)

is adjusted to achieve activity equivalent to the stated weight with 100% potency. The actual mass and volume fraction of the antimicrobial agent in those formulations is not published. It must be assumed that their mechanical performance has been studied and that their compressive strength is above the 70 MPa standard defined by the International Organization for Standardization (ISO 5833: 2002). Caution is necessary when hand mixing similar formulations in the operating room because the activity of the aminoglycoside powder available from the hospital pharmacy may be as low as 0.5; at this level, twice the volume of powder is required to achieve the same activity. Furthermore, some antimicrobial powders are less dense than others. The density of the powder of same drug formulated by different manufacturers can vary as much as 3.5 times, and differences in the volume of powder for the same weight and activity can be important.[37] A 36% loss of mechanical strength was reported for ALBC made with a higher volume powder; the degradation in mechanical strength was attributed to hand mixing, but the higher volume fraction of the powder is more likely to be the cause of the decrease in mechanical strength.[93] When hand-mixed low-dose formulations are used for implant fixation, the volume of the generic antibiotic powder is of considerable importance because the effect on the mechanical properties of the ALBC may be sufficient to compromise the performance of the implant. Definitive data are not available to establish the correct amounts of generic antimicrobial powder to be used in low-dose ALBC.

The antimicrobial loading in high-dose ALBC is sufficient to cause degradation of compressive strength to values considerably below the ISO standard. In clinical use, spacers made with high-dose ALBC have not mechanically failed during periods of 1 to more than 5 years if they are made with adequate metal reinforcing.[68] The temporary use of spacers made with high-

dose ALBC appears to carry an acceptable risk, considering the beneficial effects on wound status and patient functioning provided by mechanical stability from the spacer.

Clinical Applications of ALBC

ALBC in Bulk, Beads, or Chips

The high-dose ALBC used to deliver high concentrations of antimicrobial agents to a resected infection site generally is in bulk or bead form. Antimicrobial delivery is a surface-related phenomenon; therefore, depots with low surface-to-volume ratio could be considered undesirable. A bead is a sphere, which has the lowest possible surface-to-volume ratio. To improve the surface-to-volume ratio, some surgeons use thin layers instead of beads. However, if the ALBC is formulated with sufficient poragen to render it highly porous, the large increase in the internal surface area of the pores overwhelms the inherent limitation of low surface-to-volume ratio for beads or bulk applications. Other considerations may be important when determining the form into which ALBC should be shaped for use. Fabrication of beads requires using a mold, and it can be more challenging than expected for occasional users.[94] Beads usually become entrapped in scar tissue, where they are difficult to identify and retrieve, especially in intramedullary locations. Thin sheets placed between tissue planes or layered in dead spaces are easier to locate and remove. These thin sheets, sometimes called chips, are 1 to 2 mm thick by a couple of centimeters wide and several centimeters long (Figure 2). Smooth rods can be used in intramedullary locations (Figure 3).

Antimicrobial Spacers

High-dose ALBC is used to deliver high concentrations of antimicrobial agents to control residual contamination following resection. The wound usually has dead space that can be managed using beads, sheets, chips, rods, or bulk ALBC. If structurally important bone, such as a diaphyseal segment or a joint, was removed during the resection, mechanical instability will occur, causing tissue shear, extremity instability, and functional limitation. Beads, thin layers, rods, and even bulk filler do not provide mechanical stability. Mechanical stability can be provided when bulk ALBC is molded into a structural shape. The mechanical strength of high-dose ALBC is significantly decreased, but it has sufficient mechanical integrity for shaping around a metal core to form a spacer. The essential feature of a so-called antimicrobial spacer is that it replaces the structural function of the resected bone or joint until a second-stage reconstruction. Although the mechanical considerations vary with the individual resection site, several general principles apply to most sites. All spacers must maintain their primary purpose, which is antimicrobial delivery (Table 2).

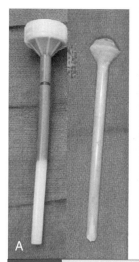
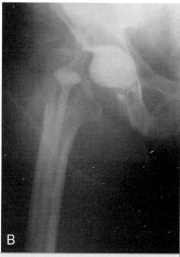

Figure 3 **A,** Photograph of an ALBC intramedullary rod *(right)* made using a cement gun nozzle *(left).* This is a reliable method of making a nonstructural intramedullary ALBC rod. **B,** AP radiograph showing an ALBC rod placed in the intramedullary canal of the proximal femur after removal of an infected arthroplasty. The bulk ALBC in the acetabulum increases local antimicrobial delivery and controls the dead space. (Courtesy of Tad Mabry, MD, Rochester, MN.)

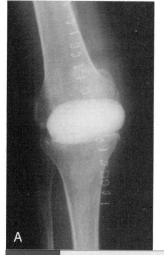
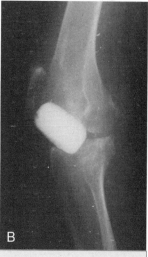

Figure 4 AP **(A)** and lateral **(B)** radiographs showing a hockey puck ALBC spacer placed after removal of an infected total knee replacement. This type of spacer is not acceptable because the absence of constraint in all planes fails the mechanical requirement of a spacer; immediate postoperative bone destruction is seen here. ALBC impingement places the patellar tendon at risk of disruption, and possible dislocation of an unstable disk of ALBC in any direction places all nearby structures at risk **(B).**

Table 2

The Functions of an Antimicrobial Spacer

Deliver high local levels of antimicrobial agents

Fill dead space

Prevent tissue shear

Preserve working space for implants and grafts needed for secondary reconstruction

Maintain tissue length of critical soft tissue, such as collateral ligaments

Maintain limb length

Provide mechanical limb stability

Control postoperative pain

Allow functional rehabilitation for activities of daily living

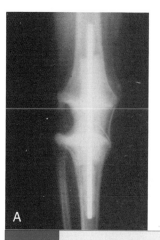
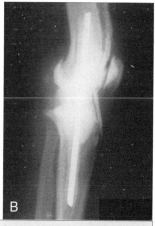

Figure 5 AP **(A)** and lateral **(B)** radiographs of a static ALBC knee spacer reinforced with a Rush rod showing stability at the spacer-bone interface as well as a stable limb and soft-tissue envelope. The soft tissues are out to length, and most of the dead space is filled with ALBC. ALBC in the recesses behind the posterior condyles, in the medial gutter, and in the suprapatellar pouch maintain these tissue planes and also should have been placed in the lateral gutter. This type of static knee spacer is durable and allows early, full weight bearing.

The fabrication of the spacer must ensure stability at the spacer-bone interface. Instability leads to unacceptable bone destruction (**Figure 4**). Intramedullary extensions usually are required for this purpose; they require mechanical reinforcement, often with Rush rods or heavy Kirschner wires that pass into or through the body of the spacer.

The spacer should have sufficient volume and dimensions to maintain the length and shape of the soft tissues. The collateral ligaments should be held at full length, and the volume of missing tissue should be filled to provide working space for the implant and graft material to be used in the reconstruction. Limb stability provides considerable pain control and allows functional rehabilitation, thereby facilitating recovery from both the first-stage resection and the second-stage reconstruction (**Figure 5**).

3: Approach to Treatment

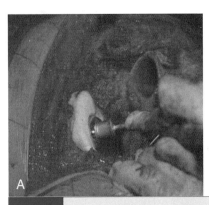
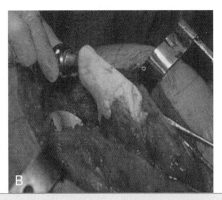
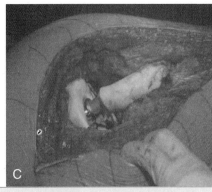

Figure 6 Intraoperative photographs of an articulating ALBC hip spacer. The proximal femur is spanned with a prosthetic component that has the entire stem completely covered with a single batch of ALBC, leaving only the neck and head exposed. **A,** The acetabular spacer is fabricated from a double batch of ALBC in the late-dough phase; the femoral head is used to mold the acetabular articular surface. **B,** ALBC in the late-dough phase is used to grout the stem into place about the proximal end and a few centimeters of the intramedullary region. **C,** The durable final construct allows full weight bearing and sedentary activity.

For hips, the femoral spacer is reinforced with a new, small, low-demand hip stem. Usually the femoral spacer is grouted into place using a separate batch of ALBC placed in the metaphyseal region during the late-dough phase. The acetabular spacer is a mass of high-dose ALBC placed into the acetabular defect during the late-dough phase; the articular surface is molded with the head of the femoral component (**Figure 6**). Antibiotic spacers of the hip using ALBC for both articulating surfaces were first described using the term "high-friction arthroplasty"; an ALBC–tibial intramedullary nail composite was used to span the deficit remaining after resection of the upper half of the femur for infection, in a manner similar to that shown in **Figure 7, A** and **B.** The femoral head was shaped using an acetabular total hip trial, and the acetabulum was shaped using a total hip femoral head trial. The articulation was ALBC on ALBC, and it squeaked audibly with movement. It functioned well with the patient non–weight bearing for 6 weeks until the reconstruction was performed. Other surgeon-directed designs with smaller reinforcement are structurally inadequate. Large-head femoral spacers that do not have an acetabular component (**Figure 7, C**) can function without causing excessive acetabular bone loss; however, they must be properly sized in a congruent acetabular fossa and cannot be used for complex nonspherical defects. The preferable alternative to a large-head femoral spacer, which articulates directly with the acetabular bone, is a stable acetabular spacer to articulate with the femoral spacer (**Figure 6, C** and **Figure 7, D**).

Handmade spacers are completely custom, and therefore all structural issues can be addressed. However, there is an art to fabricating spacers if the structural defect is complex. The use of a femoral component to reinforce a hip femoral spacer has resolved the issue of spacer fracture with weight bearing. Patients are fully functional for sedentary activities, usually without assistive devices, for as long as is needed for the periarticular healing response to completely mature

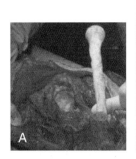
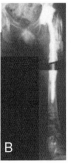
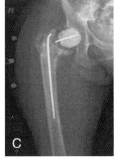
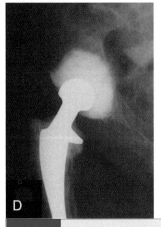
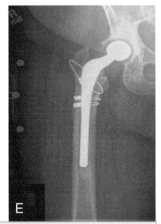

Figure 7 Intraoperative photograph **(A)** and postoperative AP radiograph **(B)** showing an articulating hip spacer from 1990, hand made intraoperatively with ALBC articulating surfaces and a tibial rod to reinforce the femoral stem. **C,** AP radiograph showing a handmade large-head articulating ALBC hip spacer with ALBC articulating directly with acetabular bone. The spacer is fractured because the metal reinforcement is inadequate. **D,** AP radiograph showing a contemporary handmade hip spacer. **E,** AP radiograph showing a PROSTALAC hip spacer. (*C* and *E*, courtesy of M. Spangehl, MD, Scottsdale, AZ.)

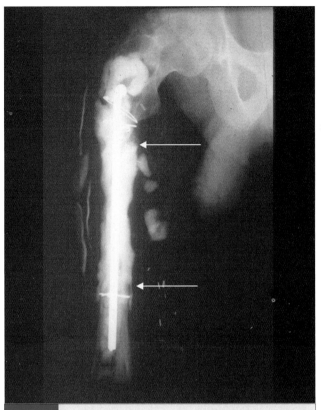

Figure 8 | AP radiograph of a femur showing a static diaphyseal ALBC spacer of the middle three fifths of the diaphysis (*arrows*). The spacer was reinforced using a 0.25-inch Rush rod. Cerclage wires were placed to prevent iatrogenic fracture of the remaining metaphyseal segments. This is a somewhat extreme example of the use of an ALBC spacer to stabilize a large diaphyseal resection site.

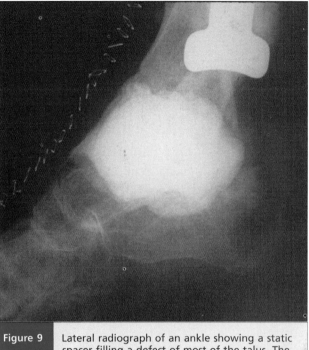

Figure 9 | Lateral radiograph of an ankle showing a static spacer filling a defect of most of the talus. The foot position and adjacent osteopenic bone required the patient to avoid bearing weight until reconstruction.

and all medical issues to be stabilized. A commercial hip spacer system (PROSTALAC, DuPuy, Warsaw, IN) has molds and reinforcing stems for the femur that mechanize the fabrication of the hip spacer stem. A thin ultra-high molecular weight polyethylene acetabular liner is embedded in ALBC for the articulation surface. All of the complexities of the resected wound still must be addressed, and the postoperative care is the same as with the handmade spacer (**Figure 7, E**).

Although first-generation cementing technique is used for fixation, radiolucent zones do not develop about high-dose ALBC spacers, perhaps because there are no bacteria to induce a fibrohistiocytic response. Previously it was considered acceptable to sterilize an infected implant and reuse it for fracture fixation or as the reinforcing core in an arthroplasty spacer. This practice has been abandoned because adherent glycocalyx increases the vulnerability of the surface to repopulation by infecting organisms.

When possible, the spacer should be static to minimize tissue shear and maximize the local host status. Static spacers are effective for long bone resections and

for small joints about the foot, ankle, wrist, or hand, where a temporary absence of motion is acceptable (**Figures 8** and **9**). The stability of an antibiotic spacer is paramount, but determining the structural capabilities of a spacer is somewhat subjective. Significant metal reinforcement is required for long lever arms and heavy limbs (**Figure 10**). The intramedullary extensions should be a couple of bone diameters long in sound bone and well grouted for stability at the spacer-bone interface. Patient compliance is essential. If there is unresolved concern about the durability of the spacer, alternative fixation should be considered.

Static spacers generally are unsuitable for major joints, except for the knee, because of long lever arms and functional demands. Spacers that allow stable movement at the joint, called articulating spacers, are used for the shoulder (**Figure 10**), the elbow (**Figure 11**), the hip (**Figure 6; Figure 7, C** and **D**), and often the knee (**Figure 12**). Articulating spacers of the elbow and shoulder are hand made by shaping the articular surfaces from ALBC and articulating with the opposite matching surface made of ALBC (for the elbow) or bone of the opposing resected glenoid surface (for the shoulder). The expectation is that the spacer will function for sedentary activities until the second-stage reconstruction is performed.

The knee is a special situation. Both a static spacer and an articulating spacer are acceptable. A static spacer for the knee is equivalent to a temporary ALBC fusion (**Figure 5**). The soft-tissue envelope is not subject to shear from movement following resection. Patients function independently, and knee motion reliably

3: Approach to Treatment

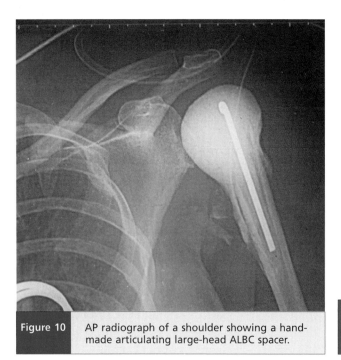

Figure 10 | AP radiograph of a shoulder showing a hand-made articulating large-head ALBC spacer.

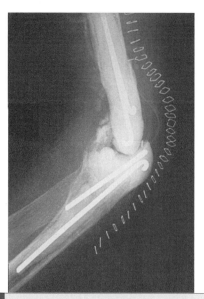

Figure 11 | Lateral radiograph of an elbow showing a hand-made articulating ALBC spacer placed after complete resection.

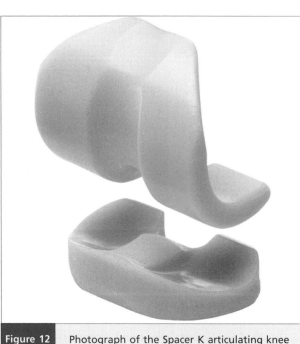

Figure 12 | Photograph of the Spacer K articulating knee spacer for use in a patient without extensive bone loss. (Courtesy of Tecres, Verona, Italy.)

recovers after reconstruction without the need for a quadricepsplasty. The desire of surgeons to attain a functional range of motion before reconstruction has led to the development of articulating spacers for the knee. Articulating knee spacers can be made by hand or with a commercial mold, or commercially prefabricated ALBC components can be used (**Figure 12**). The results of using articulated knee spacers have been excellent.[47,48,66] A novel, custom-made ball-and-socket spacer was reported to have good results.[50]

The choice of a static or articulating spacer for the knee is largely a matter of surgeon preference. The arguments in favor of one or the other often are based on a comparison of well-made spacers of one type with poorly executed spacers of the other type. A static knee spacer may be preferable if the soft-tissue envelope is very tenuous. Placing a knee with an articulating spacer in a brace until the soft tissues heal does not prevent motion. Tissue shear from 10° to 30° of motion in the brace can compromise the local host status and healing response.

Several commercial systems are available to aid in antimicrobial spacer fabrication. They include a hip spacer system consisting of a mold, a reinforcing stem, and a polyethylene acetabular component (PROSTA-LAC); silicone molds for the hip and knee (Stage One Hip and Knee Cement Sparer Molds, Biomet, Warsaw, IN); and prefabricated hip and knee spacers made from gentamicin-loaded bone cement (Spacer G and Spacer K, Tecres, Verona, Italy). The use of prefabricated large-head hip spacers, in which the ALBC surface articulates directly with the acetabulum, has led to concern about acetabular bone erosion; however, the results of more than 10 years' clinical use have not borne out this concern. When the spacer is constructed intraoperatively using a mold, ALBC can be formulated with patient-specific antimicrobial agents. However, high-dose ALBC is too stiff to be formed in the mold, and intermediate-dose ALBC must be used (containing, for example, 3.6 g of tobramycin and 1.5 g of vancomycin per batch of bone cement). Four months following implantation of a PROSTALAC hip spacer using 3.6 g of tobramycin and 1.5 g of vancomycin, the gentamicin level in synovial fluid was measured at concentrations above the break point susceptibility limit.[36]

The advantage of using a commercial system is the ease of successfully fabricating the spacer components. These systems do not simplify the implantation of the spacer components or the management of complex defects.

Implant Fixation With ALBC

When used for implant fixation, ALBC takes the shape of the interval between the implant and the prepared site. The interval typically is a few millimeters thick, with a high surface-to-volume ratio. However, the low-dose ALBC that is used for implant fixation has limited permeability, and most of the contained antimicrobial agent remains entrapped in the PMMA for the lifespan of the fixation. The benefits of using low-dose ALBC for fixation are believed to be short-term protection of the implant, PMMA surfaces, and, possibly, adjacent bone (to a limited extent). The cement-host interface is very narrow, with the ALBC either in direct contact or a few micrometers away in the acute postimplantation wound. The fluid volume in the interface is extremely small, with almost no flow. Although antimicrobial levels have not been directly measured in the cement-bone interface, local levels have the potential to be extremely high. With biointegration, the PMMA surface is separated from the host with a thin fibrous membrane that does not have a fibrohistiocytic component. The levels of antimicrobial agents in a mature interface are unknown, but the synovial fluid levels and levels in connective tissue found after total hip replacements fixed with low-dose ALBC suggest that high levels persist for months.[10,36,65]

Commercially available low-dose ALBC containing 500 mg to 1 g of active aminoglycoside per batch is similar in dosage to the gentamicin-loaded Palacos originally used in 1970.[4] Pharmacokinetic data on patients undergoing total hip replacement with these formulations showed drain levels averaging from 30 to 100 µg/mL; 7% of the gentamicin load was recovered in the drain fluid and urine.[9] In other reports, gentamicin levels in joint fluid were detectable for almost 9 months in patients with a total hip replacement.[36,65]

Data from a 1978 study showed that when 7-mm beads were formulated with approximately 1,350 mg of gentamicin per batch and used to treat osteomyelitis, wound drain levels ranged from 30 to 650 µg/mL on postoperative day 1 and ranged from 5 to 269 µg/mL on postoperative day 4.[9] Measurable tissue and bone levels of gentamicin were recorded at 116 days in a canine model.[9] However, Septopal beads were used in this study, and the results must not be confused with release from beads made from the low-dose ALBC available in the United States. To achieve release performance equivalent to that of Septopal, hand-mixed ALBC must be high dose. The antimicrobial delivery associated with low-dose ALBC is not considered acceptable for treatment of active infection, and it should be used only for prophylaxis or for implant fixation after an infection has been controlled.

Clinical Outcomes Using ALBC for Implant Fixation

Reported infection rates are approximately 2% to 3% lower when low-dose ALBC is used than when it is not used in revision surgery for aseptic loosening of a total hip or knee prosthesis (for example, a decrease from 4% to 2%).[5,6,50] The reported infection rates after second-stage reconstruction following control of an established infection are 10% to 20% lower when ALBC is used than when it is not used.[5,6,50] The outcomes of single-stage treatment of an infected arthroplasty using ALBC were surprisingly similar to those of a two-stage regimen, when meticulous attention was paid to patient selection and surgical technique.[6]

Low-dose ALBC used for prophylaxis in the initial procedure is associated with a 0.5% to 1% decrease in infection; however, the results are not always statistically significant, even in large numbers from national registries. In some studies, ALBC was found to be effective only when used in combination with perioperative antimicrobial agents.[27,34]

Studies of the results of using high-dose ALBC are difficult to analyze because of differing protocols, but the consensus is that established orthopaedic infections should be treated with high antimicrobial levels delivered locally. The long-term control of infection is universally reported to be approximately 90%. Continuing infection was found in 28% of patients when ALBC was not used in a second-stage reimplantation and in 5% of patients when it was used.[5,6,50]

ALBC Beads in Open Fractures

An ALBC bead pouch can be used to manage the dead space in a postdébridement wound following an open fracture. The wound is left open but sealed with an adhesive incision drape to cover the beads and isolate the wound from nosocomial microbes. The ALBC beads elute a high concentration of antimicrobial agents into the wound site. A suction drain is placed into the wound space, and the bead pouch is changed during repeat débridements every 48 to 72 hours until wound closure. In the original description, the beads were made of ALBC using 2 g of tobramycin per batch of Simplex P PMMA. The tobramycin levels in the bead pouch were measured at 7.2 to 258 µg/mL.[95,96] The reported rate of infection rate was 3.7% when a bead pouch was used with débridement and systemic antimicrobial agents, in comparison with 12% when a bead pouch was not used.[95,97] The improvement in outcomes was statistically significant for acute infection following a grade IIIB or IIIC fracture and for late osteomyelitis following a grade II or IIIB fracture.

Following complete débridement of an infected fracture, with or without nonunion and with or without fixation (including fixation with an intramedullary rod), antimicrobial agents can be locally delivered in ALBC beads[46] or in an ALBC rod formed inside a chest tube of a diameter appropriate for the intramedullary canal. For an unstable diaphyseal segment, the ALBC

3: Approach to Treatment

Table 3

Essentials of Local Antimicrobial Treatment

The biology of biofilm-based orthopaedic infections requires delivery of higher antimicrobial levels than can be achieved systemically.

Local delivery is capable of delivering the required antimicrobial levels (at least 100 times the MIC).

Many delivery materials and preparation methods have been investigated. Bone cement, bone graft, and (to a lesser extent) calcium sulfate are the materials currently in clinical use.

Pharmacokinetic and pharmacodynamic performance is important. Pharmacokinetic data are acquired through elution studies that require standardized protocols and sound engineering principles to allow comparison of one system with another. Pharmacodynamic data to guide the concentration and duration of release are largely extrapolated from data related to planktonic organisms. The data acquired directly from biofilm-specific investigations are limited.

Drug release is by diffusion from deep inside the delivery material, and material permeability (porosity) therefore is important.

ALBC porosity is achieved by adding a poragen.

Surface-bonded systems can protect the material or implant surface but are not yet in clinical use.

Drug-release systems deliver antimicrobial agents to the wound fluid and adjacent tissues at levels above those required to treat biofilm-based bacteria.

Local delivery desensitizes a patient with an allergy to the antimicrobial agent.

ALBC is used in beads, rods, and thin layers for soft-tissue and dead space management and in bulk form for structural spacers.

Local delivery of antimicrobial agents improves clinical outcomes by 1% to 3% when used for prophylaxis and 10% to 20% when used for treatment of an infection.

Bacteria present at revision surgery after ALBC was used are likely to be resistant to the antimicrobial agent used in the ALBC.

rod must be formed over a large Rush rod or a solid titanium nail to provide structural integrity and prevent rod fracture.[98] To avoid sticking during fabrication, the ALBC-rod composite can be rolled on the backing from an incision drape in the dough phase of polymerization or formed with metal reinforcing inside the chest tube used to make the ALBC rod.

Local Delivery Pumps

External pumps and implantable osmotic pumps have been used for local delivery of antimicrobial agents through a catheter tunneled subcutaneously to the infection site. Distribution of the antimicrobial agent depends on wound fluid flow and diffusion into the postresection hematoma. The possible concerns include bacterial adherence to the catheter and altered antimicrobial distribution with hematoma organization and wound healing. An implantable pump requires removal, usually during the second-stage reconstruction. Despite good results, pumps have not gained clinical acceptance. Long-term control of infection was achieved in 11 of 14 patients (79%) with an implanted pump[99] and in 8 of 9 patients (89%) with an external pump.[100]

Antimicrobial Drains

Wound drains are frequently used following orthopaedic procedures. Commensal organisms in the dermis can colonize the drain catheter at the exit site, however, and over time the developing biofilm can extend progressively more deeply. Recent data show that 21% of orthopaedic drains are colonized 2 to 4 cm deep to the skin when they are removed 1 to 3 days after surgery.[101] If the resection is under a thin soft-tissue envelope, a drain is important to prevent a tense collection of postoperative fluid and blood, but there is a risk that microbes will advance along a drain catheter to the surgical site. Clinical concern about retrograde infections along drains has led to inappropriate continuance of prophylactic antimicrobial agents until drain removal. Probably it is preferable to deliver antimicrobial agents locally at the drain catheter surface. The technology is not yet available for surgical drains, but effective minocycline- and rifampin-coated intravenous catheters are in clinical use, as are chlorhexidine- and silver sulfadiazine–impregnated urinary catheters.[17] Surgical drains made with antimicrobial-impregnated materials should be available soon.

Summary

Important aspects of local antimicrobial treatment are summarized in Table 3. The extreme antimicrobial concentrations necessary to kill bacteria in biofilm are clinically achievable by local delivery, but there is a risk of misapplication if the principles are not thoroughly understood. It is not possible to treat established infections with local antimicrobial delivery alone, and orthopaedic infections should never be treated with local antimicrobial delivery instead of complete surgical resection. Local delivery is intended to control residual bacteria in the wound space and protect the exposed surfaces from bacteria that can reestablish biofilm. Any formulation, fabrication, or implantation process that does not optimize delivery of the antimicrobial agent from its vehicle is of secondary importance or counterproductive.

Locally delivered antimicrobial concentrations cannot be assumed to extend more than a few millimeters beyond the local wound space, and local antimicrobial delivery does not treat remote disease. The prudent use of perioperative systemic antimicrobial agents is an important independent variable in clinical outcome.

Many drugs, dosages, delivery materials, and clinical applications have been studied. Extensive treatment regimen and outcomes reports not only support the use of locally delivered antimicrobial agents but also reveal the need for more data on release performance and clinical outcomes.

Annotated References

1. Wainwright M: Moulds in folk medicine. *Folklore* 1989;100:162-166.

2. Broughton G II, Janis JE, Attinger CE: A brief history of wound care. *Plast Reconstr Surg* 2006;117:6S-11S.

   The history of wound care is reviewed.

3. Becker RO, Spadaro JA: Treatment of orthopaedic infections with electrically generated silver ions: A preliminary report. *J Bone Joint Surg Am* 1978;60:871-881.

4. Buchholz HW, Engelbrecht H: Uber Die Depotwirkung Einiger Antibiotica Bei Vermischung mit dem Kunstharz Palacos. *Chirurg* 1970;41:511-515.

5. Hanssen AD: Local antibiotic delivery vehicles in the treatment of musculoskeletal infection. *Clin Orthop Relat Res* 2005;437:91-96.

   Local antibiotic delivery vehicles are discussed, including materials to deliver extremely high levels of local antibiotics without systemic toxicity. The gold standard is ALBC. Some biodegradable alternate materials also promote bone regeneration. Local toxicity to bone healing is dose dependent.

6. Joseph TN, Chen AL, Di Cesare PE: Use of antibiotic-impregnated cement in total joint arthroplasty. *J Am Acad Orthop Surg* 2003;11:38-47.

   This comprehensive review of ALBC, from antimicrobial agents and PMMA to associated in vitro and in vivo data and clinical applications, includes outcomes data associated with ALBC use. The consensus is that ALBC improves outcomes of orthopaedic infections.

7. Klemm K: The use of antibiotic-containing bead chains in the treatment of chronic bone infections. *Clin Microbiol Infect* 2001;7:28-31.

8. Klemm KW: Antibiotic bead chains. *Clin Orthop Relat Res* 1993;295:63-76.

9. Wahlig H, Dingeldein E, Bergmann R, Reuss K: The release of gentamicin from polymethylmethacrylate beads: An experimental and pharmacokinetic study. *J Bone Joint Surg Br* 1978;60:270-275.

10. Wahlig H, Dingeldein E: Antibiotics and bone cements: Experimental and clinical long-term observations. *Acta Orthop Scand* 1980;51:49-56.

11. McLaren AC: Alternative materials to acrylic bone cement for delivery of depot antibiotics in orthopaedic infections. *Clin Orthop Relat Res* 2004;427:101-106.

    Alternatives to PMMA for antimicrobial delivery are under investigation. The stimulus is the desire to avoid second surgeries for ALBC removal. None of these protein-based, bone or bone graft substitute, or polymer materials are FDA approved for antimicrobial delivery. The clinical application of bone and calcium sulfate is described.

12. Hoad-Reddick DA, Evans CR, Norman P, Stockley I: Is there a role for extended antibiotic therapy in a two-stage revision of the infected knee arthroplasty? *J Bone Joint Surg Br* 2005;87:171-174.

    A retrospective case series evaluated the use of prolonged systemic antimicrobial therapy to manage infected total knee arthroplasties. The results were satisfactory when only short-duration postoperative systemic antimicrobial agents were used.

13. Chuard C, Vaudaux P, Waldvogel FA, Lew DP: Susceptibility of staphylococcus aureus growing on fibronectin-coated surfaces to bactericidal antibiotics. *Antimicrob Agents Chemother* 1993;37:625-632.

14. Stewart PS, Costerton JW: Antibiotic resistance of bacteria in biofilms. *Lancet* 2001;358:135-138.

15. Nelson CL, Hickmon SG, Skinner RA: Treatment of experimental osteomyelitis by surgical debridement and the implantation of bioerodable, polyanhydride-gentamicin beads. *J Orthop Res* 1997;15:249-255.

16. Parvizi J, Antoci V Jr, Hickok NJ, Shapiro IM: Selfprotective smart orthopedic implants. *Expert Rev Med Devices* 2007;4:55-64.

    This is a review of the emerging technology in which antimicrobial agents are bound to the surface of biomaterials to protect the surface from bacterial adherence and prevent infection.

17. Rupp ME, Lisco SJ, Lipsett PA, et al: Effect of a second-generation venous catheter impregnated with chlorhexidine and silver sulfadiazine on central catheter-related infections: A randomized, controlled trial. *Ann Intern Med* 2005;143:570-580.

    A multicenter, randomized, controlled trial examined the clinical tolerance and efficacy of second-generation, antiseptic-coated central venous catheters.

18. Justinger C, Moussavian MR, Schlueter C, Koppa B, Kollmar O, Schilling MK: Antibiotic coating of abdominal closure sutures and wound infection. *Surgery* 2009; 145:330-334.

    A lower infection rate was found in abdominal incision closures with triclosan-coated polyglactin 910 sutures, compared with sutures having no antimicrobial coating.

19. Haverich A, Hirt S, Karck M, Siclari F, Wahlig H: Prevention of graft infection by bonding of gentamycin to Dacron prostheses. *J Vasc Surg* 1992;15:187-193.

3: Approach to Treatment

20. Lawson MC, Bowman CN, Anseth KS: Vancomycin derivative photopolymerized to titanium kills S. epidermidis. *Clin Orthop Relat Res* 2007;461:96-105.

A laboratory study reported the bactericidal surface protection of vancomycin–poly(ethylene glycol) covalently bonded to the surface of titanium alloy using photopolymerization.

21. Antoci V Jr, King SB, Jose B, et al: Vancomycin covalently bonded to titanium alloy prevents bacterial colonization. *J Orthop Res* 2007;25:858-866.

A laboratory study found that vancomycin can be bound to a titanium alloy surface and prevent colonization by *S aureus*.

22. Ketonis C, Aiyer A, Adams CS, Shapiro IM, Hickok NJ, Parvizi J: Abstract: Bone graft modification with antibiotics confers protection from bacteria. *18th Open Scientific Annual Meeting*. Rochester, MN, Musculoskeletal Infection Society, 2008. http://www.msis-na.org/id242.htm. Accessed April 20, 2009.

In a laboratory study, vancomycin was covalently bonded to morcellized human bone, leading to decreased colonization on exposure to *S aureus* without altering the surface appearance or biocompatibility of the bone.

23. Neut D, van de Belt H, van Horn JR, van der Mei HC, Busscher HJ: Residual gentamicin-release from antibiotic-loaded polymethylmethacrylate beads after 5 years of implantation. *Biomaterials* 2003;24:1829-1831.

This case report of ALBC retrieved after 5 years in situ found continued gentamicin release and the presence of gentamicin-resistant bacteria.

24. Thomes B, Murray P, Bouchier-Hayes D: Development of resistant strains of Staphylococcus epidermidis on gentamicin-loaded bone cement in vivo. *J Bone Joint Surg Br* 2002;84:758-760.

25. Czock D, Keller F: Mechanism-based pharmacokinetic-pharmacodynamic modeling of antimicrobial drug effects. *J Pharmacokinet Pharmacodyn* 2007;34:727-751.

A common mathematical model is proposed as the basis for antimicrobial pharmacokinetics-pharmacodynamics.

26. Mouton JW, Vinks AA: Pharmacokinetic/pharmacodynamic modeling of antibacterials in vitro and in vivo using bacterial growth and kill kinetics: The minimum inhibitory concentration versus stationary concentration. *Clin Pharmacokinet* 2005;44:201-210.

A laboratory study compared the time-kill curves for three antimicrobial agents against *Pseudomonas*, relating the MIC to the stationary concentration from concentration-dependent and independent antimicrobial agents.

27. Amorena B, Gracia E, Monzoin M: Antibiotic susceptibility assay for staphylococcus aureus in biofilms developed in vitro. *J Antimicrob Chemother* 1999;44:43-55.

28. Anwar H, Strap JL, Costerton JW: Establishment of aging biofilms: Possible mechanism of bacterial resistance to antimicrobial therapy. *Antimicrob Agents Chemother* 1992;36:1347-1351.

29. Tam VH, Kabbara S, Vo G, Schilling AN, Coyle EA: Comparative pharmacodynamics of gentamicin against Staphylococcus aureus and Pseudomonas aeruginosa. *Antimicrob Agents Chemother* 2006;50:2626-2631.

A laboratory study found limited concentration-dependent killing of *S aureus* and strong concentration-dependent killing of *Pseudomonas* by gentamicin.

30. Roberts JA, Kruger P, Paterson DL, Lipman J: Antibiotic resistance: What's dosing got to do with it? *Crit Care Med* 2008;36:2433-2440.

This is a review of the literature on antibiotic resistance related to antibiotic dosing, with a discussion of the clinical application of the findings.

31. Schafer JA, Hovde LB, Rotschafer JC: Consistent rates of kill of Staphylococcus aureus by gentamicin over a 6-fold clinical concentration range in an in vitro pharmacodynamic model (IVPDM). *J Antimicrob Chemother* 2006;58:108-111.

An in vitro pharmacodynamics study found that gentamicin killing of planktonic *S aureus* does not increase with concentrations above 5 mg/L.

32. Bertazzoni Minelli E, Benini A, Magnan B, Bartolozzi P: Release of gentamicin and vancomycin from temporary human hip spacers in two-stage revision of infected arthroplasty. *J Antimicrob Chemother* 2004;53:329-334.

A laboratory study measured the elution of antimicrobial agents from industrially manufactured hip spacers following explantation.

33. Evans RP, Nelson CL: Gentamicin-impregnated polymethylmethacrylate beads compared with systemic antibiotic therapy in the treatment of chronic osteomyelitis. *Clin Orthop Relat Res* 1993;295:37-42.

34. Frutos P, Diez-Peña E, Frutos G, Barrales-Rienda JM: Release of gentamicin sulphate from a modified commercial bone cement: Effect of (2-hydroxyethyl methacrylate) comonomer and poly(N-vinyl-2-pyrrolidone) additive on release mechanism and kinetics. *Biomaterials* 2002;23:3787-3797.

35. Goodell JA, Flick AB, Hebert JC, Howe JG: Preparation and release characteristics of tobramycin impregnated polymethylmethacrylate beads. *Am J Hosp Pharm* 1986;43:1454-1460.

36. Masri BA, Duncan CP, Beauchamp CP: Long-term elution of antibiotics from bone-cement: An in vivo study using the prosthesis of antibiotic-loaded acrylic cement (PROSTALAC) system. *J Arthroplasty* 1998;13:331-338.

37. McLaren RL, McLaren AC, Vernon BL: Generic tobramycin elutes from bone cement faster than proprietary tobramycin. *Clin Orthop Relat Res* 2008;466:1372-1376.

A laboratory study measured the release of proprietary and generic tobramycin from bone cement, finding a greater release using the generic tobramycin, which had a greater volume of powder per gram of drug.

38. Murray WR: Use of antibiotic-containing bone cement. *Clin Orthop Relat Res* 1984;190:89-95.

39. Nelson CL, Griffin FM, Harrison BH, Cooper RE: In vitro elution characteristics of commercially and noncommercially prepared antibiotic PMMA beads. *Clin Orthop Relat Res* 1992;284:303-309.

40. Seligson D, Popham GJ, Voos K, Henry SL, Paguri M: Antibiotic leaching from polymethylmethacrylate beads. *J Bone Joint Surg Am* 1993;75:714-720.

41. Von Frauhofer JA, Polk HC Jr, Seligson D: Leaching of tobramycin from PMMA bone cement beads. *J Biomed Mater Res* 1985;19:751-756.

42. Walenkamp GHIM: *Gentamicin-PMMA Beads: A Clinical, Pharmacokinetic and Toxicological Study.* Darmstadt, Germany, Merck, 1983.

43. Adams K, Couch L, Cierny G, Calhoun J, Mader JT: In vitro and in vivo evaluation of antibiotic diffusion from antibiotic-impregnated polymethylmethacrylate beads. *Clin Orthop Relat Res* 1992;278:244-252.

44. Walenkamp GH, Vree TB, van Rens TJ: Gentamicin-PMMA beads: Pharmacokinetic and nephrotoxicological study. *Clin Orthop Relat Res* 1986;205:171-183.

45. Blaha JD, Calhoun JH, Nelson CL, et al: Comparison of the clinical efficacy and tolerance of gentamicin PMMA beads on surgical wire versus combined and systemic therapy for osteomyelitis. *Clin Orthop Relat Res* 1993;295:8-12.

46. Calhoun JH, Henry SL, Anger DM, Cobos JA, Mader JT: The treatment of infected nonunions with gentamicin-polymethylmethacrylate antibiotic beads. *Clin Orthop Relat Res* 1993;295:23-27.

47. Fehring TK, Odum S, Calton TF, Mason JB: Articulating versus static spacers in revision total knee arthroplasty for sepsis. *Clin Orthop Relat Res* 2000;380:9-16.

48. Hofmann AA, Kane KR, Tkack TK, Plaster RL, Camargo MP: Treatment of infected total knee arthroplasty using an articulating spacer. *Clin Orthop Relat Res* 1995;321:45-54.

49. Nelson CL, Evans RP, Blaha JD, Calhoun J, Henry SL, Patzakis MJ: A comparison of gentamicin-impregnated polymethylmethacrylate bead implantation to conventional parenteral antibiotic therapy in infected total hip and knee arthroplasty. *Clin Orthop Relat Res* 1993;295:96-101.

50. Cui Q, Mihalko WM, Shields JS, Ries M, Saleh KJ: Antibiotic-impregnated cement spacers for the treatment of infection associated with total hip or knee arthroplasty. *J Bone Joint Surg Am* 2007;89:871-882.

This current concepts review covers the classification of total joint arthroplasty infections and two-stage revision for late chronic infection. An articulating or static spacer is chosen based on the amount of bone loss, condition of the soft tissues, need for joint motion, availability of prefabricated spacers or molds, and antibiotic selection.

51. Bruce AS, Kerry RM, Norman P, Stockley I: Fluconazole-impregnated beads in the management of fungal infection of prosthetic joints. *J Bone Joint Surg Br* 2001;83:183-184.

52. Goss B, Lutton C, Weinrauch P, Jabur M, Gillett G, Crawford R: Elution and mechanical properties of antifungal bone cement. *J Arthroplasty* 2007;22:902-908.

A laboratory study found increased compressive strength of the bone cement but no release of amphotericin when 200 mg of amphotericin was mixed into bone cement.

53. McLaren AC, McLaren SG, McLemore R, Vernon BL: Particle size of fillers affects permeability of polymethylmethacrylate. *Clin Orthop Relat Res* 2007;461:64-67.

This is a report of a laboratory study of the effect of particle size on permeability of bone cement loaded with a soluble particulate poragen.

54. Seldes RM, Winiarsky R, Jordan LC, et al: Liquid gentamicin in bone cement: A laboratory study of a potentially more cost-effective cement spacer. *J Bone Joint Surg Am* 2005;87:268-272.

An elution study on gentamicin-loaded bone cement using liquid gentamicin found a 49% loss of compressive strength and eluent levels averaging 26.4 µg/mL during the first 24 hours.

55. Hsieh PH, Tai CL, Lee PC, Chang YH: Liquid gentamicin and vancomycin in bone cement: A potentially more cost-effective regimen. *J Arthroplasty* 2009;24:125-130.

This is a report of a laboratory study of the elution and mechanical strength of ALBC made with combinations of liquid gentamicin and powdered vancomycin.

56. Dovas S, Liakopoulos V, Papatheodorou L: Acute renal failure after antibiotic-impregnated bone cement treatment of an infected total knee arthroplasty. *Clin Nephrol* 2008;69:207-212.

Renal toxicity associated with gentamicin-loaded bone cement was reported in two patients.

57. Patrick BN, Rivey MP, Allington DR: Acute renal failure associated with vancomycin and tobramycin laden cement in total hip arthroplasty. *Ann Pharmacother* 2006;40:2037-2042.

Two patients developed acute renal failure associated with the use of tobramycin-loaded bone cement.

58. Castells M: Desensitization for drug allergy. *Curr Opin Allergy Clin Immunol* 2006;6:476-481.

3: Approach to Treatment

The current state of knowledge related to desensitization for drug allergies is described in an expert narrative review.

59. Tidwell BH, Cleary JD, Lorenz KR: Antimicrobial desensitization: A review of published protocols. *Hosp Pharm* 1997;32:1362-1369.

60. Richter-Hintz D, Rieker J, Rauch L, Homey B: Sensitivity to constituents of bone cement in a patient with joint prosthesis. *Hautarzt* 2004;55:987-989.

    This case report describes a patient with delayed hypersensitivity to PMMA, which required removal of the PMMA and conversion to an implant that did not use PMMA for fixation.

61. Edin ML, Miclau T, Lester GE, Lindsey RW, Dahners LE: Effect of cefazolin and vancomycin on osteoblasts in vitro. *Clin Orthop Relat Res* 1996;333: 245-251.

62. Isefuku S, Joyner CJ, Simpson AH: Gentamicin may have an adverse effect on osteogenesis. *J Orthop Trauma* 2003;17:212-216.

    This is a report of a cell culture study of the inhibition of osteoblast metabolism, thymidine incorporation, and total DNA when cells were cultured in concentrations of gentamicin greater than 100 µg/mL.

63. Miclau T, Edin ML, Lester GE, Lindsey RW, Dahners LE: Bone toxicity of locally applied aminoglycosides. *J Orthop Trauma* 1995;9:401-406.

64. Nelson CL, McLaren AC, McLaren SG, Johnson JW, Smeltzer MS: Is aseptic loosening truly aseptic? *Clin Orthop Relat Res* 2005;437:25-30.

    A narrative expert discussion of the evidence suggests that bacteria may play a role in the loosening process in at least some loose arthroplasties.

65. Kostamo T, Biring GS, Masri BA, Garbuz DS, Duncan CP: Abstract: Two-stage hip revision for infection. A 10-15 year follow-up in 103 patients. *75th Annual Meeting Proceedings*. Rosemont, IL, American Academy of Orthopaedic Surgeons, 2008, p 391.

    This is an observational report of the results from treating infected hip arthroplasties with PROSTALAC.

66. Evans RP: Successful treatment of total hip and knee infection with articulating antibiotic components: A modified treatment method. *Clin Orthop Relat Res* 2004; 427:37-46.

    This observational retrospective review reports the results of a single surgeon's experience with articulating spacers used in two-stage management of prosthetic joint infections.

67. McLaren AC, Spooner CE: Abstract: Antibiotic levels in drain fluid following antibiotic spacer insertion. *64th Annual Meeting Proceedings*. Rosemont, IL: American Academy of Orthopaedic Surgeons, 1997, p 199.

68. McLaren AC, Spooner CE: Abstract: Antibiotic spacer arthroplasty in the staged treatment of infected total joint replacements. *63rd Annual Meeting Proceedings*. Rosemont, IL: American Academy of Orthopaedic Surgeons, 1996, p 181.

69. Orhan Z, Cevher E, Mulazimoglu L, et al: The preparation of ciprofloxacin hydrochloride-loaded chitosan and pectin microspheres: Their evaluation in an animal osteomyelitis model. *J Bone Joint Surg Br* 2006;88: 270-275.

    A laboratory study investigated the release of ciprofloxacin from chitosan and pectin microspheres, reporting a slower release from the chitosan microspheres.

70. Laurencin CT, Gerhart T, Witschger P, et al: Bioerodible polyanhydrides for antibiotic drug delivery: In vivo osteomyelitis treatment in a rat model system. *J Orthop Res* 1993;11:256-262.

71. Turner TM, Urban RM, Gitelis S, Kuo KN, Andersson GB: Radiographic and histologic assessment of calcium sulfate in experimental animal models and clinical use as a resorbable bone-graft substitute, a bone-graft expander, and a method for local antibiotic delivery: One institution's experience. *J Bone Joint Surg Am* 2001;83(suppl 2):8-18.

72. Winkler H, Janata O, Berger C, Wein W, Georgopoulos A: In vitro release of vancomycin and tobramycin from impregnated human and bovine bone grafts. *J Antimicrob Chemother* 2000;46:423-428.

73. McLaren AC, Miniaci A: In vivo study to determine the efficacy of cancellous bone graft as a delivery vehicle for antibiotics. *Transactions of the Twelfth Annual Meeting*. Mt. Laurel, NJ, Society for Biomaterials, 1986, p 102.

74. McLaren AC: Antibiotic impregnated bone graft: Post-op levels of vancomycin and tobramycin. *J Orthop Trauma* 1989;3:171.

75. Witso E: Antibiotic impregnated bone grafts: What do we know? in Meani E, Romanò C, Crosby L, Hofmann G, Calonego G (eds): *Infection and Local Treatment in Orthopedic Surgery*. Berlin, Germany, Springer, 2007, pp 154-159.

    This narrative expert opinion about the local treatment of orthopaedic infections includes a discussion of antibiotic-loaded MCB.

76. McLaren AC: Abstract: Antibiotic bone graft for reconstruction following established bone infection. *Annual Meeting Proceedings*. Westmount, QC, Canadian Orthopaedic Research Society, 1990, p 47.

77. Buttaro M, Comba F, Piccaluga F: Vancomycin-supplemented cancellous bone allografts in hip revision surgery. *Clin Orthop Relat Res* 2007;461:74-80.

    A laboratory study and clinical observational case series reported the incorporation of graft, elution of vancomycin, and control of infection associated with vancomycin-supplemented cancellous bone allografts.

78. Khoo PPC, Michalak KA, Yates PJ, Megson SM, Day RE, Wood DJ: Iontophoresis of antibiotics into segmental allografts. *J Bone Joint Surg Br* 2006;88:1149-1157.

This observational review of 31 patients undergoing massive allograft reconstruction reported the infection rate associated with a novel iontophoresis method used to load the allograft with antimicrobial agents.

79. Patzakis MJ, Mazur K, Wilkins J, Sherman R, Holtom P: Septopal beads and autogenous bone grafting for bone defects in patients with chronic osteomyelitis. *Clin Orthop Relat Res* 1993;295:112-118.

80. McLaren AC, Nelson CL, McLaren SG, DeClerk GR: The effect of glycine filler on the elution of gentamicin from acrylic bone cement. *Clin Orthop Relat Res* 2004;427:25-27.

This is a report of a laboratory study of the use of glycine as a soluble particulate filler to increase the release of antimicrobial agents from hand-mixed ALBC.

81. Bridgens J, Davies S, Tilley L, Norman P, Stockley I: Orthopaedic bone cement: Do we know what we are using? *J Bone Joint Surg Br* 2008;90:643-647.

A laboratory study found a decrease in antibiotic elution of the current formulation of Palacos bone cement, compared with the old formulation.

82. Sterling GJ, Crawford S, Potter JH, Koerbin G, Crawford R: The pharmacokinetics of Simplex-tobramycin bone cement. *J Bone Joint Surg Br* 2003;85:646-649.

The serum, urine, and wound drain levels of tobramycin in patients undergoing total hip replacement using low-dose ALBC were reported.

83. McLaren AC, Nelson CL, McLaren SG, Wassell DL: Phenolphthalein used to assess permeability of antibiotic-laden polymethylmethacrylate: A pilot study. *Clin Orthop Relat Res* 2005;439:48-51.

This laboratory study reports the effect on permeability of adding soluble particulate fillers loaded in bone cement using a novel method with phenolphthalein.

84. Cierny G III: Chronic osteomyelitis: Results of treatment. *Instr Course Lect* 1990;39:495-508.

85. Kydonieus A: *Treatise on Controlled Drug Delivery.* New York, NY, Marcel Dekker, 1991.

86. Ensing GT, Hendriks J, Jongsma JE, van Horn JR, van der Mei HC, Busscher HJ: The influence of ultrasound on the release of gentamicin from antibiotic-loaded acrylic beads and bone cements. *J Biomed Mater Res* 2005;75:1-5.

An in vitro laboratory study found enhanced release of gentamicin and increased porosity following release from Septopal beads but not from commercially prepared low-dose ALBC using ultrasonography.

87. Ensing GT, Neut D, van Horn JR, van der Mei HC, Busscher HJ: The combination of ultrasound with antibiotics released from bone cement decreases the viability of planktonic and biofilm bacteria: An in vitro study with clinical strains. *J Antimicrob Chemother* 2006;58:1287-1290.

A laboratory study found greater bacterial kill in suspension and in biofilm when pulsed ultrasonography was used with ALBC.

88. Naraharisetti PK, Guan Lee HC, Fu YC, Lee DJ, Wang CH: In vitro and in vivo release of gentamicin from biodegradable disks. *J Biomed Mater Res B Appl Biomater* 2006;77:329-337.

An in vitro, in vivo, and computer modeling study measured gentamicin release from biodegradable polylactic-polyglycolic copolymers.

89. Göğüş A, Akman S, Göksan SB, Bozdağ E: Mechanical strength of antibiotic-impregnated bone cement on day 0 and day 15: A biomechanical study with surgical Simplex P and teicoplanin. *Acta Orthop Traumatol Turc* 2002;36:63-71.

90. Lewis G, Bhattaram A: Influence of a pre-blended antibiotic (gentamicin sulfate powder) on various mechanical, thermal, and physical properties of three acrylic bone cements. *J Biomater Appl* 2006;20:377-408.

A laboratory study found no meaningful change in multiple physical properties of three different bone cements when low-dose gentamicin was added.

91. Gambhir AK, Hanson B, Wroblewski BM, Kay PR: The mechanical properties of modern additional antibiotics in acrylic bone cement. *J Bone Joint Surg Br* 2002;84 (suppl 2):152-153.

92. Lautenschlager EP, Jacobs JJ, Marshall GW, Meyer PR Jr: Mechanical properties of bone cements containing large doses of antibiotic powders. *J Biomed Mater Res* 1976;10:929-938.

93. DeLuise M, Scott CP: Addition of hand-blended generic tobramycin in bone cement: Effect on mechanical strength. *Orthopedics* 2004;27:1289-1291.

A laboratory comparison of the mechanical strength of commercially premixed and hand-mixed tobramycin-loaded bone cement found a 36% decrease in the mechanical strength of the hand-mixed ALBC but did not take into account the volume fraction of the generic tobramycin formulation.

94. Cunningham A, Demarest G, Rosen P, DeCoster TA: Antibiotic bead production. *Iowa Orthop J* 2000;20:31-35.

95. Henry SL, Ostermann PAW, Seligson D: The antibiotic bead pouch technique: The management of severe compound fractures. *Clin Orthop Relat Res* 1993;295:54-62.

96. Henry SL, Ostermann PA, Seligson D: The prophylactic use of antibiotic impregnated beads in open fractures. *J Trauma* 1990;30:1231-1238.

97. Seligson D, Mehta S, Voos K, Henry SL, Johnson JR: The use of antibiotic-impregnated polymethylmethacrylate beads to prevent the evolution of localized infection. *J Orthop Trauma* 1992;6:401-406.

98. Ohtsuka H, Yokoyama K, Higashi K, et al: Use of antibiotic-impregnated bone cement nail to treat septic nonunion after open tibial fracture. *J Trauma* 2002;52: 364-366.

99. Perry CR, Rice S, Ritterbusch JK, Burdge RE: Local administration of antibiotics with an implantable osmotic pump. *Clin Orthop Relat Res* 1985;192:284-290.

100. Meani E, Romanõ C: Treatment of osteomyelitis by local antibiotics using a portable electronic micropump. *Rev Chir Orthop Reparatrice Appar Mot* 1994;80: 285-290.

101. Schneiderbauer MM: Abstract: Surgical drains. A potential risk for infection in orthopaedic patients. *18th Open Scientific Annual Meeting.* Rochester, MN, Musculoskeletal Infection Society, 2008. http://www. msis-na.org/id256.htm. Accessed April 20, 2009.

    In a case series, bacterial colonization of orthopaedic wound drains with coagulase-negative *Staphylococcus* was found in 7 of 33 drains 4 cm deep to the skin.

Systemic Antimicrobial Treatment

Camelia E. Marculescu, MD, MSCR   Douglas R. Osmon, MD, MPH

Introduction

Success in treating a musculoskeletal infection often requires both an optimal surgical approach and optimally targeted antimicrobial therapy. The type of infection, the virulence and antimicrobial susceptibilities of the involved microorganism, the adverse effects of the proposed antimicrobial therapy, alternative antimicrobial therapies, and the patient's general health should be considered before a musculoskeletal infection is treated. Many musculoskeletal infections require prolonged systemic antimicrobial therapy, often administered on an outpatient basis under the guidance of an infectious disease specialist in close collaboration with an orthopaedic surgeon.

Selection of Antimicrobial Therapy

An infectious disease specialist can advise the orthopaedic surgeon as to the necessary initial culturing of a musculoskeletal infection and can arrange for specialized culturing, obtain details of any earlier microbiologic culturing as well as earlier medical or surgical treatment, and select the optimal type and dosage of antimicrobial therapy. To ensure an adequate growth of microorganisms for culturing, empiric antimicrobial therapy usually should be withheld for at least 10 to 14 days before surgical débridement of a chronic infection.[1] However, a blood or aspirated tissue specimen should be obtained immediately if hemodynamic instability or soft-tissue infection is suspected, and empiric antimicrobial therapy should be initiated regardless of other considerations. The most efficacious antimicrobial agent can be chosen after determining the microorganism causing the infection as well as the results of any in vitro susceptibility tests, available clinical data or experience supporting the use of the agent for treating the particular infection, and the clinical status of the patient (including comorbidities, antimicrobial allergies or intolerances, and renal and hepatic function).[2] Table 1 lists intravenous antimicrobial drugs commonly used for outpatient treatment. If possible, a patient being treated on an outpatient basis should receive an agent that requires relatively infrequent administration.

Antimicrobial Agents

Methicillin-Susceptible Staphylococcal Infection

Nafcillin or cefazolin is the drug of choice for the treatment of a methicillin-susceptible staphylococcal musculoskeletal infection. Cefazolin can be used, for example, if the patient does not have concomitant infectious endocarditis or central nervous system infection; it should be used at a higher dosage in a patient who weighs more than 80 kg.[3] The reliability of cephalosporin therapy in treating a significant methicillin-susceptible *Staphylococcus aureus* (MSSA) infection continues to be controversial. The failure of cefazolin therapy in certain MSSA infections may be attributable to type A β-lactamase production by the infected strain. However, cefazolin therapy led to a favorable outcome, despite the presence of type A β-lactamase in MSSA-infected prosthetic joint isolates, when used with a two-stage exchange and an antimicrobial-impregnated spacer.[4] Nafcillin has been successfully used with an electronic ambulatory infusion pump.[5,6] Vancomycin can be used for a patient with a severe type I β-lactam allergy manifested as laryngeal edema, immediate

Table 1

Intravenous Antimicrobial Drugs Commonly Used for Outpatient Treatment of Musculoskeletal Infection

Drug Class	Drug
β-lactam–β-lactamase inhibitor combination	Piperacillin-tazobactam
Carbapenems	Glycopeptide
	Meropenem
	Vancomycin
Cephalosporins	Cefazolin
	Cefepime
	Ceftriaxone
Penicillins	Penicillin G

(Adapted with permission from Osmon DR, Berbari EF: Outpatient intravenous antimicrobial therapy for the practicing orthopaedic surgeon. *Clin Orthop Relat Res* 2002;403:80-86.)

3: Approach to Treatment

urticaria, or bronchospasm. It may be helpful to use penicillin skin testing to determine whether the patient has a true penicillin allergy.[7] Vancomycin is inferior to nafcillin or cefazolin for treating methicillin-susceptible staphylococci, and it should be the first choice for such an infection only if an adverse effect or severe allergic reaction precludes the use of other agents.[2]

A combination of a quinolone and rifampin can be used to treat an implant-associated staphylococcal infection. Rifampin has bactericidal activity against slow-growing, surface-adhering, biofilm-producing microorganisms. Its activity against staphylococci has been tested in in vitro animal models and clinical studies.[8-10] After initial treatment with intravenous flucloxacillin or vancomycin (in lieu of ciprofloxacin), 33 patients with staphylococcal infection of a stable prosthesis or internal fixation device were randomly assigned to 3 to 6 months of oral treatment with ciprofloxacin or ciprofloxacin plus rifampin. All 12 patients treated with the ciprofloxacin-rifampin regimen and 7 of the 12 who did not receive rifampin (58%) were cured without removal of the device.[11,12] The use of rifampin is limited by gastrointestinal and other adverse effects as well as its potential for interaction with other drugs. Rifampin should not be used as the sole antimicrobial agent because doing so often leads to the emergence of resistance. To minimize the development of resistance, it is recommended that rifampin be started after surgery when the results of susceptibility testing are known, surgical drains are removed, and adequate trough levels of vancomycin are obtained.

Methicillin-Resistant Staphylococcal Infection

The treatment of methicillin-resistant *S aureus* (MRSA) is challenging. Recent data suggest that prosthetic joint infections caused by MRSA may have worse outcomes than those caused by MSSA.[13] Although vancomycin is the traditional drug of choice to treat MSRA infection, the clinical success rate is low and inversely correlated with vancomycin minimum inhibitory concentration (MIC).[14] In the treatment of MRSA bacteremia, a significant risk of vancomycin treatment failure begins to emerge with an increase in vancomycin MIC that is well within the susceptible range. For example, vancomycin successfully treated MRSA isolates having a vancomycin MIC of less than 0.5 µg/mL in 55.6% of patients with bacteremia; in contrast, vancomycin was effective in only 9.5% of patients if the vancomycin MIC for MRSA was 1 to 2 µg/mL.[15] The implications of increasing vancomycin MIC for the treatment of musculoskeletal infection is not yet known. In addition, renal insufficiency is a significant risk factor for vancomycin failure.[14]

The alternatives to vancomycin for treating an MRSA infection include linezolid, daptomycin, teicoplanin, trimethoprim-sulfamethoxazole, quinupristin-dalfopristin, and tigecycline. However, no other drug has been proved superior to vancomycin in therapeutic effect. Although linezolid is promising for use in treating staphylococcal osteomyelitis,[16-18] long-term administration may be inadvisable because of adverse effects including bone marrow suppression and neuropathy.[18] Daptomycin, a cyclic lipopeptide antibiotic, was found to be rapidly bactericidal in vitro against a broad spectrum of gram-positive bacteria, including MRSA; studies using a rabbit or rat model of osteomyelitis achieved an encouraging level of MSRA eradication from infected bone.[18] The clinical data conflict as to the usefulness of daptomycin for bone or joint infection,[19,20] and evaluation of its usefulness in prosthetic joint infection is under way. Tigecycline, a tetracycline-like bacteriostatic antibiotic, reaches a higher concentration in infected bone than in uninfected bone. The results of experimental studies of tigecycline in MRSA osteomyelitis have been promising.[21] Tigecycline and daptomycin have not yet been approved by the US Food and Drug Administration for the treatment of bone and joint infection.

Streptococcal and Enterococcal Infection

The use of cephalosporins such as cefazolin or ceftriaxone is recommended for outpatient treatment of musculoskeletal infection caused by a β-hemolytic streptococcus. These agents accommodate the need for relatively infrequent outpatient administration and are as efficacious as intermittently or continuously infused penicillin G.[2] The recommended drugs for the treatment of enterococcal infection are listed in Table 2. Cephalosporins are not active against enterococci, and quinolones do not reliably cover enterococci. In the absence of concomitant endocarditis or complicated enterococcal bacteremia, aminoglycosides should not be routinely used for outpatient treatment of enterococcal musculoskeletal infection because less toxic alternative drugs are available. In addition, data are lacking to support the adjunctive use of aminoglycosides; these agents are frequently administered for local treatment of musculoskeletal infection via antibiotic-impregnated polymethylmethacrylate cement.[22]

Infection Caused by Gram-Negative Microorganisms

Gram-negative microorganisms often are isolated from a nosocomial infection. The antimicrobial agents recommended for treating *Pseudomonas* and *Enterobacter* species are listed in Table 2. Depending on the susceptibility pattern of the offending microorganism, the treatment regimen for infections caused by Enterobacteriaceae includes ceftriaxone as a first-line treatment and ciprofloxacin or another quinolone as a second choice.[23] In an animal model, quinolones impaired fracture healing, and they should be avoided in patients with an infected nonunion.[24] A cumulative analysis of the bacteriologic efficacy of ciprofloxacin against 301 microorganisms found success rates of 92% and 72% against infections caused by Enterobacteriaceae or *P aeruginosa*, respectively. Osteomyelitis caused by *P aeruginosa* or *S aureus* was associated with a four-

Table 2

Suggested Antimicrobial Therapy for the Treatment of Selected Microorganisms in Adults

Microorganism	Preferred Agent (Dosage*)	Alternative Agent (Dosage*)
Oxacillin-susceptible *Staphylococcus* species	Nafcillin sodium (1.5-2 g IV q 4 h) *or* Cefazolin (1-2 g IV q 8 h)	Vancomycin (15 mg/kg IV q 12 h) *or* Levofloxacin (500–750 mg PO or IV q 24 h) *or* Levofloxacin + rifampin (300–450 mg PO q 12 h)[†]
Oxacillin-resistant *Staphylococcus* species	Vancomycin (15 mg/kg IV q 12 h)	Linezolid (600 mg PO or IV q 12 h) *or* Levofloxacin (500–750 mg PO or IV q 24 h) *or* Levofloxacin + rifampin (300–450 mg PO q 12 h)[†]
Penicillin-susceptible *Enterococcus* species[‡]	Aqueous crystalline penicillin G (20-24 million units IV q 24 h continuously or in 6 divided doses) *or* Ampicillin sodium (12 g IV q 24 h continuously or in 6 divided doses)	Vancomycin (15 mg/kg IV q 12 h)
Penicillin-resistant *Enterococcus* species[‡]	Vancomycin (15 mg/kg IV q 12 h)	Linezolid (600 mg PO or IV q 12 h)
Pseudomonas aeruginosa[§]	Cefepime (1-2 g IV q 12 h) *or* Meropenem (1 g IV q 8 h) *or* Imipenem (500 mg IV q 6-8 h)	Ciprofloxacin (750 mg PO or 400 mg IV q 12 h) *or* Ceftazidime (2 g IV q 8 h)
Enterobacter species	Meropenem (1 g IV q 8 h) *or* Imipenem (500 mg IV q 6-8 h)	Cefepime (1-2 g IV q 12 h) *or* Ciprofloxacin (750 mg PO or 400 mg IV q 12 h)
β-hemolytic streptococci	Aqueous crystalline penicillin G (20-24 million units IV q 24 h continuously or in 6 divided doses) *or* Ceftriaxone (1-2 g IV q 24 h)	Vancomycin (15 mg/kg IV q12 h)
Propionibacterium acnes *Corynebacterium* species	Aqueous crystalline penicillin G (20-24 million units IV q 24 h continuously or in 6 divided doses) *or* Ceftriaxone (1-2 g IV q 24 h) *or* Vancomycin (15 mg/kg IV q 12 h)	Clindamycin (600-900 mg IV q 8 h)

h = hour, IV = intravenous, PO = by mouth, q = every.
*Must be adjusted for a patient with renal impairment.
[†]For a patient treated with débridement and prosthesis retention.
[‡]Considerations in choice of agent are similar to those for enterococcal endocarditis; optional addition of an aminoglycoside for bactericidal synergy.
[§]Optional addition of an aminoglycoside for bactericidal synergy.
(Adapted with permission from Sia IG, Berbari EF, Karchmer AW: Prosthetic joint infections. *Infect Dis Clin North Am* 2005;19:885-914.)

fold increase in the failure rate compared with osteomyelitis caused by other pathogens (odds ratio, 3.85; confidence interval, 95% [1.97-7.5]; $P < 0.001$).[25]

Polymicrobial Infection

Polymicrobial infections often are encountered in an open fracture or contiguous-focus osteomyelitis, with or without vascular compromise. Although *S aureus* is the most commonly isolated pathogen, coagulase-negative staphylococci, streptococci, enterococci, gram-negative bacilli, and anaerobes also are frequently isolated.[26] The factors to be considered in choosing an empiric treatment are the severity of the infection and the microorganism most likely to cause such an infection. For a patient with a severe infection, a broad-spectrum antimicrobial regimen is chosen that includes agents active against staphylococci (including MRSA), streptococci, and gram-negative bacilli. The useful regimens

Table 3

Antimicrobial Agents With Excellent Oral Bioavailability Commonly Used for Patients With a Musculoskeletal Infection

Azoles
  Fluconazole
  Itraconazole
  Voriconazole
Linezolid
Metronidazole
Quinolones
  Ciprofloxacin
  Levofloxacin
  Moxifloxacin
Rifampin
Trimethoprim-sulfamethoxazole

(Adapted with permission from Osmon DR, Berbari EF: Outpatient intravenous antimicrobial therapy for the practicing orthopaedic surgeon. *Clin Orthop Relat Res* 2002;403:80-86.)

include ampicillin and sulbactam, piperacillin and tazobactam, and a carbapenem and an antimicrobial agent with MRSA activity. A gangrenous or foul-smelling wound is treated with antianaerobic agents. If cultures and susceptibility testing are available, the regimen can be narrowed to cover the offending microorganism.

Candida Infection

Candida musculoskeletal infection, including risk factors, epidemiology, and treatment, is discussed in chapter 18.

Other Considerations in Antimicrobial Therapy

Oral Administration

Oral and parenteral routes of antibiotic administration are equally efficacious, provided that adequate serum and bone concentrations can be achieved. Oral administration can be used for a drug that has excellent bioavailability, as long as the microorganism is susceptible

Table 4

Suggested Route of Administration and Duration of Systemic Antimicrobial Therapy for Selected Musculoskeletal Infections

Infection	Route	Duration
Septic arthritis	Parenteral	2-4 weeks May include a period of stepdown oral therapy
Osteomyelitis	Parenteral	4-6 weeks May include a period of stepdown oral therapy
Bone or joint infection in patient with diabetes mellitus		
Postsurgical, with no residual infected tissue (such as postamputation)	Parenteral or oral	2-5 days
Postsurgical, with residual infected soft tissue but no infected bone	Parenteral or oral	2-4 weeks
Postsurgical, with residual infected but viable tissue	Initially parenteral	4-6 weeks Oral therapy may be considered after initial parenteral course.
Postsurgical, with residual dead bone	Initially parenteral	3 months Oral therapy may be considered after initial parenteral course.
No surgery performed	Initially parenteral	3 months Oral therapy may be considered after initial parenteral course.
Prosthetic joint infection		
Positive intraoperative cultures	Initially parenteral	4-6 weeks Chronic oral suppressive therapy may be added.
Infection within 1 month of arthroplasty or acute late infection treated with débridement and prosthesis retention	Initially parenteral	2-6 weeks (rifampin) Chronic oral suppressive therapy may be added.
Infection later than 1 month after arthroplasty, treated with resection and delayed reimplantation	Parenteral	4-6 weeks

Table 5		

Adverse Effects of Antimicrobial Therapy

Drug	Adverse Effects	Cautions
β-lactams	Antibiotic-associated diarrhea Pseudomembranous colitis Genital moniliasis Hepatic dysfunction	
Fluconazole	Hepatotoxicity Prolongation of QT interval	Propensity for drug-drug interaction.
Fluoroquinolones	Phototoxicity Tendon rupture Arrhythmia (very rare) Disturbance in blood glucose level (possible) Lower seizure threshold (possible)	Should not be taken with antacids.
Linezolid	Myelosuppression Peripheral and optic neuropathy	Tyramine-containing food should be avoided. May interact with adrenergic or serotonergic agents.
Metronidazole	Peripheral neuropathy Ataxia Disulfiram-like reaction	Concurrent use with oral anticoagulant can increase risk of bleeding.
Minocycline	Photosensitivity Skin discoloration Permanent tooth discoloration in young children Drug-induced lupus Dizziness, light-headedness, vertigo Pseudotumor cerebri (rare)	Should not be taken with antacids or iron-containing preparations. Concurrent use with oral anticoagulant can increase risk of bleeding. Decreases effectiveness of contraceptive drugs.
Rifampin	Orange discoloration of body secretions Hepatotoxicity	Propensity for drug-drug interaction. Requires increased dosage of anticoagulant drugs. May decrease effectiveness of contraceptive drugs.
Trimethoprim-sulfamethoxazole	Myelosuppression Elevated creatinine level Nephrotoxicity Crystalluria Disulfiram-like reaction (possible)	May enhance hypoglycemic effect of sulfonylureas.

(Adapted with permission from Sia IG, Berbari EF, Karchmer AW: Prosthetic joint infections. *Infect Dis Clin North Am* 2005;19:885-914.)

to the agent, the patient has a functional gastrointestinal tract, no known drug-drug interaction will decrease the drug's efficacy, the patient is willing to comply with the regimen, and the drug's use for the specific indication is supported by clinical data or experience. These oral agents are listed in Table 3.

Duration
Table 4 lists the suggested duration of systemic antimicrobial therapy for specific types of musculoskeletal infections.[22,27-33]

Adverse Effects and Monitoring
The most important adverse effects of the antimicrobial drugs commonly used for the treatment of musculoskeletal infection are listed in Table 5. It is important to inform patients of the signs and symptoms of drug toxicity, and patients should be instructed to inform the physician if a possible complication occurs. The common complications include rash, nausea, vomiting, and diarrhea; ototoxicity (from vancomycin use) is less common.[2] Hematologic, renal, dermatologic, and some other adverse effects tend to occur approximately 1 month after antimicrobial therapy begins.[34] Vancomycin or a β-lactam antimicrobial agent was found to be the most common cause of leukopenia. Nephrotoxicity occurred in 8% of 269 patients and was most commonly associated with amphotericin B.[34] Recent increases in the failure rate of vancomycin as used for eliminating MRSA strains with high MIC led to a recommendation that the vancomycin target trough be increased to between 15 and 20 μg/mL. However, higher vancomycin troughs are associated with an increase in nephrotoxicity. In a recent prospective cohort study of 95 patients with an MRSA infection, nephrotoxicity occurred in 12% of those with a high vancomycin trough (15 μg/mL or higher).[35] In accordance with the

3: Approach to Treatment

Infectious Diseases Society of America guideline, patients undergoing intravenous antimicrobial therapy should be evaluated weekly for complete blood count and differential as well as serum electrolyte and serum creatinine levels.[36] Liver function tests should be done weekly for a patient receiving ceftriaxone, nafcillin, oxacillin, or a carbapenem, and creatine phosphokinase testing should be done weekly for a patient receiving daptomycin. A high-risk patient or a patient requiring an aminoglycoside or amphotericin B may require more frequent or additional laboratory monitoring.

Chronic Oral Antimicrobial Suppression

Recommendations for chronic oral antimicrobial suppression are based on expert opinion and small cohort studies rather than randomized clinical trials.[37-40] Indefinite long-term suppressive therapy can be used to treat some patients with a prosthetic joint infection or an implant-associated early postsurgical spinal infection[41] and is used for many patients after successful débridement with prosthesis retention.[38,39,42,43] Long-term suppressive therapy may be appropriate if prosthesis removal is anticipated to lead to a poor functional result or if the prosthesis is well fixed and difficult to remove.[1] In addition, long-term suppressive therapy is useful if surgery is not feasible because the patient is in poor health or refuses to undergo an additional surgical procedure. The goal of long-term suppression is not to cure the infection but rather to relieve its symptoms, maintain a functional joint, and prevent the systemic spread of infection. The prerequisites for a successful outcome include the presence of an infection caused by a highly susceptible microorganism, an absence of systemic infection, the availability of highly bioavailable oral antimicrobial drugs for the microorganism, patient compliance and tolerance of the regimen, the acceptability of any drug-drug interaction, and the presence of a well-fixed and functional prosthesis. When these criteria were met, the success of chronic oral antimicrobial suppression was found to range from 23% to 86%, depending on study design, patient selection, the microorganism, surgical therapy, and the definitions of success and failure.[37-40,42] The ideal regimen and optimal duration of chronic oral antimicrobial suppression therapy have not yet been established.

Summary

Successfully treating a musculoskeletal infection requires both the best surgical technique and targeted antimicrobial therapy. Intraoperative culture specimens, obtained whenever possible in the absence of antimicrobial therapy, are crucial for identifying and appropriately treating the offending microorganism. The physician should consider the virulence and antimicrobial susceptibilities of the pathogen as well as possible drug interactions and the patient's overall health, projected longevity, and comorbid conditions. The treatment must be individualized for the patient and the infection. Close collaboration between the orthopaedic surgeon and the infectious disease specialist is required to achieve an optimal outcome.

Annotated References

1. Sia IG, Berbari EF, Karchmer AW: Prosthetic joint infections. *Infect Dis Clin North Am* 2005;19:885-914.

    Treatment of an infected orthopaedic prosthesis must be individualized. The best surgical technique is determined by the type of infection, condition of the bone stock and soft tissue, virulence and antimicrobial susceptibility of the pathogen, general health and projected longevity of the patient, and experience of the surgeon. Long-term oral antimicrobial suppression is an alternative to surgery for maintaining a functioning prosthesis.

2. Osmon DR, Berbari EF: Outpatient intravenous antimicrobial therapy for the practicing orthopaedic surgeon. *Clin Orthop Relat Res* 2002;403:80-86.

3. Weed HG: Antimicrobial prophylaxis in the surgical patient. *Med Clin North Am* 2003;87:59-75.

    The prophylactic use of antimicrobial agents requires balancing potential benefits against risks. In the absence of randomized, controlled trials or detailed, patient-specific information for precisely estimating the balance, general guidelines can help the clinician choose the best treatment.

4. Shuford JA, Piper KE, Hein M, Trampuz A, Steckelberg JM, Patel R: Lack of association of Staphylococcus aureus type A beta-lactamase with cefazolin combined with antimicrobial spacer placement prosthetic joint infection treatment failure. *Diagn Microbiol Infect Dis* 2006;54:189-192.

    The prevalence of β-lactamase gene types among 23 MSSA isolates associated with prosthetic joint infection treated with cefazolin was determined using polymerase chain reaction, and clinical and microbiologic outcomes were assessed. In all eight patients with type A β-lactamase–producing *S aureus* who underwent reimplantation, the prosthesis was in place at a median 798-day follow-up.

5. Gilbert DN, Dworkin RJ, Raber SR, Leggett JE: Outpatient parenteral antimicrobial-drug therapy. *N Engl J Med* 1997;337:829-838.

6. Mortlock NJ, Schleis T: Outpatient parenteral antimicrobial therapy technology. *Infect Dis Clin North Am* 1998;12:861-878.

7. Marculescu CE, Osmon DR: Antibiotic prophylaxis in orthopedic prosthetic surgery. *Infect Dis Clin North Am* 2005;19:931-946.

    Antimicrobial prophylaxis remains the most effective method of reducing the likelihood of infection after total joint arthroplasty. Postsurgical prophylaxis can protect the prosthetic joint against hematogenous seeding from oral, urologic, skin, or gastrointestinal sources. Dental and urologic advisory statements recommend antimicrobial prophylaxis for high-risk patients undergoing a high-risk procedure after total joint arthroplasty.

8. Chuard C, Herrmann M, Vaudaux P, Waldvogel FA, Lew DP: Successful therapy of experimental chronic foreign-body infection due to methicillin-resistant Staphylococcus aureus by antimicrobial combinations. *Antimicrob Agents Chemother* 1991;35:2611-2616.

9. Chuard C, Vaudaux P, Waldvogel FA, Lew DP: Susceptibility of Staphylococcus aureus growing on fibronectin-coated surfaces to bactericidal antibiotics. *Antimicrob Agents Chemother* 1993;37:625-632.

10. Zimmerli W, Trampuz A, Ochsner PE: Prosthetic-joint infections. *N Engl J Med* 2004;351:1645-1654.

    The current concepts of diagnosis and treatment of prosthetic joint infection are described.

11. Zimmerli W, Widmer AF, Blatter M, Frei R, Ochsner PE: Role of rifampin for treatment of orthopedic implant-related staphylococcal infections: A randomized controlled trial. Foreign-Body Infection (FBI) Study Group. *JAMA* 1998;279:1537-1541.

12. Zavasky DM, Sande MA: Reconsideration of rifampin: A unique drug for a unique infection. *JAMA* 1998;279:1575-1577.

13. Salgado CD, Dash S, Cantey JR, Marculescu CE: Higher risk of failure of methicillin-resistant Staphylococcus aureus prosthetic joint infections. *Clin Orthop Relat Res* 2007;461:48-53.

    In a retrospective cohort study, the presence of MRSA was an independent risk factor for failure in the treatment of prosthetic joint infection, compared with the presence of MSSA.

14. Moise-Broder PA, Sakoulas G, Eliopoulos GM, Schentag JJ, Forrest A, Moellering RC Jr: Accessory gene regulator group II polymorphism in methicillin-resistant Staphylococcus aureus is predictive of failure of vancomycin therapy. *Clin Infect Dis* 2004;38:1700-1705.

    In 87 patients treated with vancomycin, 122 MRSA isolates were evaluated. Of 36 clinically evaluable patients with accessory gene regulator group II polymorphism, 31 failed to respond to vancomycin. This finding suggests that glycopeptide-intermediately resistant *S aureus* and hetero–glycopeptide-intermediately resistant *S aureus* clinical isolates are enriched for the accessory gene regulator group II polymorphism. An intrinsic survival advantage may exist for some *S aureus* clones with this genetic marker under vancomycin-selective pressure.

15. Sakoulas G, Moise-Broder PA, Schentag J, Forrest A, Moellering RC Jr, Eliopoulos GM: Relationship of MIC and bactericidal activity to efficacy of vancomycin for treatment of methicillin-resistant Staphylococcus aureus bacteremia. *J Clin Microbiol* 2004;42:2398-2402.

Elucidating the mechanisms involved in intermediate-level glycopeptide resistance in *S aureus* begins by examining bacteria that show changes in vancomycin susceptibility before the development of obvious resistance. Prognostic information on vancomycin treatment outcome in MRSA bacteremia also can be obtained by testing the in vitro bactericidal potency of vancomycin.

16. Rao N, Ziran BH, Hall RA, Santa ER: Successful treatment of chronic bone and joint infections with oral linezolid. *Clin Orthop Relat Res* 2004;427:67-71.

    Oral linezolid was found to produce long-term remission in a prospective study of 11 consecutive adult patients (9 with osteomyelitis, 2 with prosthetic joint infection). All patients had remission at a mean 27-month follow-up.

17. Rayner CR, Baddour LM, Birmingham MC, Norden C, Meagher AK, Schentag JJ: Linezolid in the treatment of osteomyelitis: Results of compassionate use experience. *Infection* 2004;32:8-14.

    Oral or intravenous linezolid was successful in treating patients with osteomyelitis caused by a resistant gram-positive organism and patients who did not tolerate or respond to other treatments.

18. Razonable RR, Osmon DR, Steckelberg JM: Linezolid therapy for orthopedic infections. *Mayo Clin Proc* 2004;79:1137-1144.

    Oral linezolid may be an effective therapy for orthopaedic infection caused by linezolid-susceptible gram-positive bacteria in patients who do not tolerate or respond to other treatments.

19. Finney MS, Crank CW, Segreti J: Use of daptomycin to treat drug-resistant gram-positive bone and joint infections. *Curr Med Res Opin* 2005;21:1923-1926.

    Eight of nine patients were successfully treated for a gram-positive bone or joint infection by using daptomycin for at least 8 days. Daptomycin was well tolerated for as long as 44 days.

20. Rao N, Regalla DM: Uncertain efficacy of daptomycin for prosthetic joint infections: A prospective case series. *Clin Orthop Relat Res* 2006;451:34-37.

    The efficacy of daptomycin (4 mg/kg/day) is uncertain in patients with prosthetic joint infection, especially if hardware is retained. Further study is needed to explain the failure of in vitro data to predict clinical success or to determine any benefit from higher dosages. Level of evidence: IV.

21. Yin L-Y, Lazzarini L, Li F, Stevens CM, Calhoun JH: Comparative evaluation of tigecycline and vancomycin, with and without rifampicin, in the treatment of methicillin-resistant Staphylococcus aureus experimental osteomyelitis in a rabbit model. *J Antimicrob Chemother* 2005;55:995-1002.

    Tigecycline may be an effective alternative to vancomycin for the treatment of MRSA osteomyelitis.

22. Steckelberg JM, Osmon DR: Prosthetic joint infections, in Bisno AL, Waldvogel FA (eds): *Infections of Indwelling Prosthetic Devices*. Washington, DC, American Society for Microbiology, 2000, pp 173-209.

3: Approach to Treatment

23. Berbari EF, Osmon DR, Steckelberg JM: Osteomyelitis and infectious arthritis, in Baddour LM, Gorbach SL (eds): *Therapy of Infectious Diseases*. Philadelphia, PA, Elsevier, 2003, pp 331-342.

24. Huddleston PM, Steckelberg JM, Hanssen AD, Rouse MS, Bolander ME, Patel R: Ciprofloxacin inhibition of experimental fracture healing. *J Bone Joint Surg Am* 2000;82:161-173.

25. Lew DP, Waldvogel FA: Quinolones and osteomyelitis: State-of-the-art. *Drugs* 1995;49(suppl 2):100-111.

26. Mader JT, Calhoun JC, Lazzarini L: Adult long bone osteomyelitis, in Calhoun JS, Mader JT (eds): *Musculoskeletal Infections*. New York, NY, Marcel Dekker, 2003, pp 149-177.

27. Calhoun JH, Manring MM: Adult osteomyelitis. *Infect Dis Clin North Am* 2005;19:765-786.

   Adult osteomyelitis is difficult to treat and carries considerable morbidity and cost. The treatment includes culture-directed antibiotic therapy and surgical débridement. The clinician and patient must understand the goals of treatment and potential difficulties.

28. Goldenberg DL: Septic arthritis. *Lancet* 1998;351: 197-202.

29. Haas DW, McAndrew MP: Bacterial osteomyelitis in adults: Evolving considerations in diagnosis and treatment. *Am J Med* 1996;101:550-561.

30. Lew DP, Waldvogel FA: Osteomyelitis. *N Engl J Med* 1997;336:999-1007.

31. Lipski BA, Berendt AR, Deery HG, et al: Diagnosis and treatment of diabetic foot infections. *Plast Reconstr Surg* 2006;117:212-238.

   This review article addresses common problems and pitfalls in the diagnosis and treatment of diabetic foot infection.

32. Mader JT, Shirtliff ME, Bergquist SC, Calhoun J: Antimicrobial treatment of chronic osteomyelitis. *Clin Orthop Relat Res* 1999;360:47-65.

33. Ross JJ: Septic arthritis. *Infect Dis Clin North Am* 2005;19:799-817.

   The US incidence of septic arthritis is increasing, especially among older patients with a chronic illness, who are more susceptible to drug-resistant organisms. Successful treatment requires a high diagnostic suspicion, empiric antibiotic treatment, and joint drainage. Inoculation into blood culture bottles is more successful for a bacteriologic diagnosis than plating on solid media.

34. Hoffman-Terry ML, Fraimow HS, Fox TR, Swift BG, Wolf JE: Adverse effects of outpatient parenteral antibiotic therapy. *Am J Med* 1999;106:44-49.

35. Hidayat LK, Hsu DI, Quist R, Shriner KA, Wong-Beringer A: High-dose vancomycin therapy for methicillin-resistant Staphylococcus aureus infections: Efficacy and toxicity. *Arch Intern Med* 2006;166:2138-2144.

   The prevalence of clinical MRSA strains with an elevated vancomycin MIC (2 µg/mL) requires that aggressive empirical vancomycin dosing be used to achieve a trough greater than 15 µg/mL. Combination or alternative therapy should be considered for an invasive infection caused by these strains.

36. Tice AD, Rehm SJ, Dalovisio JR, et al: Practice guidelines for outpatient parenteral antimicrobial therapy: IDSA guidelines. *Clin Infect Dis* 2004;38:1651-1672.

   The current guidelines of the Infectious Diseases Society of America are provided.

37. Brandt CM, Sistrunk WW, Duffy MC, et al: Staphylococcus aureus prosthetic joint infection treated with debridement and prosthesis retention. *Clin Infect Dis* 1997;24:914-919.

38. Rao N, Crossett LS, Sinha RK, Le Frock JL: Long-term suppression of infection in total joint arthroplasty. *Clin Orthop Relat Res* 2003;414:55-60.

   At a mean 5-year follow-up, 86.2% of patients treated with long-term suppressive antibiotic therapy for prosthetic joint infection had a functioning prosthesis. The success rate for S aureus infection was 69%. Age, joint location, symptom duration, or time of infection onset did not predict outcome.

39. Segreti J, Nelson JA, Trenholme GM: Prolonged suppressive antibiotic therapy for infected orthopedic prostheses. *Clin Infect Dis* 1998;27:711-713.

40. Tsukayama DT, Wicklund B, Gustilo RB: Suppressive antibiotic therapy in chronic prosthetic joint infections. *Orthopedics* 1991;14:841-844.

41. Kowalski TJ, Berbari EF, Huddleston PM, Steckelberg JM, Mandrekar JN, Osmon DR: The management and outcome of spinal implant infections: Contemporary retrospective cohort study. *Clin Infect Dis* 2007;44: 913-920.

   Early-onset spinal implant infections were successfully treated using débridement, implant retention, and parenteral antimicrobial therapy followed by oral suppressive therapy. Implant removal is associated with successful outcomes in late-onset infections.

42. Goulet JA, Pellicci PM, Brause BD, Salvati EM: Prolonged suppression of infection in total hip arthroplasty. *J Arthroplasty* 1988;3:109-116.

43. Marculescu CE, Berbari EF, Hanssen AD, et al: Outcome of prosthetic joint infections treated with debridement and retention of components. *Clin Infect Dis* 2006;42:471-478.

   In prosthetic joint infection, the risk factors independently associated with failure of débridement and prosthesis retention include the presence of a sinus tract and predébridement symptom duration of at least 8 days.

Section 4

Specific Situations

SECTION EDITORS:

MICHAEL J. PATZAKIS, MD
MONTRI D. WONGWORAWAT, MD

Chapter 11

Open Fractures

Charalampos G. Zalavras, MD   Michael J. Patzakis, MD

Introduction

Open fractures are complex injuries that involve both the skeleton and the surrounding soft tissues. Severe open fractures threaten the limb, and they are associated with considerable physical disability as well as depression.[1-3]

Assessment and Classification

An open fracture usually is the result of high-energy trauma and may be accompanied by other injuries. Careful evaluation and appropriate resuscitation of the patient are therefore necessary. The injured extremity should be assessed for the presence of neurovascular injury or compartment syndrome. The status of the soft-tissue envelope is important. The size and location of the wound, the extent of muscle damage, and the presence of contamination should be evaluated; fracture characteristics, including anatomic location (diaphyseal, metaphyseal, or intra-articular), comminution, and bone loss, also should be evaluated.

The most widely used classification of open fractures is the system devised by Gustilo and Anderson,[4] as modified by Gustilo, Mendoza, and Williams.[5] Type I is characterized by a puncture wound of 1 cm or less, with minimal contamination or muscle crushing. In type II, there is a laceration more than 1 cm long, with moderate soft-tissue damage and crushing; bone coverage is adequate, and fracture comminution is minimal. In type IIIA, extensive soft-tissue damage is present, often caused by a high-energy injury with a severe crushing component. The wound is massively contaminated. The fracture is severely comminuted or segmented, with adequate bone coverage. In type IIIB, there is extensive soft-tissue damage with periosteal stripping and bone exposure. Severe contamination and bone comminution are present, and flap coverage is required. Type IIIC is an arterial injury compromising perfusion of the extremity and requiring repair for limb salvage.

The reliability of the Gustilo classification system has been questioned because agreement among observers is moderate to poor.[6] The extent of contamination and soft-tissue crushing is important in classifying an open fracture and may be overlooked if the wound is small. An open fracture therefore should be classified only during surgical wound exploration and débridement.

Risk of Infection

The risk of clinical infection after an open fracture depends on the severity and location of the injury, patient characteristics, and treatment variables. Reported infection rates were 1.5% after a type I open fracture (7 of 497 fractures), 3.6% after a type II open fracture (25 of 695 fractures), and 22.7% after a type III open fracture (45 of 198 fractures). The infection rate after open tibial fractures was twice as high as the rate after open fractures at other locations.[7]

Patient characteristics such as medical comorbidities and smoking are also important. A recent study found that the presence of one or two comorbidities increased a patient's risk of infection approximately threefold, and the presence of three or more comorbidities increased the risk approximately sixfold.[8] Another recent study found that smoking increased the risk of osteomyelitis and the time to union in patients with a limb-threatening open tibial fracture.[9]

Early and appropriate antibiotic therapy, wound débridement, soft-tissue coverage, and fracture stabilization can reduce the infection rate after open fractures.[7] Tetanus prophylaxis is required unless the patient is already immunized. The infection rate does not appear to be significantly affected by the duration of antibiotic therapy, the elapsed time from injury to surgery, or the type of wound closure.[7,10,11]

Antibiotic Therapy

The role of antibiotics was established in a prospective randomized study that found a decreased infection rate when cephalosporin was administered before débridement. Infection developed in 2% of fractures (2 of 84 fractures) after antibiotic administration, compared with 14% (11 of 79 fractures) when antibiotics were not administered.[12]

Choice of Antibiotics

Open fractures may be contaminated with both gram-positive and gram-negative organisms. Antibiotics are therefore used not for prophylaxis but for treatment of wound contamination; they should be effective against both types of pathogens.[13]

Cephalosporin has been proposed for use as a single

agent in type I and II open fractures.[14] However, cephalosporin does not provide coverage against contaminating gram-negative organisms, and misclassification of a type IIIA open fracture because of small wound size could lead to inappropriate treatment with a single agent. A commonly used antibiotic regimen combines a first-generation cephalosporin such as cefazolin, which is active against gram-positive organisms, with an aminoglycoside such as gentamicin or tobramycin, which is active against gram-negative organisms. Another antibiotic with gram-negative coverage can be substituted for aminoglycoside.[15] Systemic administration of an aminoglycoside may not be necessary if aminoglycoside-impregnated beads are used for local antibiotic delivery.

Clostridial myonecrosis (gas gangrene) is of particular concern in open fracture wounds that are contaminated with anaerobic organisms (as in many farm injuries) or vascular wounds, which may create conditions of ischemia and low oxygen tension. Ampicillin or penicillin should be added to the antibiotic regimen for such injuries to provide coverage against anaerobes.

Timing and Duration of Antibiotic Therapy

Antibiotics should be administered immediately after the injury because a delay of more than 3 hours has been associated with an increased risk of infection.[7] The recommended duration of therapy is 3 days, although a shorter duration may be sufficient after a low-energy open fracture. [7,13,14] For subsequent surgical procedures such as wound coverage or bone grafting, antibiotics should be administered for 24 to 72 hours.

Local Delivery of Antibiotics

Antibiotic-impregnated polymethylmethacrylate cement can be used after open fracture for local delivery of antibiotics to complement systemic antibiotic therapy.[16] Patients with an open fracture who were treated using antibiotic beads in combination with systemic antibiotics had an overall infection rate of 3.7%; patients treated only with systemic antibiotics had an overall infection rate of 12%.[16] However, the decreased incidence of infection was statistically significant only in patients with a type III fracture (6.5% compared with 20%).

Aminoglycosides are commonly chosen for antibiotic therapy because of their broad spectrum of activity, heat stability, and low allergenicity. Vancomycin is not recommended for use as an initial agent because of concerns that overuse may lead to the development of antibiotic-resistant microorganisms.

The advantages of the bead pouch technique include a high local concentration of antibiotics and minimal systemic toxicity. In addition, the semipermeable barrier seals the wound from the external environment, thereby preventing secondary contamination by nosocomial pathogens while maintaining an aerobic wound environment.

Wound Treatment

Irrigation and Débridement

The optimal volume, delivery method, and solution to be used for irrigation remain controversial. High-pressure pulsatile irrigation can damage the bone and propel bacteria into soft tissue.[17] Low-pressure pulsatile or gravity flow irrigation therefore may be preferable. Antiseptic solutions are toxic to host cells and should be avoided. Although antibiotic solutions are used in clinical practice, there are no data on their efficacy; detergent solutions help remove bacteria and are a promising alternative. A recent study found no significant difference in infection rate after irrigation of open fracture wounds with an antibiotic solution or a nonsterile soap solution.[18]

Radical, sharp débridement is essential after irrigation. All nonviable bone and soft tissue should be resected because retained nonviable tissue and foreign material enhance microorganism growth, serve as a nidus for biofilm formation, and eventually lead to persistent infection. If the injury wound is too small to allow an assessment of tissue viability and débridement, it should be surgically extended. Viable muscle can be identified by color, consistency, contractility, and bleeding. Bone fragments without any soft-tissue attachment should be discarded, even if doing so will result in a large bone defect. Articular fragments, however, should be preserved. If necessary because of extensive comminution and soft-tissue damage, repeat débridement can be performed 24 to 48 hours later. Fasciotomies facilitate wound inspection and release compromised muscle compartments.

The infection rate after open fracture does not appear to be associated with the timing of débridement and surgical treatment.[7,10,19-21] Children who were treated for open fracture within 6 hours had a 3% infection rate (12 of 344 patients), compared with a 2% rate (4 of 210 patients) among those treated more than 6 hours after the injury.[10]

Cultures

Wound cultures often fail to identify an organism that subsequently causes an infection.[15,22,23] Wound cultures obtained before wound débridement have an especially low predictive value, probably because new pathogens cause nosocomial contamination when the wound is left exposed. Obtaining wound cultures before débridement therefore is no longer recommended. However, the results of postdébridement cultures and sensitivity testing can be helpful in selecting the best antibiotic agents for use in later procedures or in treating a possible early infection.

Wound Closure

The optimal timing of wound closure is controversial. Primary wound closure after thorough débridement is not associated with an increased rate of infection and

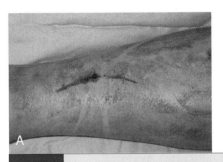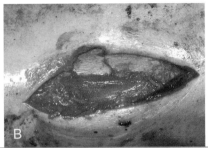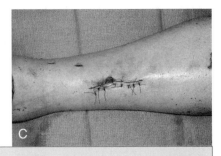

Figure 1 **A,** A small (less than 1 cm) traumatic wound resulting from a type I open fracture of the tibia. The surgical extension of the wound necessary for débridement is marked on the skin. **B,** After surgical excision of the wound, the open fracture site is débrided, and the fracture is fixed. **C,** The partial closure technique, in which the surgical extension of the wound is closed and the traumatic wound is left open, minimizes the risk of gas gangrene but does not require a second surgical procedure for wound closure. (Reproduced from Zalavras CG, Marcus RE, Levin LS, Patzakis MJ: Management of open fractures and subsequent complications. *Instr Course Lect* 2008;57:53.)

may prevent secondary contamination.[7] However, gas gangrene can occur after the primary closure of wounds contaminated with clostridial organisms, especially in the absence of adequate débridement.

The partial closure technique, in which the original wound is left open but any surgical wound extension is closed, is recommended for a type I or II open fracture wound (**Figure 1**); a type III wound should be left open.[24] Delaying wound closure for 3 to 7 days prevents the formation of anaerobic conditions, allows repeat débridement after 24 to 48 hours, and allows use of the antibiotic bead pouch technique.

Soft-Tissue Reconstruction

Severe soft-tissue damage, as in a type IIIB open fracture, requires reconstruction of the soft-tissue envelope to achieve wound coverage; prevent tissue desiccation; seal the wound from the external environment; and enhance vascularity, healing, and delivery of antibiotics. The location and magnitude of the soft-tissue defect determine the coverage method. Soft-tissue reconstruction is usually achieved using local or free muscle transfers. Fasciocutaneous flaps are useful if dead space is minimal; they are pliable, facilitate tendon gliding, and may restore sensation to the affected area if the flap remains innervated. A plan for soft-tissue reconstruction must be formulated during the initial wound assessment and fracture fixation.

Local pedicle muscle flaps include the gastrocnemius for proximal third tibial fractures and the soleus for middle third tibial fractures. However, muscle that is traumatized, crushed, or affected by a compartment syndrome should not be transferred. The rectus abdominis, gracilis, and latissimus dorsi are used for free muscle flaps in distal third tibial fractures.

Soft-tissue reconstruction should be performed within the first 7 days after the injury. Delays beyond this period are associated with increased rates of complications related to the flap or infection under the flap.[23] Some researchers promote flap coverage within 72 hours of injury.[25,26] A failure rate of less than 1% (1 of 134 patients) and an infection rate of 1.5% (2 pa-

tients) was reported after flap coverage performed within 72 hours, compared with a 12% failure rate (20 of 167 patients) and a 17.5% infection rate (29 patients) when flap closure was performed 4 to 90 days after surgery.[25] Deep infection developed in 6% of type IIIB and IIIC open fractures (4 of 63 fractures) that were covered within 72 hours, compared with 29% (6 of 21 fractures) of those covered more than 72 hours after injury.[25,26] However, an antibiotic bead pouch was not used in these studies, and secondary contamination may have contributed to the greater infection rate in fractures with delayed coverage.[23,25,26]

The wound can be temporarily treated to prevent infection before final closure using an antibiotic bead pouch or wound vacuum-assisted closure.[27]

Fracture Treatment

An open fracture must be stabilized to prevent further soft-tissue injury from bone fragments, improve wound care, and allow early motion of adjacent joints and patient mobilization. The initial fixation may be provisional or definitive. Intramedullary nailing, external fixation, or plate fixation may be required. The selection of fixation technique depends on the location of the fracture (diaphyseal, metaphyseal, or intra-articular), the nature of the fractured bone, the extent of soft-tissue injury, the extent of contamination, and the patient's physiologic status.

Intramedullary nailing is widely used to stabilize diaphyseal fractures of the lower extremity.[28-30] Plate fixation is indicated for periarticular fractures and diaphyseal fractures of the upper extremity. External fixation is indicated if extensive contamination and soft-tissue damage are present. External fixation also is preferred for rapid fracture stabilization and for minimizing interference with the patient's physiology,[31] as is required for a patient with unstable multiple trauma or a type IIIC open fracture.

For an open fracture with a vascular injury, controversy exists as to whether fracture fixation or arterial

4: Specific Situations

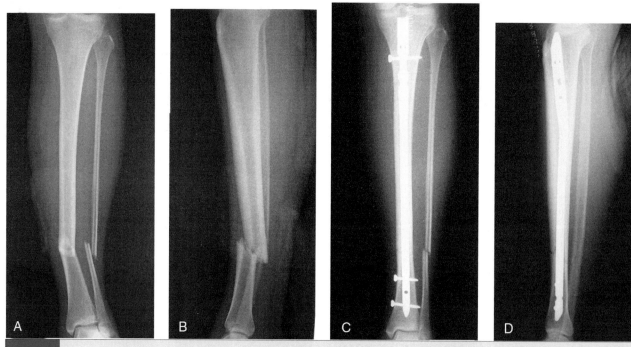

Figure 2 Presurgical AP **(A)** and lateral **(B)** radiographs of the fracture shown in Figure 1 (type I tibial fracture and fibular fracture). Postsurgical AP **(C)** and lateral **(D)** radiographs showing intramedullary nailing of the tibia. (Reproduced from Zalavras CG, Marcus RE, Levin LS, Patzakis MJ: Management of open fractures and subsequent complications. *Instr Course Lect* 2008;57:53.)

repair should be performed first. Individualized assessment is required, in consultation with a vascular surgeon. To minimize the duration of ischemia and soft-tissue damage, arterial repair should precede fracture stabilization.[32] However, microvascular anastomosis may be disrupted in the absence of skeletal stability. Definitive or provisional external fixation can be performed before arterial repair if the ischemia time is minimal.[33,34] The use of arterial intraluminal shunts allows prompt revascularization of the extremity and definitive fixation while avoiding the detrimental effects of prolonged ischemia.[35]

Open Diaphyseal Fractures of the Tibia

Both intramedullary nailing and external fixation have been successfully used to treat open tibial fractures (**Figure 2**). The severity of soft-tissue injury is the most important influence on infection and bone healing.[29] Two prospective randomized studies found no difference in infection and union rates after intramedullary nailing or external fixation.[29,30] Half-pin external fixators were associated with fracture malalignment and pin tract infections.[29] Unreamed intramedullary nailing may reduce the risk of revision, malunion, or superficial infection, compared with external fixation.[36]

Controversy exists as to whether reaming should be used with intramedullary nailing. Unreamed nailing better preserves the endosteal blood supply, although cortical circulation is gradually restored after reamed nailing.[37] Reamed nailing allows insertion of a larger diameter implant, improves stability at the fracture site,

and decreases the incidence of implant failure. Two prospective, randomized studies did not find significantly different infection rates after reamed or unreamed nailing in open tibial fractures.[38,39] Both studies found fewer screw failures after reamed nailing. A recent study of 143 open tibial fractures found unreamed nailing to be safe and effective when combined with appropriate soft-tissue treatment.[40] Two implants failed because of broken screws, and three failed because of loose screws; there were no broken nails. The low rate of implant failure was attributed to avoiding gaps at the fracture site. Minimal reaming using a reamed-to-fit technique also has been used with satisfactory results.[41]

External fixation can successfully be used as the definitive treatment. Many of the reported complications are attributable to the transition from external fixation to another form of fixation.[42,43] Delayed conversion of external fixation to intramedullary nailing resulted in infection rates as high as 50%,[23,44] whereas the infection rate after early (average, 17 days) conversion of the fixator to a nail was 5%, in the absence of pin tract infection.[45] Conversion to intramedullary nailing can be safe if the fixator has been in place no longer than 3 weeks and there is no pin tract infection. In other circumstances, external fixation should be used as the definitive treatment.[43]

Open Diaphyseal Fractures of the Femur

Reamed intramedullary nailing is the preferred technique for fixation of an open diaphyseal femoral fracture, although external fixation is an option for provisional fracture stabilization if the patient's condition is unstable.[31] No infections were found in 62 type I, II, and IIIA open femoral fractures treated with reamed intramedullary nails; infection was found in 11% of type IIIB fractures (3 of 27 fractures).[28] A recent study reported a 6% infection rate in open femoral fractures (5 of 89 fractures); the only variable significantly correlated with the presence of deep infection was the Gustilo-Anderson classification type.[46]

Open Diaphyseal Fractures of the Upper Extremity

Plate fixation is the preferred technique for an open forearm or humerus fracture.[47] Intramedullary nailing is an option for an open diaphyseal fracture of the humerus, although nonunion as well as shoulder pain and stiffness are concerns. External fixation can be useful if severe soft-tissue injury and contamination are present.[48]

Open Periarticular Fractures

Open periarticular fractures can be treated using provisional spanning external fixation. In addition, limited internal fixation with screws is used to restore articular congruency in intra-articular fractures. Definitive plate fixation is performed later.[49] Alternatively, these fractures can be treated definitively using plate fixation or fine-wire ring fixation, with limited internal fixation if necessary.[50,51] Locking plates and minimally invasive osteosynthesis techniques have had promising results in open periarticular fractures.[52]

Bone Grafting and Other Techniques to Promote Healing

Bone Grafting

Autogenous iliac crest bone graft can be used to promote the healing of open fractures when a bone defect or delayed union is a consideration. Bone grafting for a defect should not be performed during the initial procedure; it should be delayed until 6 to 8 weeks after the injury, when the soft-tissue envelope has healed and there is no infection.[23] Bone grafting may be necessary in the absence of a bone defect if no callus is apparent on radiographs 8 to 12 weeks after the injury. Bone graft can be applied at the fracture site or posterolateral to the fracture site. The decreased vascularity and contamination characteristic of open fractures are concerns in any consideration of bone substitutes.

Bone Morphogenetic Proteins

Recombinant bone morphogenetic proteins have osteoinductive properties and promote bone healing. Two prospective, randomized studies used recombinant human bone morphogenetic protein 2 (rhBMP-2) to treat open fractures. All 510 patients received intramedullary

nail fixation and routine soft-tissue treatment; those who also received an rhBMP-2 implant had significantly fewer secondary interventions before fracture union. Patients with a type III fracture had a lower infection rate.[53] Data revealed that treatment with rhBMP-2 significantly improved the outcome of type IIIA and IIIB open fractures; fewer invasive secondary interventions were required, and fewer infections occurred.[54] However, no significant differences were found between fractures treated with or without rhBMP-2 in the subgroup of fractures that were treated with reamed intramedullary nailing.[54]

Specialized Procedures

Bone defects larger than 6 cm require specialized reconstructive procedures such as distraction osteogenesis or vascularized bone grafting from the fibula or iliac crest. A free vascularized fibular graft provides the defect site with structural support and a new blood supply; it can be used for defects as large as 26 cm and is a versatile graft that can be combined with muscle, skin, and fascia grafts.[55] The Ilizarov technique, based on the principle of distraction osteogenesis, can reconstruct large bone defects and correct malalignment.[56,57] A recent study reported successful use of this technique for simultaneous reconstruction of bone and soft-tissue defects in patients who were not candidates for free flap coverage.[58]

Summary

The goals of open fracture treatment are prevention of infection, bone healing, and restoration of function. The principles of treatment include careful patient assessment, intrasurgical classification of the injury, appropriate antibiotic therapy, aggressive débridement, early soft-tissue coverage, stable fracture fixation, and early bone grafting or other supplementary procedures to achieve healing.

Annotated References

1. MacKenzie EJ, Bosse MJ, Pollak AN, et al: Long-term persistence of disability following severe lower-limb trauma. Results of a seven-year follow-up. *J Bone Joint Surg Am* 2005;87:1801-1809.

   Approximately half of 397 patients had substantial disability an average 84 months after severe lower extremity injury, regardless of whether the selected treatment was amputation or reconstruction. Level of evidence: II.

2. Gopal S, Giannoudis PV, Murray A, Matthews SJ, Smith RM: The functional outcome of severe, open tibial fractures managed with early fixation and flap coverage. *J Bone Joint Surg Br* 2004;86:861-867.

   At a mean 46-month follow-up, patients with a severe open tibial fracture had comparatively low physical and mental scores on the Medical Outcomes Study Short Form-36 Health Survey. Level of evidence: II.

3. Crichlow RJ, Andres PL, Morrison SM, Haley SM, Vrahas MS: Depression in orthopaedic trauma patients: Prevalence and severity. *J Bone Joint Surg Am* 2006;88: 1927-1933.

    The presence of an open fracture was the only injury-specific factor significantly associated with depression (odds ratio, 4.6; 95% confidence interval, 1.6-12.4). Level of evidence: II.

4. Gustilo RB, Anderson JT: Prevention of infection in the treatment of one thousand and twenty-five open fractures of long bones: Retrospective and prospective analyses. *J Bone Joint Surg Am* 1976;58:453-458.

5. Gustilo RB, Mendoza RM, Williams DN: Problems in the management of type III (severe) open fractures: A new classification of type III open fractures. *J Trauma* 1984;24:742-746.

6. Brumback RJ, Jones AL: Interobserver agreement in the classification of open fractures of the tibia: The results of a survey of two hundred and forty-five orthopaedic surgeons. *J Bone Joint Surg Am* 1994;76:1162-1166.

7. Patzakis MJ, Wilkins J: Factors influencing infection rate in open fracture wounds. *Clin Orthop Relat Res* 1989;243:36-40.

8. Bowen TR, Widmaier JC: Host classification predicts infection after open fracture. *Clin Orthop Relat Res* 2005;433:205-211.

    Medical comorbidities were significantly associated with infection in patients with open fractures. The presence of one or two comorbidities increased the infection risk 2.9 times, and the presence of three or more comorbidities increased the risk 5.7 times, compared with healthy patients. Level of evidence: II.

9. Castillo RC, Bosse MJ, MacKenzie EJ, Patterson BM: Impact of smoking on fracture healing and risk of complications in limb-threatening open tibia fractures. *J Orthop Trauma* 2005;19:151-157.

    Smoking or a history of smoking increases the time to union and the risk of osteomyelitis in patients with open fractures. Patients should be encouraged to enter a smoking cessation program. Level of evidence: II.

10. Skaggs DL, Friend L, Alman B, et al: The effect of surgical delay on acute infection following 554 open fractures in children. *J Bone Joint Surg Am* 2005;87:8-12.

    This multicenter study of open fractures in pediatric patients found no difference in the infection rate between those treated within 6 hours and those treated more than 6 hours after the injury. Intravenous antibiotics were administered upon emergency department arrival.

11. Dellinger EP, Caplan ES, Weaver LD, et al: Duration of preventive antibiotic administration for open extremity fractures. *Arch Surg* 1988;123:333-339.

12. Patzakis MJ, Harvey JP Jr, Ivler D: The role of antibiotics in the management of open fractures. *J Bone Joint Surg Am* 1974;56:532-541.

13. Zalavras CG, Patzakis MJ: Open fractures: Evaluation and management. *J Am Acad Orthop Surg* 2003;11: 212-219.

    The concepts governing open fracture treatment are reviewed.

14. Templeman DC, Gulli B, Tsukayama DT, Gustilo RB: Update on the management of open fractures of the tibial shaft. *Clin Orthop Relat Res* 1998;350:18-25.

15. Patzakis MJ, Bains RS, Lee J, et al: Prospective, randomized, double-blind study comparing single-agent antibiotic therapy, ciprofloxacin, to combination antibiotic therapy in open fracture wounds. *J Orthop Trauma* 2000;14:529-533.

16. Ostermann PA, Seligson D, Henry SL: Local antibiotic therapy for severe open fractures: A review of 1085 consecutive cases. *J Bone Joint Surg Br* 1995;77:93-97.

17. Hassinger SM, Harding G, Wongworawat MD: High-pressure pulsatile lavage propagates bacteria into soft tissue. *Clin Orthop Relat Res* 2005;439:27-31.

    This experimental study of fresh ovine muscle found that high-pressure pulsatile lavage causes deeper penetration of bacteria into soft tissue and results in greater bacterial retention, compared with low-pressure lavage.

18. Anglen JO: Comparison of soap and antibiotic solutions for irrigation of lower-limb open fracture wounds: A prospective, randomized study. *J Bone Joint Surg Am* 2005;87:1415-1422.

    A prospective, randomized study of 458 open lower extremity fractures found that antibiotic solutions used for irrigation of open fracture wounds offer no advantage over nonsterile soap solutions and may increase the risk of wound-healing problems. Level of evidence: I.

19. Khatod M, Botte MJ, Hoyt DB, Meyer RS, Smith JM, Akeson WH: Outcomes in open tibial fractures: Relationship between delay in treatment and infection. *J Trauma* 2003;55:949-954.

    This study found no difference in infection rates between open fractures treated within 6 hours after injury and those treated later. Level of evidence: II.

20. Spencer J, Smith A, Woods D: The effect of time delay on infection in open long-bone fractures: A 5-year prospective audit from a district general hospital. *Ann R Coll Surg Engl* 2004;86:108-112.

    This study found no difference in infection rates between open fractures treated within 6 hours after injury and those treated later. Level of evidence: II.

21. Charalambous CP, Siddique I, Zenios M, et al: Early versus delayed surgical treatment of open tibial frac-

tures: Effect on the rates of infection and need of secondary surgical procedures to promote bone union. *Injury* 2005;36:656-661.

This study found no difference in infection rates between open fractures treated within 6 hours after injury and those treated later. Level of evidence: II.

22. Lee J: Efficacy of cultures in the management of open fractures. *Clin Orthop Relat Res* 1997;339:71-75.

23. Fischer MD, Gustilo RB, Varecka TF: The timing of flap coverage, bone-grafting, and intramedullary nailing in patients who have a fracture of the tibial shaft with extensive soft-tissue injury. *J Bone Joint Surg Am* 1991;73: 1316-1322.

24. Patzakis MJ, Wilkins J, Moore TM: Considerations in reducing the infection rate in open tibial fractures. *Clin Orthop Relat Res* 1983;178:36-41.

25. Godina M: Early microsurgical reconstruction of complex trauma of the extremities. *Plast Reconstr Surg* 1986;78:285-292.

26. Gopal S, Majumder S, Batchelor AG, Knight SL, De Boer P, Smith RM: Fix and flap: The radical orthopaedic and plastic treatment of severe open fractures of the tibia. *J Bone Joint Surg Br* 2000;82:959-966.

27. Dedmond BT, Kortesis B, Punger K, et al: Subatmospheric pressure dressings in the temporary treatment of soft tissue injuries associated with type III open tibial shaft fractures in children. *J Pediatr Orthop* 2006;26: 728-732.

    The use of negative pressure dressings in children with a high-energy open fracture decreased the need for major soft-tissue procedures. Level of evidence: IV.

28. Brumback RJ, Ellison PS Jr, Poka A, Lakatos R, Bathon GH, Burgess AR: Intramedullary nailing of open fractures of the femoral shaft. *J Bone Joint Surg Am* 1989;71:1324-1331.

29. Henley MB, Chapman JR, Agel J, Harvey EJ, Whorton AM, Swiontkowski MF: Treatment of type II, IIIA, and IIIB open fractures of the tibial shaft: A prospective comparison of unreamed interlocking intramedullary nails and half-pin external fixators. *J Orthop Trauma* 1998;12:1-7.

30. Tornetta P III, Bergman M, Watnik N, Berkowitz G, Steuer J: Treatment of grade-IIIb open tibial fractures: A prospective randomised comparison of external fixation and non-reamed locked nailing. *J Bone Joint Surg Br* 1994;76:13-19.

31. Roberts CS, Pape HC, Jones AL, Malkani AL, Rodriguez JL, Giannoudis PV: Damage control orthopaedics: Evolving concepts in the treatment of patients who have sustained orthopaedic trauma. *Instr Course Lect* 2005;54:447-462.

    This review highlights the principles of damage-control orthopaedics. In selected patients, the injury should be

stabilized and controlled rather than repaired, while minimizing additional physiologic insult.

32. Ashworth EM, Dalsing MC, Glover JL, Reilly MK: Lower extremity vascular trauma: A comprehensive, aggressive approach. *J Trauma* 1988;28:329-336.

33. Seligson D, Ostermann PA, Henry SL, Wolley T: The management of open fractures associated with arterial injury requiring vascular repair. *J Trauma* 1994;37:938-940.

34. Iannacone WM, Taffet R, DeLong WG Jr, Born CT, Dalsey RM, Deutsch LS: Early exchange intramedullary nailing of distal femoral fractures with vascular injury initially stabilized with external fixation. *J Trauma* 1994;37:446-451.

35. Nunley JA, Koman LA, Urbaniak JR: Arterial shunting as an adjunct to major limb revascularization. *Ann Surg* 1981;193:271-273.

36. Bhandari M, Guyatt GH, Swiontkowski MF, Schemitsch EH: Treatment of open fractures of the shaft of the tibia. *J Bone Joint Surg Br* 2001;83:62-68.

37. Schemitsch EH, Kowalski MJ, Swiontkowski MF, Senft D: Cortical bone blood flow in reamed and unreamed locked intramedullary nailing: A fractured tibia model in sheep. *J Orthop Trauma* 1994;8:373-382.

38. Keating JF, Blachut PA, O'Brien PJ, Meek RN, Broekhuyse H: Reamed nailing of open tibial fractures: Does the antibiotic bead pouch reduce the deep infection rate? *J Orthop Trauma* 1996;10:298-303.

39. Finkemeier CG, Schmidt AH, Kyle RF, Templeman DC, Varecka TF: A prospective, randomized study of intramedullary nails inserted with and without reaming for the treatment of open and closed fractures of the tibial shaft. *J Orthop Trauma* 2000;14:187-193.

40. Kakar S, Tornetta P III: Open fractures of the tibia treated by immediate intramedullary tibial nail insertion without reaming: A prospective study. *J Orthop Trauma* 2007;21:153-157.

    In a prospective study, unreamed nailing of open tibial fractures was found to be safe and effective. The importance of appropriate soft-tissue treatment and gap avoidance at the fracture site is emphasized. Level of evidence: IV.

41. Ziran BH, Darowish M, Klatt BA, Agudelo JF, Smith WR: Intramedullary nailing in open tibia fractures: A comparison of two techniques. *Int Orthop* 2004;28:235-238.

    Minimal reaming in open fractures of the tibia decreased the number of secondary procedures required to achieve union, compared with unreamed nailing. Level of evidence: III.

42. Edwards CC, Simmons SC, Browner BD, Weigel MC: Severe open tibial fractures: Results treating 202 injuries

with external fixation. *Clin Orthop Relat Res* 1988; 230:98-115.

43. Marsh JL, Nepola JV, Wuest TK, Osteen D, Cox K, Oppenheim W: Unilateral external fixation until healing with the dynamic axial fixator for severe open tibial fractures. *J Orthop Trauma* 1991;5:341-348.

44. McGraw JM, Lim EV: Treatment of open tibial-shaft fractures: External fixation and secondary intramedullary nailing. *J Bone Joint Surg Am* 1988;70:900-911.

45. Blachut PA, Meek RN, O'Brien PJ: External fixation and delayed intramedullary nailing of open fractures of the tibial shaft: A sequential protocol. *J Bone Joint Surg Am* 1990;72:729-735.

46. Noumi T, Yokoyama K, Ohtsuka H, Nakamura K, Itoman M: Intramedullary nailing for open fractures of the femoral shaft: Evaluation of contributing factors on deep infection and nonunion using multivariate analysis. *Injury* 2005;36:1085-1093.

   The only variable significantly correlated with deep infection in open femoral fractures was Gustilo-Anderson classification type. The overall infection rate was 6% (5 of 89 fractures). Level of evidence: II.

47. Moed BR, Kellam JF, Foster RJ, Tile M, Hansen ST Jr : Immediate internal fixation of open fractures of the diaphysis of the forearm. *J Bone Joint Surg Am* 1986;68: 1008-1017.

48. Mostafavi HR, Tornetta P III: Open fractures of the humerus treated with external fixation. *Clin Orthop Relat Res* 1997;337:187-197.

49. Sirkin M, Sanders R, DiPasquale T, Herscovici D Jr: A staged protocol for soft tissue management in the treatment of complex pilon fractures. *J Orthop Trauma* 1999;13:78-84.

50. Watson JT: High-energy fractures of the tibial plateau. *Orthop Clin North Am* 1994;25:723-752.

51. Benirschke SK, Agnew SG, Mayo KA, Santoro VM, Henley MB: Immediate internal fixation of open, complex tibial plateau fractures: Treatment by a standard protocol. *J Orthop Trauma* 1992;6:78-86.

52. Kregor PJ, Stannard JA, Zlowodzki M, Cole PA: Treatment of distal femur fractures using the less invasive stabilization system: Surgical experience and early clinical results in 103 fractures. *J Orthop Trauma* 2004;18: 509-520.

   Locking-plate fixation was used in 103 distal femoral fractures (68 closed and 35 open fractures). There were two infections and six revisions for bone grafting in the open fractures. No loss of fixation occurred. Level of evidence: IV.

53. Govender S, Csimma C, Genant HK, et al: Recombinant human bone morphogenetic protein-2 for treatment of open tibial fractures: A prospective, controlled, randomized study of four hundred and fifty patients. *J Bone Joint Surg Am* 2002;84:2123-2134.

54. Swiontkowski MF, Aro HT, Donell S, et al: Recombinant human bone morphogenetic protein-2 in open tibial fractures: A subgroup analysis of data combined from two prospective randomized studies. *J Bone Joint Surg Am* 2006;88:1258-1265.

   This study found that rhBMP-2 significantly improves the outcome of a type IIIA or IIIB open fracture, decreasing the number of invasive secondary interventions required and the number of infections. No significant differences were found in the subgroup of fractures treated with reamed intramedullary nailing. Level of evidence: I.

55. Malizos KN, Zalavras CG, Soucacos PN, Beris AE, Urbaniak JR: Free vascularized fibular grafts for reconstruction of skeletal defects. *J Am Acad Orthop Surg* 2004;12:360-369.

   The use of vascularized fibular grafts for reconstruction of large skeletal defects is reviewed.

56. Paley D, Maar DC: Ilizarov bone transport treatment for tibial defects. *J Orthop Trauma* 2000;14:76-85.

57. Mekhail AO, Abraham E, Gruber B, Gonzalez M: Bone transport in the management of posttraumatic bone defects in the lower extremity. *J Trauma* 2004;56: 368-378.

   Bone transport was used in treating posttraumatic bone defects in 19 patients. The mean length of regenerated bone was 5.7 cm and the mean time in external fixation was 13.8 months. There were two transtibial amputations and four fractures at the docking site. Level of evidence: IV.

58. Rozbruch SR, Weitzman AM, Watson JT, Freudigman P, Katz HV, Ilizarov S: Simultaneous treatment of tibial bone and soft-tissue defects with the Ilizarov method. *J Orthop Trauma* 2006;20:197-205.

   The Ilizarov method was successfully used for simultaneous reconstruction of bone and soft-tissue defects in patients who were not candidates for free flap coverage. Level of evidence: IV.

Chapter 12
Adult Osteomyelitis

*George Cierny III, MD   Doreen DiPasquale, MD

Introduction

The treatment of chronic osteomyelitis in adult patients is directed by careful consideration of anatomic, physiologic, and socioeconomic parameters including the site and extent of disease involvement, the functional impairment caused by disease, the condition of the patient host, the physician's experience, and institutional resources. The complex interplay of these factors determines whether the treatment is palliative or curative, simple or complex, limb sparing or ablative.

With time and opportunity, an acute infection becomes chronic (refractory) by a process that follows the fundamental mechanisms of microbial colonization. Reactions between surface macromolecules form at the pathogen-substrate interfaces and lead to the formation of a resilient microzone of attachment. Phenotypic pathogen transformations occur, and colony-forming units secrete a protective matrix (biofilm), which offers an enhanced mode of growth and protection from antimicrobial agents and host defenses.[1,2] To resolve a biofilm infection, the biofilm colony and all of its substrates for attachment (inert and nonviable surfaces) must be surgically removed[3] (**Figure 1**).

Historical Perspectives

Before 1976, the principles of sepsis surgery[4-8] emphasized sequential débridement, healing by secondary intention, bypass or open bone grafting,[9-11] prolonged antibiotic therapy,[12] and long-term external support using orthotics or casts. Because the methods of restoring hard- and soft-tissue deficits were unreliable, bone infection, unlike cancer, was tolerated. Surgeons were reluctant to completely remove infected segments for fear of causing fracture, loss of function, or death. As a result, the patient selection criteria for limb salvage were restrictive, and débridement was intralesional only. Wound-healing deficiencies and persistent infections contributed to the low rates of treatment success (50% to 72%).[4,7,13,14]

*George Cierny III, MD or the department with which he is affiliated has received miscellaneous nonincome support, commercially derived honoraria, or other nonresearch-related funding from Kimberly-Clark; has received royalties from Wright Medical; and holds stock or stock options in Royer Biomedical.

During the past three decades, the treatment of osteomyelitis has evolved with improvements in knowledge, experience, science, and technology.[15-23] Methods developed to counter the mechanisms inherent to pathogen colonization of wounds have become the foundation of modern treatment protocols.[19,24-29] Currently, treatment with limb salvage protocols is successful in more than 90% of patients with chronic osteomyelitis, even though there has been an increase in the number of patients with multiple comorbidities that affect wound healing. Versatile external fixation devices have enhanced the care of massive injuries and supported gentle methods of deformity correction and composite tissue restoration.[30,31] Innovative technologies have led to new fixation strategies, such as locking plates and retrograde nails; methods to detect and isolate biofilm pathogens;[32-35] antimicrobial agents for resistant pathogen strains; and new approaches to open wound treatment, such as vacuum-assisted closure.[36,37] The clinical application of vascular territories,[38] new methods of tissue transfer,[16,30,31,39-43] and the local delivery of antibiotics by implantable depots[44-46] have broadened the selection criteria for treatment and provided a basis for limb salvage following débridement.[47]

As a result of these advances, wounds could become stable, vigorous, and resilient. Both hard- and soft-tissue deficits could be managed. Dirty wounds were converted to clean wounds able to tolerate any method of reconstruction.[48] Opportunities opened for using massive bone grafts, internal fixation strategies, and prosthetic total joints.[45-47,49]

Success in using antibiotic depot protocols before final reconstruction has led to a new era of treating musculoskeletal sepsis with staged treatment protocols.[47,50,51] The process parallels the staging and treatment of musculoskeletal tumors and requires the same precision and foresight.[52] Discovery, precise preoperative planning, and cross referencing of treatment options with patient and wound parameters are carefully conducted and confirmed to ensure the efficient use of host reserves and institutional resources.

This new prospect of a successful reconstruction following infection has overcome orthopaedic surgeons' earlier fear of treatment failure and provided the confidence to perform thorough débridements.[53] Maintenance or restoration of a competent soft-tissue envelope facilitates reexposure, contains and concentrates locally released antibiotics, revascularizes bone and

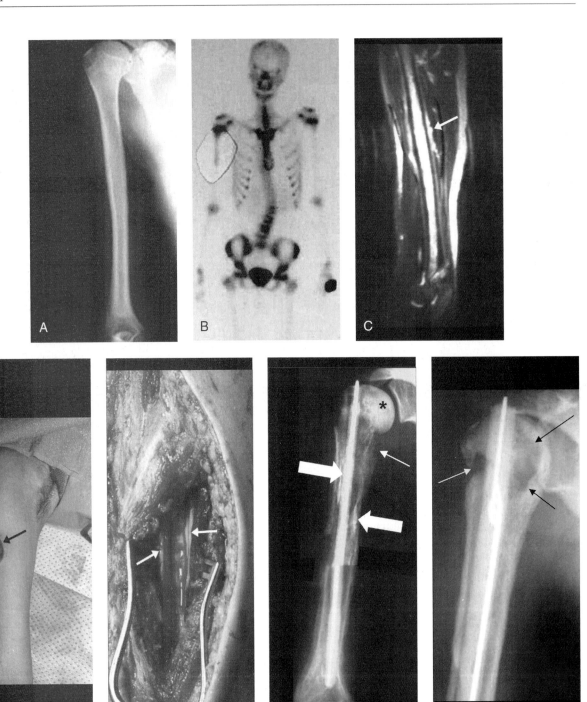

Figure 1 Diagnosis and treatment of infection in a malnourished 16-year-old girl who had fever, malaise, and right upper extremity pain for 2 weeks before admission to the hospital. **A,** AP radiograph of the right humerus, revealing no obvious lesions. **B,** Bone scan showing a mild hyperconcentration of radiotracer in the proximal diaphysis *(circled).* **C,** T2-weighted sagittal MRI study of the humerus, showing an intense medullary signal, an effusion in the right elbow, and inflammation *(arrow)* within investing soft tissues along the diaphysis. **D,** After 6 weeks of parenteral antibiotics, cultures from an open biopsy *(arrow)* revealed a polymicrobial, anaerobic infection, confirming the diagnosis of a diffuse hematogenous osteomyelitis. **E,** Photograph taken during débridement showing surgical unroofing of the proximal half of the lesion. Dead marrow elements and sequestered cortical bone *(arrows)* were found along the length of the diaphysis. Distal to the unroofing, the bone was débrided using medullary reamers. **F,** AP radiograph showing dead cortical fragments *(large arrows),* which were gradually removed during six serial débridements at intervals of 2 to 3 weeks. This method encouraged consolidation of an involucrum *(small arrow)* while bone was being removed and stabilized with an antibiotic-coated medullary rod. During treatment, necrosis within the humeral head *(*)* was diagnosed. **G,** AP radiograph showing the surgical approach *(white arrow)* used to débride the subchondral bone *(black arrows)* and implant antibiotic-loaded beads (OsteoSet pellets, Wright Medical, Memphis, TN). *(Continued on page 137.)*

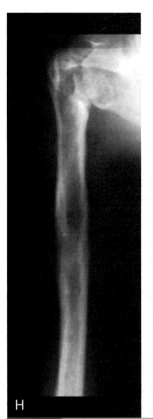
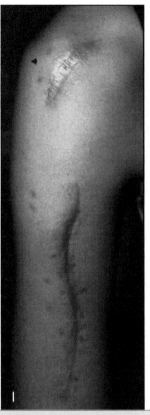
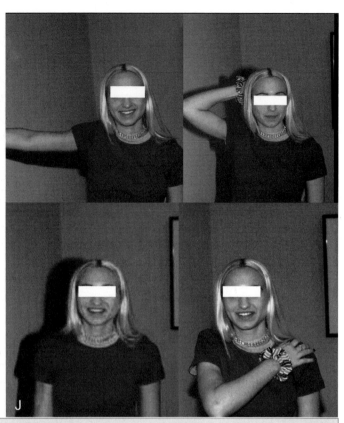

Figure 1	*(Continued from page 136.)* **H,** The involucrum eventually reconstituted the patient's humeral diaphysis without bone grafting, as shown in an AP radiograph. At 5-year follow-up, the patient was infection free **(I)** and had an excellent range of motion **(J),** despite aseptic collapse of the humeral head.

tendon grafts, and prevents secondary colonization of the wound. A treatment algorithm for chronic osteomyelitis is presented in Figure 2. Local antibiotic depots preserve length, safeguard an early wound closure, maintain working dead space, and prepare the wound for reconstruction using methods including vascularized bone flaps, bone transport, compression-distraction, total joint arthroplasty or mega-arthroplasty, and fixation-assisted cancellous grafting.[54-60]

Classification of the Host and Disease

The Cierny-Mader classification of chronic osteomyelitis[3,19] in 1983 became the first classification system to articulate the natural history of osteomyelitis with treatment and outcomes.[13,61] Three host cohorts and four anatomic types of infection are described and sequentially ordered to denote disease and treatment complexity as well as the risk of failure.

Clinical Staging

In the Cierny-Mader classification system,[19] clinical staging defines the nidus of infection, the physiologic capacity of the host patient, and the best surgical treatment approach. The physiologic status of the host (class A, B, or C) and the anatomic extent of bony disease (type I, II, III, or IV) are combined to designate 1 of the 12 stages of adult osteomyelitis (for example, stage IVB osteomyelitis). Clinical staging establishes a format for comparing outcomes in host cohorts and developing new treatment protocols.

The Host

The physiologic status of the host ultimately determines patient selection. A candidate for treatment must have the physiologic ability to impede infection; heal surgical wounds; and tolerate the metabolic and psychologic stresses of sequential procedures, significant blood loss, and prolonged hospitalization. The health of the host and the disability caused by the disease are combined into a single physiologic class based on the risks and benefits of treatment. A healthy patient with a normal response to stress, trauma, and infection is classified as an A-host; a patient with comorbidities that inherently compromise wound healing and response to treatment is classified as a B-host (Table 1).

The goal of treatment is to improve the patient's quality of life. The factors that guide patient selection are the impact of the infection on the patient's physiologic well-being and the level of physical disability caused by the disease itself. Pain resulting in dysfunction and recurrent episodes of sepsis are strong indications for surgical intervention. If the treatment will lead

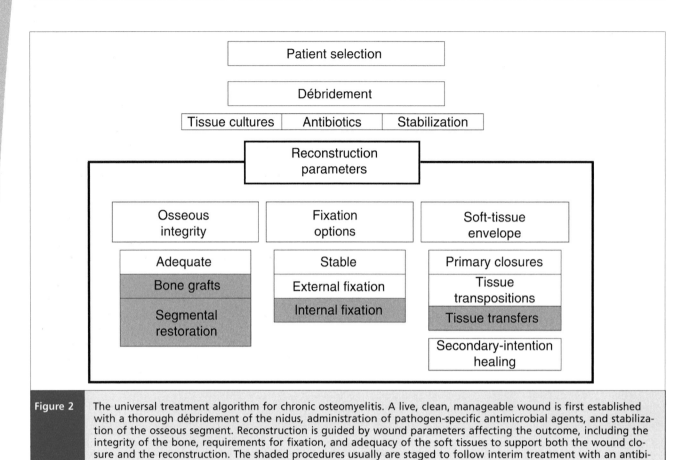

Figure 2 The universal treatment algorithm for chronic osteomyelitis. A live, clean, manageable wound is first established with a thorough débridement of the nidus, administration of pathogen-specific antimicrobial agents, and stabilization of the osseous segment. Reconstruction is guided by wound parameters affecting the outcome, including the integrity of the bone, requirements for fixation, and adequacy of the soft tissues to support both the wound closure and the reconstruction. The shaded procedures usually are staged to follow interim treatment with an antibiotic depot. (Courtesy of G Cierny III, MD, San Diego, CA.)

to morbidity or loss of function exceeding the impact of the disease on the patient's quality of life, the patient is classified as a C-host and is offered observation or palliation alone.[59,62,63] For a C-host, asymptomatic infection, persistent drainage, abnormal laboratory values, or limb deformity may not require treatment. However, if the condition worsens over time or a new technology can offer an outcome that favors treatment over restraint, a C-host may be reconsidered for treatment and reclassified as an A-host or B-host.

The Disease

Because a thorough débridement is the unchallenged cornerstone of successful therapy for osteomyelitis, the Cierny-Mader classification system articulates with surgical procedures.[29] Anatomic types I through IV match the natural history of osteomyelitis to specific treatment modalities, in increasing order of complexity (**Figure 3**).

Type I: Medullary Osteomyelitis

In type I osteomyelitis, the sequestered nidus is confined to the endosteum and is associated with ischemic scar or granulations, sequestered bone (trabeculae, endosteal cortex), or medullary implants. The investing soft-tissue envelope may be involved. In an adult, the hematogenous variant of type I osteomyelitis occurs primarily in immunocompromised hosts, tends to be

more diaphyseal than metaphyseal, and accounts for fewer than 5% of the cases of type I osteomyelitis listed in the authors' registry since 1981.

Type II: Superficial Osteomyelitis

Type II is the contiguous-focus form of osteomyelitis.[61] The biofilm nidus is an exposed, bony surface at the base of an atrophic soft-tissue defect. The nidus involves only the superficial part of an otherwise healthy osseous segment and does not extend into the medullary canal. Type II osteomyelitis commonly occurs at the base of a pressure or stasis ulcer and with breakdown of wounds closed by secondary intention, such as with Papineau bone grafts.[11]

Type III: Localized Osteomyelitis

The hallmark of type III osteomyelitis is a full-thickness cortical sequestrum located inside or juxtaposed to a stable osseous segment. The canal is involved, as in type I; the soft-tissue envelope may be deficient, as in type II; and a foreign body (such as indwelling hardware) is common. Type III osteomyelitis most commonly is seen as an infected fracture union with sequestration of an end cortex (a butterfly fragment). In these patients, the entire lesion can be excised with a cuff of viable tissue while preserving the integrity and stability of the involved segment (**Figures 4** and **5**).

Table 1.

Comorbidities Associated With Wound-Healing Deficiencies in Adult Patients Undergoing Treatment for Chronic Osteomyelitis or Periprosthetic Total Joint Infection

Local Factors Affecting the Vascular Status of the Wound

Arteritis

Chronic edema

Extensive scar

Foreign body excess*

Large vessel disease

Obesity

Radiation fibrosis

Venous stasis

Systemic Factors Compromising the Patient's General Health and Well-Being

Bleeding diathesis

Diabetes

Drug inhibitors†

Hypoxia

Immune deficiency

Intravenous drug abuse

Malignancy

Malnutrition

Nicotine abuse

Age older than approximately 70 years

Organ failure

Skin colonization with *Staphylococcus aureus*

*Unavoidably incomplete removal of foreign material (such as scattered shotgun pellets, suture materials) during salvage or infection control
†For example, dilantin and ciprofloxacin, which inhibit bone formation

Type IV: Diffuse Osteomyelitis

Type IV osteomyelitis is a permeative, through-and-through infection having the characteristics of types I, II, and III osteomyelitis and the additional feature of instability (Figure 6). The lesions are intrinsically unstable, as with fracture nonunions or a refractory septic arthritis; or they will become unstable following débridement, as with a periprosthetic total joint infection or permeative diaphyseal osteomyelitis of hematogenous origin. An intercalary resection is required to establish an infection-free surgical margin following débridement.

Case Presentation and Discussion

Presentation

An 80-year-old man has an infected nonunion (type IV osteomyelitis) of the distal-third tibia. He is lethargic and weak and has drainage from an anteromedial soft-tissue deficit (2.5 cm × 7 cm) at the fracture site. The work-up reveals myocardial ischemia, mild congestive heart failure, and significant peripheral vascular disease. He is unable to bear weight without the use of a walker, and his condition has not improved on parenteral antibiotic therapy.

Discussion

The patient is classified as a B-host (stage IVB osteomyelitis) on the basis of his age and cardiovascular status. He is a candidate for treatment because of the impact of the infection (weakness) and the disability associated with the disease (immobility). However, the options for management are limited to ablation because of the morbidity and mortality associated with a limb salvage attempt in so compromised a host. An amputation offers him the best treatment outcome.

On the other hand, if the patient had been treated with and responded favorably to oral rather than parenteral antibiotic agents, and if he had become functional with the use of a short leg brace, he would have satisfied the criteria for palliation as a C-host (stage IVC osteomyelitis).[54,58,61,62]

Approach to Treatment

The treatment format is selected based on the clinical stage of disease, the anatomic site of the infection, wound parameters, and the experience of the health care team. When curative treatment is contraindicated, untimely, or too debilitating for the patient, palliative and suppressive therapies are used to improve the patient's well-being.[3,64,65] To justify the morbidity and risk associated with limb salvage, its potential outcomes must be distinctly better than those of amputation. Limb ablation is indicated if neither limb salvage nor palliation is safe and feasible. The selection process is heavily influenced by intrinsic conditions (host comorbidities) affecting the health of the patient, which increase the risk of treatment failure. These risk factors (Table 1) lead to metabolic deficiencies, skin and wound breakdown, immune deficiencies, bacteremia, and complications related to excessive bleeding. Furthermore, the effects of multiple comorbidities compound the risk.[3,58,61,62,65]

After the work-up establishes that a patient is at risk due to the presence of comorbidities, every effort should be made to solicit intervention to optimize the host response, regardless of the treatment format selected[66,67] (Table 2). The preoperative reversal of wound-healing deficiencies can convert the potential outcomes for a B-host to resemble those for an A-host.[55] Similar results can be obtained by using methods that have a low surgical morbidity, such as atraumatic exposures, staged treatment protocols, and reconstructions that are unlikely to require surgical implants[68-74] (Table 3). If internal stabilization is an absolute requirement, the final reconstruction may best be staged to follow an

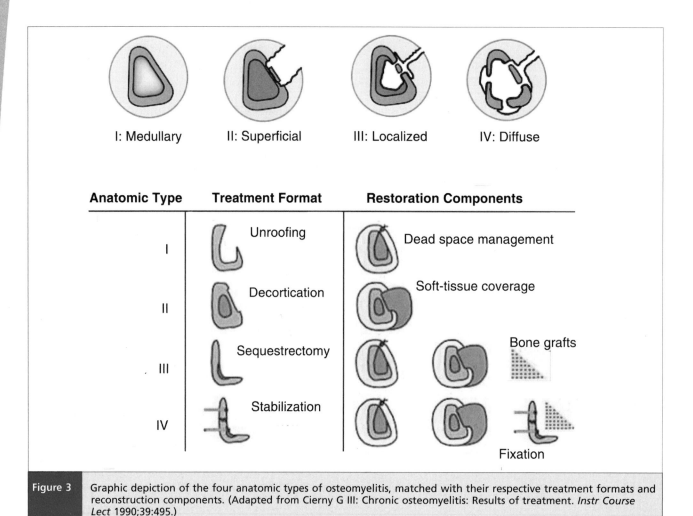

Anatomic Type	Treatment Format	Restoration Components

I: Medullary   II: Superficial   III: Localized   IV: Diffuse

I — Unroofing — Dead space management

II — Decortication — Soft-tissue coverage

III — Sequestrectomy — Bone grafts

IV — Stabilization — Fixation

Figure 3 Graphic depiction of the four anatomic types of osteomyelitis, matched with their respective treatment formats and reconstruction components. (Adapted from Cierny G III: Chronic osteomyelitis: Results of treatment. *Instr Course Lect* 1990;39:495.)

interval of local antibiotic therapy. The use of an antibiotic depot lessens the morbidity of treatment and decreases the strain on host defenses by clearing residual pathogens and separating a wound's restoration from its reconstruction.[46,75,76]

Case Discussion *(continued)*

For the previously described 80-year-old man with stage IVB osteomyelitis of the tibia, the low-risk protocols include a below-knee amputation or an acute permanent shortening of the limb. An open bone transport would present moderate risk. The high-risk treatments include external fixation, osteocutaneous free fibula grafting, and an interpositional tumor prosthesis with free flap coverage.

Clinical Evaluation

The patient's medical and surgical history is reviewed, and a complete physical examination is performed to document the patient's general health, the integrity of the musculoskeletal system, and the location of the pathologic process. The quality and quantity of the soft-tissue envelope are assessed with respect to the surgical approach, wound closure, and fixation strate-

gies. Joint contractures, axial deformities, and joint arcs of motion are considered as part of the selection process.

Laboratory test results are scrutinized for information pertaining to the patient's systemic response to infection and comorbidities affecting metabolic, immune, or hematopoietic function. Clinical suspicion and signs and symptoms of vascular compromise guide the adjuvant use of angiography, sonography, and transcutaneous oxygen tension measurement.

Diagnostic radiology is used to delineate the inflammatory nidus (Figures 1 and 4). Plain radiographs can disclose hardware, alignment, fracture, and instability. Nuclear scans can confirm cellular activity and osseous viability. CT scans show sequestra, the status of a union, and bony integrity and volume; they also provide guidance on the best surgical approach. MRI studies can define inflammatory margins and skip lesions within bone, marrow, and surrounding soft tissues.[77,78]

Pathogen Identification and Antibiotic Selection

The organism or organisms responsible for the infection are isolated from preoperative tissue samples, specimens

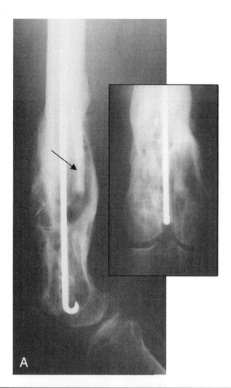

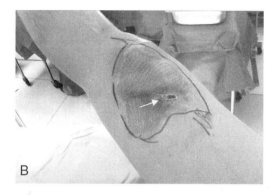

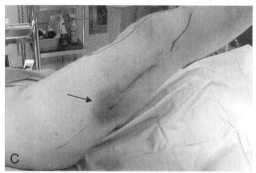

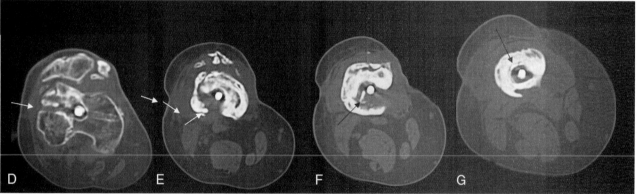

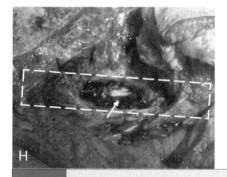

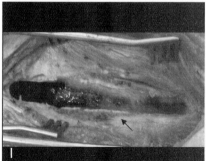

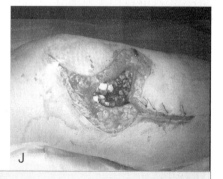

4: Specific Situations

Figure 4   Stage IIIA osteomyelitis. **A**, Lateral *(left)* and AP *(right)* radiographs showing an infected fracture union of the distal femur with indwelling hardware and sequestered cortex *(arrow)*. **B**, Photograph of a type II component found anteromedially *(outlined)*, with atrophic, woody soft tissues and a draining, fistulous tract *(arrow)*. **C**, Photograph of an acute abscess *(arrow)* forming at the apex of a lateral incision that was initially used to stabilize the fracture with a blade plate and screws. **D**, CT scan showing the tract of a blade plate passing through the femoral condyles *(arrow)* and communicating with a medullary abscess surrounding the hardware (a type I component). **E**, CT scan showing the cloaca associated with the abscess *(arrows)* seen in *C*. **F**, CT scan showing a cortical sequestrum *(arrow)* at the base of the fistula seen in *B*. **G**, CT scan showing evidence of sequestered cortex *(arrow)* more proximally. **H**, Intraoperative photograph showing the sequestrum seen in *A* and *F* *(arrow)* as well as the intended exposure *(broken line)* for unroofing the nidus. **I**, Intraoperative photograph showing the full cortical window used for nidus exposure and access for reaming the proximal diaphysis. **J**, Clinical photograph taken 3 days after the débridement showing the loosely approximated wound sealed with a transparent dressing to create an antibiotic bead pouch.

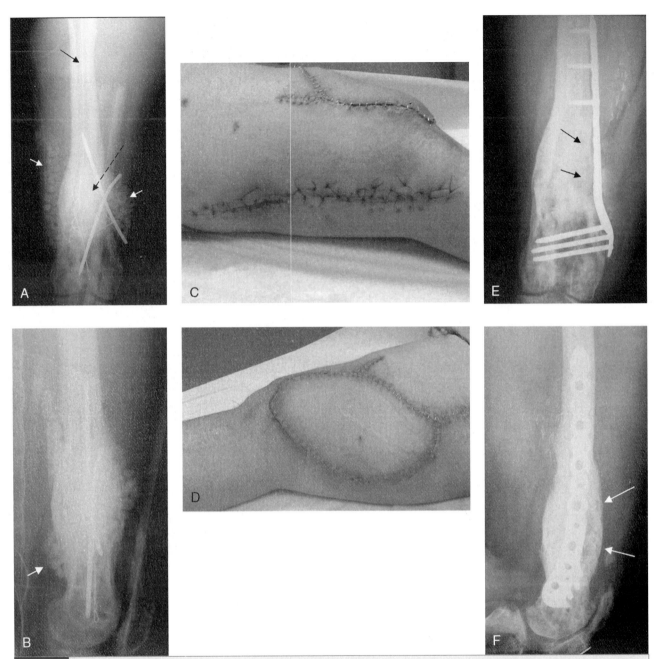

Figure 5 **A,** Postoperative AP **(A)** and lateral **(B)** radiographs showing the débridement defect in Figure 4, which was managed using an antibiotic spacer with rebar *(dashed black arrow)*, antibiotic beads in chains *(white arrows)*, and antibiotic beads on a wire *(solid black arrow)*. Clinical photographs taken at discharge show the lateral incision **(C)** used to débride the condyles, the abscess, and the proximal cloaca seen in Figure 4, *E*; and the rectus abdominis myocutaneous free flap **(D)** used to cover the medial wound. Three months later, the free flap was lifted to reconstruct the femur using a locking plate and cancellous bone grafts. AP **(E)** and lateral **(F)** radiographs taken at 2-year follow-up show plate fixation and consolidation of the bone grafts that restored continuity to medial *(black arrows)* and anterior *(white arrows)* cortices of the débridement defect.

collected during débridement, or both. The samples are collected from loculated fluids, inflamed tissues, and foreign bodies.[79,80] Compared with swab cultures, tissue blocks and actual fluid collections increase the yield of wound pathogens and provide substance for storage and revaluation as the treatment proceeds.

Frozen section biopsies are used to confirm the pres-

ence of an acute or chronic infection and facilitate the diagnosis of other pathologic processes, such as granulomatous inflammation and neoplasms mimicking infection. The microbiology laboratory is asked to perform 14-day cultures and sensitivity testing for aerobic and anaerobic bacterial species;[81] mycobacterial (acid-fast) and fungal cultures (if granulomas are seen on fro-

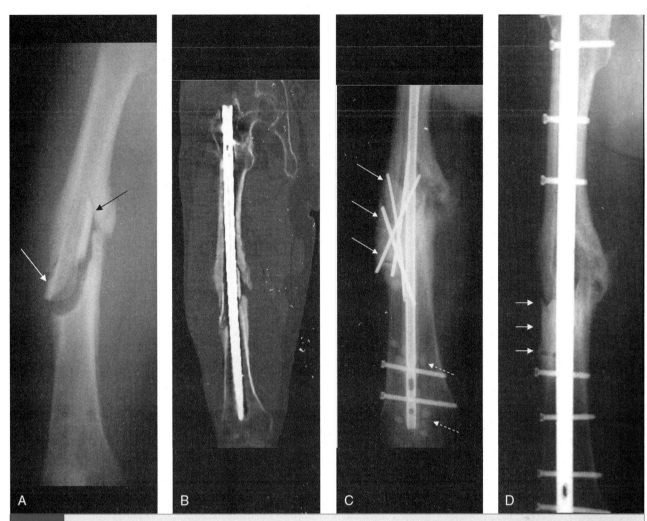

Figure 6	Stage IVA osteomyelitis. **A,** AP radiograph of an infected nonunion of the right femur. The fracture site is unstable, and multiple end sequestra can be seen *(arrows)*. **B,** AP radiograph showing the fracture as originally stabilized with a medullary rod. **C,** AP radiograph of the femur after a débridement that included unroofing at the non-union site, sequestrectomy, and both proximal and distal reaming of the medullary canal. Stability was established with a locked, antibiotic-coated nail. Residual dead space was managed with acute shortening, an antibiotic spacer *(solid arrows)*, and biodegradable antibiotic beads *(dashed arrows)*. A staged reconstruction took place 3 months later using a custom locked rod, an antibiotic spacer, and cancellous grafts. **D,** AP radiograph taken at 6-month follow-up, showing union of the femur, incorporation of the bone grafts, and the permanent antibiotic-loaded PMMA spacer along the lateral cortex *(arrows)*. The spacer was used to augment stability while the bone grafts and fracture site consolidated. At 3-year follow-up, the patient remained functional and infection free.

zen section); and vortex sonication cultures of foreign bodies, implants, and bony sequestra.[35] If a neoplasm is discovered on biopsy, additional tissue can be sent for specific processing.

After adequate tissue samples are secured for processing, broad-spectrum antibiotics are initiated based on the medical history, frozen sections, and most likely pathogens. Coverage is thereafter tailored to the sensitivities of the wound isolates. The ideal antibiotic coverage maintains a 1:1 ratio between a pathogen's mean inhibitory concentration and mean bactericidal concentration; serum concentrations are kept at least six times the mean bactericidal concentration.[3] No difference has been reported in the outcomes of oral and intravenous antibiotic regimens, providing the regimen is

bactericidal and covers all wound isolates. The duration of coverage varies with the anatomic site, the condition of the host, and the methods used.

Local Antibiotic Depots

Significant numbers of planktonic bacteria and microscopic fragments of the biofilm colony (sessile cells) persist after débridement, despite copious lavage. The high local concentrations of antimicrobial agents achieved in the seroma following implantation of an antibiotic depot are capable of killing residual pathogen phenotypes. In the United States, the use of antibiotic depots to treat infection is limited to handmade antibiotic beads and antibiotic spacers. To push the elution kinetics in favor of very high antibiotic concentrations, only high-dose

Table 2

Protocol for the Treatment of Adult Osteomyelitis

I. Evaluation

A. Medical History Related to Injury
- Mechanism and time of injury
- Treatment history (surgical procedures, cultures, sensitivities, antibiotic regimens)

B. Overall Medical History, Health, and Functional Status
- Comorbidities
- Cognitive and functional status
- Allergies
- Medications

C. Physical Examination
- Body habitus, gait, ambulatory aids
- Anatomic site (wounds, scars, tissue defects)
- Extremity status
- Neurovascular status

II. Preoperative Testing
- Laboratory values: full metabolic panel, complete blood cell count with differential, coagulation panel, urinalysis, erythrocyte sedimentation rate (ESR), C-reactive protein (CRP) level
- Diagnostic tests: vascular indices, angiography, ultrasonography, tissue oxygen tension measurements
- Radiographic studies: Plain radiography, MRI, CT, nuclear scanning, positron emission tomography
- Tissue biopsies

III. Clinical Staging
- Anatomic type: I, medullary; II, superficial; III, localized; IV, diffuse
- Physiologic class: A-host, B-host, C-host

IV. Treatment Format
- Limb salvage
- Amputation
- Palliation or suppression (no treatment for cure)

V. Host Optimization
- Reversal of amenable comorbidities
- Selection of low-risk procedures (for B-hosts)

VI. First Surgery

A. Single-Stage Treatment
- Débridement, biopsy, cultures, stabilization, systemic antibiotics
- Dead space management
  - Wound management (secondary-intention healing, primary closure, delayed closure)
  - Antibiotic depots (beads, gels)

B. First Stage of Two- or Three-Stage Treatment
- Débridement, biopsy, cultures, systemic antibiotics
  Double setup (new instruments, repreparation, redraping, new gowns and gloves)
- Temporary fixation
- Dead space management
  - Wound management (secondary-intention healing, primary closure, delayed closure)
  - Antibiotic depots (beads, spacers, gels, impregnated implants)

VII. Outpatient Follow-Up
- Monitoring of wound healing
- Laboratory values: ESR, CRP, albumin, prealbumin
- Physical rehabilitation

VIII. Second Surgery

A. Second Stage of Two-Stage Treatment: Definitive Reconstruction
- Prophylactic antibiotics
- Débridement, cultures, biopsy (with no evidence of acute infection)
  Double setup (new instruments, repreparation, redraping, new gowns and gloves)
- Reconstruction
  - Bone grafts, internal or external fixation, prosthetic implants
  - Antibiotic depots (beads, spacers, gels)

B. Second Stage of Three-Stage Treatment
- Prophylactic antibiotics
- Débridement, cultures, biopsy (with positive evidence of acute infection)
  Double setup (new instruments, repreparation, redraping, new gowns and gloves)
- Temporary fixation
- Dead space management
  - Wound management (secondary-intention healing, primary closure, delayed closure)
  - Antibiotic depots (beads, spacers, gels, impregnated implants)

IX. Third Surgery

A. Third Stage of Three-Stage Treatment: Definitive Reconstruction
- Prophylactic antibiotics
- Débridement, cultures, biopsy (with no evidence of acute infection)
  Double setup (new instruments, repreparation, redraping, new gowns and gloves)
- Reconstruction
  - Bone grafts, internal or external fixation, prosthetic implants
  - Antibiotic depots (beads, spacers, gels)

B. Third Stage of Four-Stage Treatment
- Prophylactic antibiotics
- Débridement, cultures, biopsy (with positive evidence of acute infection)
  Double setup (new instruments, repreparation, redraping, new gowns and gloves)
- Temporary fixation
- Dead space management
  - Wound management (secondary-intention healing, primary closure, delayed closure)
  - Antibiotic depots (beads, spacers, gels, impregnated implants)

X. Fourth Surgery
Biologic solutions (such as fusion, amputation, resection arthroplasty)

XI. Outpatient Follow-Up
- Monitoring of wound healing
- Laboratory values: ESR, CRP (at 3-month follow-up)
- Twice-yearly follow-up for 2 years

Table 3

Initial Success Rates After Reconstruction of Débridement Defects Using Procedures Associated With a High or Low Rate of Surgical Morbidity

Procedure	Number of Procedures	Successful Initial Outcome (%)	
		A-Host (Noncompromised Patient)	B-Host (Compromised Patient)
High Morbidity*			
Muscle flap[68]	130	95	75
Cancellous graft[69]	150	94	79
Papineau graft[70]	20	80	20
Free fibula flap[68,71]	42	83	59
Revision prosthesis[59]	74	96	76
Osteosynthesis[72]	458	96	75
Low Morbidity†			
Bone transposition[73]	78	98	92
Simple closure[59,74]	142	96	91
Bone transport[56]	120	76	72
Permanent spacers[55]	44	93	88

*Procedures performed through June 2004.
†Procedures performed through January 2007.
(Adapted from Cierny G III, DiPasquale D: Treatment of chronic infection. *J Am Acad Orthop Surg* 2006;14:S109.)

antibiotic mixtures are used in the composites.[68,82-86] Commercially available antibiotic-loaded bone cements contain low-dose antibiotic mixtures and are intended only for prophylactic use in revision total joint arthroplasty. Polymethylmethacrylate (PMMA) is the material most commonly used in local-depot beads and spacers. Palacos bone cement (Zimmer, Warsaw, IN) is the preferred PMMA carrier because of its superior release kinetics. Following implantation, the antibiotic implants can be left in place indefinitely; removed during a separate procedure; or exchanged for bone grafts, flaps, or hardware[75,85,87] (**Figure 1, G; Figure 5, E and F;** and **Figure 6, C and D**).

The use of biodegradable calcium sulfate beads (OsteoSet, Wright Medical, Memphis, TN; Stimulan, Biocomposites, Wilmington, NC) obviates any concerns about leaving permanent acrylic depots in situ, but these beads have their own limitations. They are not sturdy enough to act as structural spacers; the amounts and types of antibiotics they can deliver are limited due to interactions altering their set-time characteristics; and wound fistulas may develop because of a voluminous by-product of degradation.[84]

Stage-Directed Treatment Protocols

Type I: Medullary Osteomyelitis

Medical treatment should be used alone for type I osteomyelitis only in three specific clinical scenarios:

asymptomatic, hematogenous lesions coincidentally discovered during evaluation of a patient with fever, weight loss, or bacteremia; hematogenous infection caused by sensitive microbacteria or fungi; or hematogenous vertebral osteomyelitis caused by sensitive pathogens.[3,19] Otherwise, type I osteomyelitis is a surgical disease requiring débridement (**Figure 1**).

The medullary nidus is approached through a cortical window, either directly by excising the cortex to unroof the lesion or indirectly by reaming from above or below. For reaming, the disease must be confined to an isthmus; otherwise, a combination of reaming and unroofing is necessary to treat the truncated medullary abscess found at a metaphyseal-diaphyseal junction. The procedures used to treat type I osteomyelitis also are applicable for type III or IV infections with a medullary component.

Because soft tissues are rarely compromised in type I osteomyelitis, the dead space after débridement usually is limited to the canal. The treatment of choice is implantation of an acrylic or biodegradable antibiotic depot (see chapter 9). If the organism is known and the soft tissues are supple, the wound can be closed primarily without concern. Otherwise, a 3- to 5-day delay in closure is indicated. Reactive soft-tissue involvement usually responds to a brief course of systemic antibiotics. Soft-tissue flaps are rarely necessary. The surgical site may require protection for 3 to 6 months following débridement to allow the bone and the host to recover and prevent an insufficiency fracture. Protection can be provided by using an ambulatory aid, external fixation device, or internal splint such as a rod or plate coated with antibiotic-impregnated composite.

Type II: Superficial Osteomyelitis

Because the etiology of a type II lesion is compromise to the soft-tissue envelope, preoperative planning must focus on restoration of the soft tissue. Angiograms, transcutaneous oxygen tension measurements, and vascular indices are used to assess the deficit and locate available portals for the reconstruction. The nidus itself is best mapped with a MRI study defining the zone of injury. If concomitant medullary infection is discovered, the lesion is classified as type III or IV osteomyelitis.

Treatment begins with resection of the soft tissue to viable, supple margins. The bony débridement is tangential, with an end point of uniform haversian bleeding (the paprika sign).[88] The soft-tissue management requires the surgeon to have considerable experience with tissue transfers, the clinical application of vascular territories, and the interpretation of vascular studies to predict wound healing. Transpositions, free flap transfers, and open bone transport[30,31] are the methods most commonly used in the restoration process.[89,90] Despite high rates of success, flaps sometimes fail or cannot be used.[91] In this regard, negative pressure wound therapy using vacuum-assisted closure (V.A.C. Therapy, KCI, San Antonio, TX) is a powerful option if no further reconstruction is needed.[92-94]

Type III: Localized Osteomyelitis

The treatment of type III osteomyelitis requires complete resection of the cortical sequestrum. Techniques for treating type I and type II lesions can be used. The débrided wound often is a composite defect involving both hard and soft tissues. If the osseous resection is extensive enough to threaten the integrity of the remaining osseous segment, measures should be taken to prevent an insufficiency fracture. The limb may be stabilized before débridement with a bypass bone graft, an external fixator, or both.[95-97] Alternatively, in situ stabilization can be performed immediately after the débridement, using an antibiotic-coated implant or spacer (Figure 1, G; Figure 5, A and B; and Figure 6, C).

Type II components found in type III osteomyelitis usually are treated with tissue transpositions or transfers. If an osseous reconstruction is indicated or a significant dead space will exist after closure, an antibiotic depot is implanted and a two- or three-stage reconstruction is planned. Otherwise, a primary closure is indicated, with or without a depot.

Type IV: Diffuse Osteomyelitis

Débridement of a type IV lesion creates an unstable wound with all or some of the characteristics of type I, II, and III osteomyelitis. An extended zone of injury and concomitant comorbidities (for example, previous compartment syndrome, vascular injury or disease, radiation injury) create obstacles to restoring the soft-

tissue envelope. Ipsilateral deformities and bone loss limit fixation options. As a result, type IV treatment protocols are diverse and challenging (Figure 7). More than 50% of these lesions require a staged, soft-tissue, or dead space restoration before osseous reconstruction. Following débridement, the goal is restorative: the limb is stabilized, a supple soft-tissue envelope is re-established, and residual dead space is maintained and treated with antibiotic depots (beads, spacers). If the soft tissues are adequate, the first stage can be completed at the same time as the débridement. Otherwise, completion may be delayed to enable the coverage teams to achieve complex tissue transpositions and/or microvascular transfers (Figure 4, J and Figure 5, B).[73,98] Once the wounds have healed and the patient is able to tolerate further surgery, osseous reconstruction is done as the second stage, using external or internal fixation, bone graft, a prosthetic total joint, or allograft composite.

Hard- and soft-tissue defects can be simultaneously restored and reconstructed. Following débridement and stabilization, composite defects can be eliminated by interposing a composite bone flap (for example, with microvascular transfer of a free fibula graft with an attached skin paddle). Using the methods of Ilizarov, a newly created segment of healthy bone and its attached soft-tissue envelope can be pulled or pushed (transported) along the axis of the limb and into a resection defect using an external fixator. The process is similar to the manner in which orthodontic braces move and align teeth in the oral cavity. Here, a transport segment is created by performing a subperiosteal transverse osteotomy (corticotomy) through a healthy portion of the bone, somewhere between its defect end and the joint and either above or below the débridement defect. The size of the transport piece is determined by the length of bone required for secure purchase of all bony segments using fixation wires and half pins. The fixator construct itself is engineered to permit controlled movements of all segments relative to one another. Constructs can be fashioned to accommodate compression (shortening); compression and distraction (shortening and lengthening); single or multiple bone transports; and simultaneous compression, distraction, and transport. Movement of the bone away from its corticotomy site usually is limited to between 0.5 mm and 1.0 mm per day (the rate of distraction) to allow new bone (regenerate) to form in the wake of the moving segment. The new bone is created by the process of distraction osteogenesis, in which host tissues in the corticotomy site make new columns of bone when they are exposed to the slow, controlled tension forces created by the fixator as it moves the transport segment away from the corticotomy and toward the defect. Transport is complete when this segment crosses the defect and is compressed against the opposing surface as an osteosynthesis. Bony continuity thus is restored while in the fixator; the defect is eliminated by the transport segment, and intrinsic stability is restored when the osteosynthesis heals and the regenerate consolidates to corti-

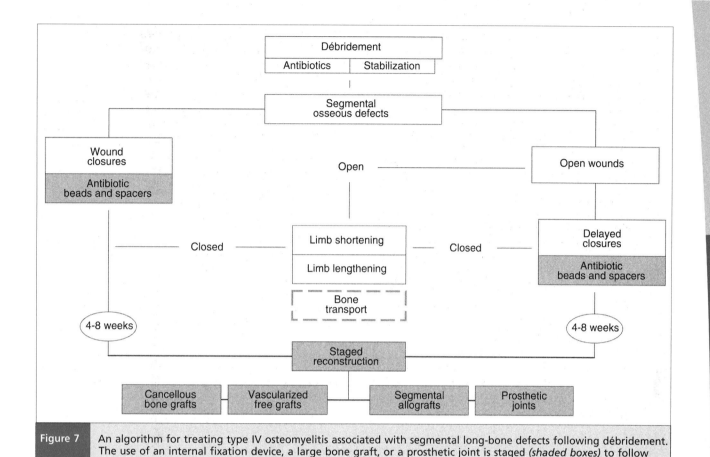

Figure 7 An algorithm for treating type IV osteomyelitis associated with segmental long-bone defects following débridement. The use of an internal fixation device, a large bone graft, or a prosthetic joint is staged *(shaded boxes)* to follow coverage and implantation of antibiotic-impregnated beads and spacers. Bone transport can be staged to follow the same coverage and antibiotic-bead protocols; however, there appears to be no statistical difference in treatment outcomes between open and closed transport methods, provided that cancellous bone grafts are used to support healing at the docking site.[56] (Adapted from Cierny G III, DiPasquale D: Treatment of chronic infection. *J Am Acad Orthop Surg* 2006;14:S108.)

cal bone. Pin capture of the soft tissues with the transport segment allows composite hard- and soft-tissue defects to be eliminated from within the injured limb segment, obviating the need for complex technical methods of harvesting and transferring living tissues from distant anatomic sites.[56]

Acute shortening can be accomplished using some of these principles. An advantage of shortening is that both osteosynthesis and closure can be accomplished quickly. Shortening of 3 to 4 cm can be tolerated acutely; larger defects require a more gradual approximation to avoid compromise to perfusion and lymphatic drainage. The shortened limb is accepted as an end point of the reconstruction or is subsequently lengthened using these distraction principles.[57] Figure 8 is a historical profile of the authors' methods for reconstructing segmental defects in the long bones of adults with osteomyelitis.

Results of Treatment

In a 15-year chronological study, 1,966 patients with chronic osteomyelitis were evaluated at the authors' centers.[55] Of these patients, 104 (5%) were classified as

C-hosts and initially received palliative treatment alone. Limb salvage protocols were offered to 1,651 patients (84%), and 216 (11%) underwent a primary partial- or whole-limb ablation. With success defined as survival with an infection-free segment that met all functional expectations, the success rate following the first attempt at treatment was 84%, including 96% of the A-hosts and 73% of the B-hosts. No significant differences were found between the outcomes of patients treated using an internal or external fixation strategy, patients with a monomicrobial or polymicrobial infection, or patients with a sensitive or resistant pathogen.[48] The infection-free survival rates were similar after all biologic treatment methods, including bone transport and lengthening, bypass bone grafting, microvascular transfer of segmental bone grafts, and massive cancellous bone grafts. However, success rates decreased an average of 6% if internal hardware was used both for the method of fixation and the form of reconstruction, as is done with intercalary allograft, prosthetic total joint arthroplasty, and permanent PMMA spacers.

The initial treatment failed in 315 (16%) of the 1,966 patients, including 22 (22%) of the C-hosts,

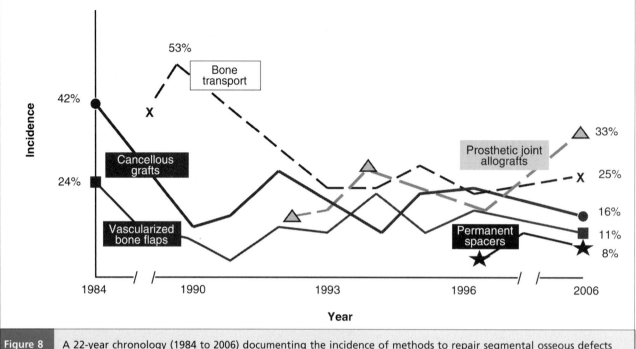

Figure 8	A 22-year chronology (1984 to 2006) documenting the incidence of methods to repair segmental osseous defects following débridement for infection. From 1993 to 1996, utilization patterns converged after each method was matched to a specific set of wound, host, and experience-based parameters. The introduction of permanent antibiotic-loaded PMMA spacers in 1996 added a salvage option for the treatment of severely compromised hosts with disabling musculoskeletal infections (Figure 6, *D*). By 2006, the primary amputation rate had fallen to 6%, and the incidence of C-hosts (nontreatment candidates) had fallen to 2%. (Adapted from Cierny G III, DiPasquale D: Treatment of chronic infection. *J Am Acad Orthop Surg* 2006;14:S107.)

19 (9%) of the patients undergoing ablation, and 274 (17%) of the patients undergoing a limb salvage attempt. The reasons for treatment failure included aseptic nonunion (43%), recurrent sepsis (12%), unexpected functional impairment (15%), wound breakdown (28%), and unrelated death within the first year (2%). A retreatment to achieve cure was attempted in 275 of the 308 surviving patients, and a retreatment success rate of 82% boosted the overall 2-year success rate to 95%[55,98] (Table 4).

Summary

Chronic osteomyelitis is refractory to nonsurgical treatment because a resilient infective nidus harbors sessile, matrix-protected pathogens bound to substrate surfaces. The clinical stage of the disease determines the surgical planning, defines the candidates for treatment, and establishes a means of comparing outcomes. Curative treatment mandates the physical removal of the entire biofilm colony. Thereafter, the limb is stabilized, residual pathogens are eliminated by using local and systemic antibiotics, and every effort is made to optimize the host response. The reconstruction is guided by wound parameters affecting outcomes such as bone integrity, fixation requirements, and soft-tissue adequacy to support both the wound closure and the reconstruction.

Table 4		

Success Rates for Adult Chronic Osteomyelitis, by Clinical Stage (Minimum 2-Year Follow-Up)

Stage	Number of Patients	Success Rate (%)
A-Host (47%)		
IA	49	100
IIA	89	100
IIIA	206	98
IVA	586	99
Total	930	99
B-Host (53%)		
IB	58	95
IIB	159	88
IIIB	115	94
IVB	704	90
Total	1,036	91
Total	**1,966**	**95**

Annotated References

1. Gristina AG: Biomaterial-centered infection: Microbial adhesion versus tissue integration. *Science* 1987;237: 1588-1595.

2. Costerton JW, Stewart PS, Greenberg EP: Bacterial biofilms: A common cause of persistent infections. *Science* 1999;284:1318-1322.

3. Cierny G III, Mader JT: The surgical treatment of adult osteomyelitis, in Evarts C, McCollister MD (ed): *Surgery of the Musculoskeletal System*. New York, NY: Churchill Livingstone, 1983, pp 4814-4834.

4. Clawson DK, Dunn AW: Management of common bacterial infections of bones and joints. *J Bone Joint Surg Am* 1967;49:164-182.

5. Taylor AR, Maudsley RH: Instillation-suction technique in chronic osteomyelitis. *J Bone Joint Surg Br* 1970;52: 88-92.

6. Burri C, Passler HH, Henkemeyer H: Treatment of posttraumatic osteomyelitis with bone, soft tissue, and skin defects. *J Trauma* 1973;13:799-810.

7. Shannon JG, Woolhouse FM, Eisinger PJ: The treatment of chronic osteomyelitis by saucerization and immediate skin grafting. *Clin Orthop Relat Res* 1973;96:98-107.

8. Kelly PJ, Wilkowske CJ, Washington JA II: Chronic osteomyelitis in the adult. *Curr Pract Orthop Surg* 1975; 6:120-127.

9. Harmon PJ: A simplified surgical approach to the posterior tibia for bone grafting and fibular transference. *J Bone Joint Surg Am* 1945;27:496-498.

10. Campanacci M, Zaanoli S: Double tibiofibular synostosis (fibula pro tibia) for non-union and delayed union of the tibia: End result review of one hundred seventy-one cases. *J Bone Joint Surg Am* 1966;48:44-56.

11. Papineau LJ: Osteocutaneous resection-reconstruction in diaphyseal osteomyelitis. *Clin Orthop Relat Res* 1974;101:306.

12. Waldvogel FA, Papageorgiou PS: Osteomyelitis: The last decade. *N Engl J Med* 1980;303:360-370.

13. Kelly PJ, Martin WJ, Coventry MB: Chronic osteomyelitis: II. Treatment with closed irrigation and suction. *JAMA* 1970;213:1843-1848.

14. Clawson DK, Davis FJ, Hansen ST Jr: Treatment of chronic osteomyelitis with emphasis on closed suction-irrigation technique. *Clin Orthop Relat Res* 1973;96: 88-97.

15. Whiteside LA, Lesker PA: The effects of extraperiosteal and subperiosteal dissection: I. On blood flow in muscle. *J Bone Joint Surg Am* 1978;60:23-30.

16. Mathes SJ, Alpert BS, Chang N: Use of the muscle flap in chronic osteomyelitis: Experimental and clinical correlation. *Plast Reconstr Surg* 1982;69:815-829.

17. Mathes SJ, Feng LJ, Hunt TK: Coverage of the infected wound. *Ann Surg* 1983;198:420-429.

18. Gristina AG, Costerton JW: Bacterial adherence and the glycocalyx and their role in musculoskeletal infection. *Orthop Clin North Am* 1984;15:517-535.

19. Cierny G, Mader JT, Pennick JJ: A clinical staging for adult osteomyelitis. *Clin Orthop Relat Res* 2003;414: 7-24.

    This a republication of a paper originally published in 1985 in a nonrefereed journal. The staging system now called the Cierny-Mader classification system for adult osteomyelitis is described. Included are the authors' theoretical approach to medical and surgical management, treatment algorithms, and outcomes of the first 192 patients treated in prospective protocols from 1981 to 1983.

20. Perry CR, Pearson RL, Miller GA: Accuracy of cultures of material from swabbing of the superficial aspect of the wound and needle biopsy in preoperative assessment of osteomyelitis. *J Bone Joint Surg Am* 1991;73: 745-749.

21. Chang CC, Merritt K: Infection at the site of implanted materials with and without pre-adhered bacteria. *J Orthop Res* 1994;12:526-531.

22. Patzakis MJ, Wilkins J, Kumar J, et al: Comparison of the results of bacterial cultures from multiple sites in chronic osteomyelitis of long bones: A prospective study. *J Bone Joint Surg Am* 1994;76:664-666.

23. Heppenstall RB, Goodwin CW, Brighton CT: Fracture healing in the presence of chronic hypoxia. *J Bone Joint Surg Am* 1976;58:1153-1156.

24. Damholt VV: Treatment of chronic osteomyelitis: A prospective study of 55 cases treated with radical surgery and primary wound closure. *Acta Orthop Scand* 1982;53:715-720.

25. Lortat-Jacob A, Guiziou B, Ramadier JO: Septic leg fractures: Value of cancellous bone grafting without skin closure, aligned on the fibula. *Rev Chir Orthop Reparatrice Appar Mot* 1985;71:515-526.

26. Esterhai JL Jr, Sennett B, Gelb H, et al: Treatment of chronic osteomyelitis complicating nonunion and segmental defects of the tibia with open cancellous bone graft, posterolateral bone graft, and soft-tissue transfer. *J Trauma* 1990;30:49-54.

27. Gayle LB, Lineaweaver WC, Oliva A, et al: Treatment of chronic osteomyelitis of the lower extremities with debridement and microvascular muscle transfer. *Clin Plast Surg* 1992;19:895-903.

28. Swiontkowski MF, Hanel DP, Vedder NB, Schwappach JR: A comparison of short- and long-term intravenous antibiotic therapy in the postoperative management of adult osteomyelitis. *J Bone Joint Surg Br* 1999; 81:1046-1050.

29. Simpson AH, Deakin M, Latham JM: Chronic osteomyelitis: The effect of the extent of surgical resection on infection-free survival. *J Bone Joint Surg Br* 2001;83: 403-407.

30. Ilizarov GA: The tension-stress effect of the genesis and growth of tissues: Part I. The influence of stability of fixation and soft tissue preservation. *Clin Orthop Relat Res* 1989;238:249-281.

31. Ilizarov GA: The tension-stress effect on the genesis and growth of tissues: Part II. The influence of the rate and frequency of distraction. *Clin Orthop Relat Res* 1989; 239:263-285.

32. Selan L, Passariello L, Rizzo L, et al: Diagnosis of vascular graft infections with antibodies against staphylococcal slime antigens. *Lancet* 2002;359:2166-2168.

33. Balaban N, Stoodley P, Fux CA, et al: Prevention of staphylococcal biofilm-associated infections by the quorum sensing inhibitor RIP. *Clin Orthop Relat Res* 2005;437: 48-54.

    Genes important to the formation of biofilm and toxin production appeared to be downregulated in all staphylococcal species by interference with quorum sensing, a complex regulatory process involved in cell-to-cell communication. Exposure to ribonucleic-acid-III-inhibiting peptide (a quorum-sensing inhibitor) prevented or enhanced resolution of implant-related staphylococcal infections.

34. McDowell A, Patrick S: Evaluation of nonculture methods for the detection of prosthetic hip biofilms. *Clin Orthop Relat Res* 2005;437:74-82.

    Immunofluorescence microscopy is an attractive and reliable method for routine detection of prosthetic hip biofilms, compared with polymerase chain reaction (PCR). The technique is relatively simple, in contrast to broad-range 16S recombinant-deoxyribonucleic-acid–based PCR. Dislodged biofilm colonies can be differentiated from skin contaminants.

35. Kobayashi M, Bauer TW, Tuohy MJ, Fujishiro T, Procop GW: Brief ultrasonication improves detection of biofilm-formative bacteria around metal implants. *Clin Orthop Relat Res* 2007;457:210-213.

    The authors sought to determine whether ultrasonication could disrupt biofilms and thereby make a sessile microorganism or its DNA available for detection. Quantitative cultures and real-time PCR were used to determine the influence of different durations of ultrasonication on bacterial adherence and viability. Sonication for 1 minute increased the yield of bacteria; sonication for more than 5 minutes led to fewer bacterial colonies on conventional culture but not PCR, suggesting lysis of the organisms with the higher exposure.

36. Greer S, Kasabian A, Thorne C, Borud L, Sims CD, Hsu M: The use of a subatmospheric pressure dressing to salvage a Gustilo grade IIIB open tibial fracture with concomitant osteomyelitis to avert a free flap. *Ann Plast Surg* 1998;41:687.

37. Webb LX: New techniques in wound management: Vacuum-assisted wound closure. *J Am Acad Orthop Surg* 2002;10:303-311.

38. McCraw JB, Dibbell DG, Carraway JH: Clinical definition of independent myocutaneous vascular territories. *Plast Reconstr Surg* 1977;60:341-352.

39. O'Brien BM, Henderson PN, Bennett RC, Crock GW: Microvascular surgical techniques. *Med J Aust* 1970;1: 722-725.

40. McLean DH, Buncke HJ: Autotransplant of omentum to a large scalp defect, with microsurgical revascularization. *Plast Reconstr Surg* 1972;49:268-274.

41. Taylor GI, Miller GD, Ham FJ: The free vascularized bone graft: A clinical extension of microvascular techniques. *Plast Reconstr Surg* 1975;55:533-544.

42. Vasconez LO, Bostwick J III, McCraw J: Coverage of exposed bone by muscle transposition and skin grafting. *Plast Reconstr Surg* 1974;53:526-531.

43. Ger R: Muscle transposition for treatment and prevention of chronic posttraumatic osteomyelitis of the tibia. *J Bone Joint Surg Am* 1977;59:784-791.

44. Klemm K: Die Behandlung Chronischer Knowcken Infektionen Mit Gentamicin PMMA Ketten und Kulgen, in Contzen HE (ed): *Gentamicin-PMMA Kette: Symposium.* Munich, Germany, Verlag fur Lehrmittel, Wissenschaft und Forschung, 1976, pp 20-22.

45. Wahlig H, Dingeldein E, Bergmann R, Reuss K: The release of gentamicin from polymethylmethacrylate beads: An experimental and pharmacokinetic study. *J Bone Joint Surg Br* 1978;60:270-275.

46. Walenkamp GH: *Gentamicin PMMA Beads: A Clinical, Pharmacokinetic and Toxicologic study.* Amsterdam, The Netherlands, Drukkerij Cliteur, 1983, pp 19-22.

47. Cierny G III: Infected tibial nonunions (1981-1995): The evolution of change. *Clin Orthop Relat Res* 1999; 360:97-105.

48. Berard F, Gandon J: Postoperative wound infections: The influence of ultraviolet irradiation of the operating room and of various other factors. *Ann Surg* 1964; 160(suppl 2):1-192.

49. Cierny G III: Managing the debridement defect, in Coombs R, Fitzgerald R (eds): *Infection in the Orthopaedic Patient.* London, England, Butterworth Publishers, 1989.

50. Hovelius L, Josefsson G: An alternative method for exchange operation of infected arthroplasty. *Acta Orthop Scand* 1979;50:93-96.

51. Salvati EA, Chekofsky KM, Brause BD, Wilson PD Jr: Reimplantation in infection: A 12-year experience. *Clin Orthop Relat Res* 1982;170:62-75.

52. Enneking WF, Spanier SS, Goodman MA: A system for the surgical staging of musculoskeletal sarcoma. *Clin Orthop Relat Res* 1980;153:106-120.

53. Klemm K, Winter-Klemm B: Unconscious guilt in the treatment of infected patients, in Coombs R, Fitzgerald R (eds): *Infection in the Orthopaedic Patient*. London, England, Butterworth Publishers, 1989.

54. Yajima H, Tamai S, Mizumoto S, Inada Y: Vascularized fibular grafts in the treatment of osteomyelitis and infected nonunion. *Clin Orthop Relat Res* 1993;293: 256-264.

55. Cierny G III, DiPasquale D: Treatment of chronic infection. *J Am Acad Orthop Surg* 2006;14:S105-S110.

    This is a 15-year chronological history of one center's experience of treating segmental, osseous, and composite defects in 1,966 adult patients with chronic osteomyelitis. Identification of a subset of low-risk surgical procedures closes the outcomes gap between healthy and compromised patients.

56. Cierny G III, Zorn K: Segmental tibial defects: Comparing conventional and Ilizarov methodologies. *Clin Orthop Relat Res* 1994;301:118-123.

57. Sen C, Kocaoglu M, Eralp L, Gulsen M, Cinar M: Bifocal compression-distraction in the acute treatment of grade III open tibia fractures with bone and soft-tissue loss: A report of 24 cases. *J Orthop Trauma* 2004;18: 150-157.

    Patients with bone defects as large as 3 cm were treated with acute shortening at the fracture site to achieve apposition of bone ends. Gradual shortening at a rate of 2 mm per day was done for patients who had bone defects larger than 3 cm. Limb-length discrepancy was overcome by lengthening at the same time through a surgically created site at a proximal or distal level, depending on fracture location. Bone assessment results were excellent in 21 and good in 3 patients. Functional assessment scores were excellent in 19, good in 4, and fair in 1 patient.

58. Younger AS, Duncan P, Masri BA: Treatment of infection associated with segmental bone loss in the proximal part of the femur in two stages with the use of an antibiotic-loaded interval prosthesis. *J Bone Joint Surg Am* 1998;80:60-69.

59. Cierny G III, DiPasquale D: Periprosthetic total joint infections: Staging, treatment, and outcomes. *Clin Orthop Relat Res* 2002;403:23-28.

60. Cobos JA, Lindsey RW, Gugala Z: The cylindrical titanium mesh cage for treatment of long bone segmental defects: Description of a new technique and report of two cases. *J Orthop Trauma* 2000;14:54-59.

61. Waldvogel FA, Medoff G, Swartz MN: Osteomyelitis: A review of clinical features, therapeutic considerations, and unusual aspects. *N Engl J Med* 1970;282:198-316.

62. McPherson EJ, Tontz WT, Patzakis M, et al: Outcome of infected total knees utilizing a staging system for prosthetic joint infection. *Am J Orthop* 1999;28: 161-165.

63. Lai K, Bohm ER, Burnell C, Hedden DR: Presence of medical co-morbidities in patients with infected primary hip or knee arthroplasties. *J Arthroplasty* 2007;22: 651-656.

    A retrospective, case-controlled study examined the individual and cumulative effects of medical comorbidities on the risk of developing a periprosthetic joint infection after surgery. Diabetes mellitus and total number of medical conditions both were associated with an increased risk of surgical site infection.

64. Patzakis MJ, Zalavras CG: Chronic posttraumatic osteomyelitis and infected nonunion of the tibia: Current management concepts. *J Am Acad Orthop Surg* 2005; 13:417-427.

    An algorithm is presented for retaining or removing an infected implant when treating acute and chronic osteomyelitis of the tibia. Bone healing, stability provided by the hardware, fracture location, and time since fracture fixation must be considered.

65. Cierny G III: Infection following open fractures, in Levin LS (ed): *Complications in Orthopaedics: Open Fractures*. Rosemont, IL, American Academy of Orthopaedic Surgeons, in press.

    Successfully applied suppression protocols shorten time to union, decrease the cost of care, and curtail patient morbidity. The details and complexity of such management depend on the clinical stage of osteomyelitis, the time since injury or intervention, and the extent of the necrotic focus. Acute and chronic treatment protocols are designed to parallel the fundamental principles of microbial colonization of biomaterials.

66. Kunisada T, Ngan SY, Powell G, Choong PF: Wound complications following pre-operative radiotherapy for soft tissue sarcoma. *Eur J Surg Oncol* 2002;28:75-79.

67. Emori TG, Gaynes RP: An overview of nosocomial infections, including the role of microbiology laboratory. *Clin Microbiol Rev* 1993;6:428-442.

68. Cierny G III: Chronic osteomyelitis: Results of treatment. *Instr Course Lect* 1990;39:495-508.

69. Cierny G III, Matava M, Zorn KE: Cancellous bone grafting in the presence of bacterial contamination: Indications, methods, long-term results. *Orthop Trans* 1990;14:633.

70. Matava M, Cierny G, Zorn KE: Papineau grafting: Still a treatment option? *Orthop Trans* 1991;15:616-617.

4: Specific Situations

71. Cierny G III, Nahai F: Dialogue: Lower extremity reconstruction. Part 2. *Perspect Plast Surg* 1988;2: 109-121.

72. Cierny G III: The classification and treatment of adult osteomyelitis, in Evarts CM (ed): *Surgery of the Musculoskeletal System*, ed 2. New York, NY, Churchill Livingstone, 1990, pp 4337-4379.

73. Cierny G III, Axelrod B, Mader JT: Ipsilateral fibular transfers in the treatment of tibial osteomyelitis defects. *Orthop Trans* 1989;13:535.

74. Cierny G III, Byrd SH, Jones RE: Primary versus delayed soft tissue coverage for severe open tibial fractures: A comparison of results. *Clin Orthop Relat Res* 1983;178:54-63.

75. Ostermann PA, Seligson D, Henry SL: Local antibiotic therapy for severe open fractures: A review of 1085 consecutive cases. *J Bone Joint Surg Br* 1995;77:93-97.

76. Engesaeter LB, Lie SA, Espehaug B, et al: Antibiotic prophylaxis in total hip arthroplasty: Effects of antibiotic prophylaxis systemically and in bone cement on the revision rate of 22,170 primary hip replacements followed 0-14 years in the Norwegian Arthroplasty Register. *Acta Orthop Scand* 2003;74:644-651.

    A study of 22,000 hip replacements produced clear data on 10-year survivorship for all types of prostheses and all reasons for revision. Using antibiotics in the cement improved survivorship when both aseptic and septic loosening were considered.

77. Erdman WA, Tamburro F, Jayson HT, et al: Osteomyelitis: Characteristics and pitfalls of diagnosis with MR imaging. *Radiology* 1991;180:533-539.

78. Gross T, Kaim AH, Regazzoni P, Widmer AF: Current concepts in posttraumatic osteomyelitis: A diagnostic challenge with new imaging options. *J Trauma* 2002;52: 1210-1210.

79. Perry CR, Pearson RL, Miller GA: Accuracy of cultures of material from swabbing of the superficial aspect of the wound and needle biopsy in the preoperative assessment of osteomyelitis. *J Bone Joint Surg Am* 1991;73: 745-749.

80. Patzakis MJ, Wilkins J, Kumar J, Holtom P, Greenbaum B, Ressler R: Comparison of the results of bacterial cultures from multiple sites in chronic osteomyelitis of long bones: A prospective study. *J Bone Joint Surg Am* 1994;76:664-666.

81. Tunney MM, Patrick S, Gorman SP, et al: Improved detection of infection in hip replacements: A currently underestimated problem. *J Bone Joint Surg Br* 1998;80: 568-572.

82. Adams K, Couch L, Cierny G III, et al: In vitro and in vivo evaluation of antibiotic diffusion from antibiotic-impregnated poly-methylmethacrylate beads. *Clin Orthop Relat Res* 1992;278:244-252.

83. Younger AS, Duncan CP, Masri BA: Treatment of infection associated with segmental bone loss in the proximal part of the femur in two stages with the use of an antibiotic-loaded interval prosthesis. *J Bone Joint Surg Am* 1998;80:60-69.

84. McKee MD, Wild LM, Schemitsch EH, Waddell JP: The use of an antibiotic-impregnated, osteoconductive, bioabsorbable bone substitute in the treatment of infected long bone defects: Early results of a prospective trial. *J Orthop Trauma* 2002;16:622-627.

85. Paley D, Herzenberg JE: Intramedullary infections treated with antibiotic cement rods: Preliminary results in nine cases. *J Orthop Trauma* 2002;16:723-729.

86. Hanssen AD: Local antibiotic delivery vehicles in the treatment of musculoskeletal infection. *Clin Orthop Relat Res* 2005;437:91-96.

    Antibiotic delivery vehicles available in the United States were reviewed. Five aminoglycoside low-dosage composites were approved by the Food and Drug Administration. The low dosage and type of antibiotics present in these composites are appropriate for prophylaxis rather than treatment of an established infection.

87. Henry SL, Seligson D: Management of open fractures and osteomyelitis with the antibiotic beads pouch technique. *South Med J* 1990;83:98-104.

88. Sachs BL, Shaffer JW: Abstract: Osteomyelitis of the tibia and femur. A critical evaluation of the effectiveness of the Papineau technique in a prospective study. *50th Annual Meeting Proceedings*. Park Ridge, IL, American Academy of Orthopaedic Surgeons, 1983.

89. Lutz DA, Hallock GG: Microsurgical transfer of vascularized tissue to close problem wounds. *AORN J* 1995; 62:234-248.

90. Kolker AR, Kasabian AK, Karp NS, Gottlieb JJ: Fate of free flap microanastomosis distal to the zone of injury in lower extremity trauma. *Plast Reconstr Surg* 1997; 99:1068-1073.

91. Archdeacon MT, Herscovici D Jr, Sanders RW: Wound care: Debridement, coverage, and antibiotic utilization. *Tech Orthop* 2001;16:398-408.

92. Argenta LC, Morykwas MJ: Vacuum-assisted closure: A new method for wound control and treatment: Clinical experience. *Ann Plast Surg* 1997;38:563-577.

93. Datiashvili RO, Knox KR: Negative pressure dressings: An alternative to free tissue transfers? *Wounds* 2005;17: 206-212.

    Negative pressure wound therapy was used in the treatment of open wounds of the extremities with relatively large areas of exposed bone. The mechanism of effectiveness was believed to be granulation tissue expanding over the exposed bone from adjacent areas of the wound, and the biomechanical properties and texture of the granulation tissue were believed to prevent joint contractures.

94. Lam WL, Garrido A, Stanley PR: Use of topical negative pressure in the treatment of chronic osteomyelitis: A case report. *J Bone Joint Surg Am* 2005;87:622-624.

    A patient with chronic osteomyelitis had recurrences with failed skin grafts, pedicled flaps, and free flaps. Topical negative pressure was successfully used as a salvage procedure before a planned amputation.

95. Harmon PJ: A simplified surgical approach to the posterior tibia for bone grafting and fibular transference. *J Bone Joint Surg Am* 1945;27:496-498.

96. Campanacci M, Zaanoli S: Double tibiofibular synostosis (fibula pro tibia) for non-union and delayed union of the tibia: End result review of one hundred seventy-one cases. *J Bone Joint Surg Am* 1966;48:44-56.

97. Fodor L, Ulmann Y, Soudry M, Calif E, Lerner A: Prophylactic external fixation and extensive debridement for chronic osteomyelitis. *Acta Orthop Belg* 2006;72: 448-453.

    A prophylactic circular external fixation frame was built on one proximal and one distal ring connected to the bone by thin wires and half pins. The frame was used to protect and support four limbs significantly weakened by a radical débridement for chronic osteomyelitis of either the femur or tibia. Bone grafting or distraction osteogenesis was unnecessary, and all wounds healed without complications.

98. Cierny G III, Fitzgerald RH: Adult osteomyelitis and septic arthritis, in Fitzgerald RH, Kaufer H, Malkani AL (eds): *Orthopaedics*. St. Louis, MO, Mosby, 2002, pp 718-727.

4: Specific Situations

Chapter 13

Septic Arthritis

Nalini Rao, MD, FACP, FSHEA   John L. Esterhai Jr, MD

Introduction

Septic arthritis is a joint inflammation caused by bacteria, viruses, fungi, or parasites. The properties of the invading organism, the premorbid condition of the joint, and the host's defense mechanisms are important in the pathophysiology of septic arthritis. Prompt recognition and correct diagnosis, followed by an organism-specific antibiotic regimen and joint decompression, are essential to avoiding disabling sequelae. Septic arthritis continues to lead to loss of function in 25% to 50% of patients, despite appropriate antibiotic and surgical therapy.

Pathophysiology

Mechanisms of Pathogenesis

Chronic arthritis, traumatic damage to soft tissue or cartilage, and certain other conditions can create a predisposition to infection. Pathogens gain access to a joint by several means, and joint sepsis can be classified by three basic mechanisms of pathogenesis or portals of entry: hematogenous dissemination, direct inoculation, and contiguous spread from adjacent osteomyelitis.

Hematogenous Dissemination

Hematogenous joint sepsis most commonly occurs when an organism is causing skin breakdown, urinary system infection, pneumonia, or another organ system condition. Between 50% and 70% of patients with intra-articular sepsis have a positive blood culture.[1] The synovial joints are vulnerable to bacterial seeding because of the rich synovial vasculature and the absence of a basement membrane between the endothelial cells. Most patients with hematogenous nongonococcal bacterial arthritis have at least one underlying chronic medical risk factor; the most common such factors are listed in chapter 1.

Direct Inoculation

Trauma or invasive treatment can lead to direct inoculation. Septic arthritis is associated with arthroscopic and open surgical procedures as well as repeated corticosteroid injections. Necrotic bone from trauma or a foreign body in or around the joint, such as nonabsorbable suture or fracture fixation hardware, can provide a nidus for bacterial adhesion and colonization. The nidus allows bacteria to form a glycocalyx biofilm, which contributes to antibiotic resistance and limits the effectiveness of the host's immune response.

Contiguous Spread

Septic arthritis from a contiguous infection spreads from the bone to the synovium and then to the joint space. The condition most often occurs in infants, who have a vascular anastomosis between the epiphysis and the metaphysis. The rapidly growing metaphyseal area of a long bone is typically affected, most frequently in the hip and knee. Direct vascular communication between metaphyseal arterioles and the epiphyseal ossicle exists before age 8 months, allowing direct hematogenous communication between an osteomyelitis of the metaphysis and the adjacent joint synovium. Between ages 8 months and 18 months, the vestiges of the nutrient artery system close down at the growth plate, obliterating the vascular anastomosis. The open physis then provides an effective barrier to the spread of infection to the joint.

Synovial Tissue and Infection

The anatomy of the joint is intricately involved in the pathogenesis of sepsis. Synovial fluid is an excellent growth medium for bacteria, and it has a relative lack of immunologic resistance. Type B synoviocytes are weakly phagocytic, but usually they are able to contain and eliminate a blood-borne bacterial inoculation. For an intra-articular infection to develop, an imbalance must exist between normal synovial cell function and the invading bacteria.

Synovial tissue is relatively resistant to infection. The synovium is infrequently colonized in joints with experimentally produced septic arthritis. A lack of ligands or a functional host resistance mechanism may help to prevent synovial colonization.

The transition zone of the synovium is rarely more than three or four cell layers thick. The synovial capillaries are superficial and relatively susceptible to trauma. Because of the lack of epithelial tissue to form a basement membrane, there is no structural barrier to the spread of bacteria from the synovium to the joint. Transient bacteremia and traumatic intra-articular hemorrhage have a role in the pathogenesis of septic arthritis.

Table 1
Microorganisms Associated With Reactive Arthritis
Campylobacter jejuni
Chlamydia trachomatis
Salmonella enteritidis
Salmonella typhimurium
Shigella flexneri
Yersinia enterocolitica
Yersinia pseudotuberculosis

Microbiology

With the exception of articular cartilage and teeth, all natural biologic surfaces are protected by epithelium, endothelium, or periosteum, which decrease bacterial adhesion by desquamation or the presence of host extracellular polysaccharide molecules. *Staphylococcus aureus* has specific surface-associated adhesins for collagen but not for enamel, and it is the natural colonizer of cartilage and collagen. The bacterial colonization of articular cartilage by any pathologic organism is unnatural and rapidly destructive.

The patient's age and physiologic status are used to predict the bacteria responsible for septic arthritis (see chapter 1). The infecting organism usually can be identified from among those that commonly cause bacteremia in the patient's age group. However, some organisms, including *Neisseria gonorrhoeae* and *S aureus*, are responsible for more incidences of septic arthritis than their bacteremial incidence suggests. *S aureus* causes 50% of nongonococcal bacterial arthritis in adult patients.[2,3] *Propionibacterium acnes* should not be dismissed as a skin contaminant. *P acnes* is an anaerobic, gram-positive bacillus found in lipid-rich areas such as hair follicles and sebaceous glands and in moist areas such as the axilla. *P acnes* frequently is responsible for shoulder sepsis, but only rarely is it the cause of other large-joint infections.

The incidence of joint infection caused by gram-negative bacilli is increasing. These infections most often occur in patients who are intravenous drug abusers, are immunocompromised,[4] or have a malignancy, diabetes, or hemoglobinopathy. *Pseudomonas* or *Serratia* species are most commonly responsible for infection in intravenous drug abusers, although the incidence of *S aureus* is increasing. *Streptococcus pneumoniae* is the most common organism in patients with chronic alcoholism or hypogammaglobulinemia. Polymicrobial infection is found in 5% to 15% of patients with septic arthritis;[5] often it is associated with an extra-articular polymicrobial infection or penetrating trauma, especially in a patient who is immunocompromised. Several unusual organisms have been implicated in articular infections, including *Kingella* species, *Aggregatibacter actinomyce-*

temcomitans, Moraxella catarrhalis, Pasteurella multocida, and *Brucella* species. Organisms associated with reactive arthritis (transient, nonpurulent arthritis occurring after infection at another site) are listed in Table 1.

Incidence

The incidence of nongonococcal acute septic arthritis among adults in the United States is 0.034% to 0.13%. The disease is monoarticular in 90% of patients: primary knee sepsis accounts for 40% to 50% of the instances; hip sepsis, 20% to 25%; and shoulder sepsis, 10% to 15%.[6-8] The incidence of septic arthritis is increasing with the aging of the population and the greater incidence of debilitating chronic disease.

Natural History

Animal studies established that direct joint inoculation with bacteria is quickly followed by synovial, bone, and cartilage changes.[9] Within minutes of inoculation, the synovium becomes inflamed. An influx of polymorphonuclear cells develops into an invading pannus, eroding and undermining the articular cartilage. Within 3 hours, a purulent exudate can be observed, and within 24 hours multiple abscesses are seen. By day 2, a simultaneous, progressive loss of glycosaminoglycan can be confirmed using safranin O staining. By day 5, synovial inflammation extends below the cartilage interface, causing erosion and loosening. Glycosaminoglycan loss is most pronounced in the marginal areas near the leading edge of the pannus. The degradation of cartilage occurs through bacterial endotoxin, prostaglandins, and cytokine-mediated events that invoke a host inflammatory response and a release of destructive enzymes by synoviocytes and leukocytes. Glycosaminoglycan is totally depleted by day 14, and the protein-polysaccharide–depleted cartilage is susceptible to degradation by collagenases released by the lysosomes. The predominant cytokine is interleukin-1, which is released by synovial macrophages and circulating monocytes. Interleukin-1 inhibits chondrocyte proliferation and decreases the expression of types II and X collagen, making the articular cartilage more friable and susceptible to bacterial adhesion.[7]

Irreversible changes occur unless the joint is sterilized within 5 days of infection. If the infection remains untreated for 7 to 10 days, cartilage fissuring and a decrease in height occur, most commonly in weight-bearing areas. Continued infection leads to joint capsule and ligament dissolution. In a rabbit model, fibrous ankylosis occurred within 5 weeks.[9]

Common Types of Clinical Septic Arthritis

Sepsis Following Arthroscopy

Arthroscopy is a clean surgical procedure, and the associated risk of infection should be low; reported rates range from 0.04% to 3.4%. The use of perisurgical antibiotics led to a fourfold decrease in the infection rate.[10] Septic arthritis occurred in four patients after 101 arthroscopic procedures done during a 3-month period. Three of the patients were being treated with intra-articular methylprednisolone. Two of the infections occurred in the glenohumeral joint and were believed to be secondary to surgical field contamination by nonsterile electrocardiography cables. The remaining two infections may have resulted from inadequate between-procedure disinfection of the arthroscope. (The equipment was soaked in 2% glutaraldehyde, sometimes for less than the required time.[11]) This study established the importance of adequate preparation of the patient as well as the equipment and operating room. If an arthroscopic procedure is followed by an open surgical procedure, as in a mini-open rotator cuff repair, the skin should be reprepared with betadine after the arthroscopy because constant arthroscopic fluid extravasation decreases the efficacy of the initial, presurgical skin preparation.

Sepsis Following Open Reduction and Internal Fixation

Internal fixation of a periarticular fracture provides an environment for bacterial adhesion and glycocalyx formation, which make an infection more difficult to eradicate. Occult infection is common after open reduction and internal fixation; its presence may be suggested by postsurgical drainage or slow incisional healing.

Septic Arthritis Superimposed on Rheumatoid Arthritis

Patients with rheumatoid arthritis have an increased susceptibility to joint sepsis,[12] and their chronic joint symptoms may delay the diagnosis of infection. Several factors can predispose a patient with rheumatoid arthritis to infection, including poor overall health; chronic, systemic use of corticosteroids or cytotoxic drugs; and intra-articular use of corticosteroids. The synovial leukocytes of a patient with rheumatoid arthritis may have less-than-normal phagocytic activity, making the joints more susceptible to sepsis.

Septic arthritis should be suspected if the clinical course of a patient with rheumatoid arthritis becomes acutely worse. Although the signs and symptoms are variable and inconsistent, the patient may have a sudden exacerbation of the usual arthritic pain, an abrupt onset of swelling, and an increased joint temperature. Erythrocyte sedimentation rate (ESR) and radiography are unreliable for diagnosis. The synovial fluid should be immediately aspirated for examination. The patient must be promptly treated with parenteral antibiotics and surgery, because septic arthritis has a high mortality rate in patients with rheumatoid arthritis.

Disseminated Gonococcal Arthritis

Disseminated gonococcal infection is the most common cause of hematogenous septic arthritis in all joints. Un-like patients with nongonococcal septic arthritis, patients with a joint infection secondary to *N gonorrhoeae* usually are young, healthy adults. The most common clinical manifestation is a migratory polyarthralgia (70%). Fever as well as tenosynovitis (67%) and dermatitis (67%) are commonly discovered on initial examination. Gram staining of joint aspirate yields a positive result only in 25% of patients, and only 50% of cultures are positive. The synovial fluid white blood cell (WBC) count is lower than that of patients with nongonococcal septic arthritis but nevertheless is higher than 50,000 WBC/mm^3. A urethral, cervical, rectal, or pharyngeal culture yields growth in 80% to 90% of patients and should be obtained from any young, sexually active patient suspected of having gonococcal arthritis.[13] The infection responds rapidly to ceftriaxone and generally is resolved within 48 to 72 hours. Most patients do not require surgical decompression because joint destruction is rare.

Clinical Evaluation

The clinical signs and symptoms of septic arthritis are variable and imprecise. The diagnosis is made through clinical history, physical examination, and laboratory studies of synovial fluid from the affected joint. The differential diagnosis of septic arthritis is presented in Table 2. More than 80% of patients have pain and limited motion in the involved joint, and 60% to 80% have fever (unless it is masked by the effect of anti-inflammatory agents or steroids).[5] A patient with septic arthritis of the sternoclavicular, acromioclavicular, sternocostal, or manubriosternal joint may have chest wall pain. A patient with infection of the sacroiliac joint may have buttock, hip, or anterior thigh pain.

Laboratory studies for the diagnosis of septic arthritis are described in chapter 5.

Imaging Studies

Conventional imaging modalities are described in chapter 6.[14] The specificity of bone scintigraphy can be increased by labeling autogenous leukocytes with indium In 111 or technetium 99m. Higher sensitivity and resolution can be obtained with single photon emission CT, in which the radioactivity of an inflamed joint or bone is differentiated from that of overlying normal soft tissue.

Diagnostic Arthroscopy

If the patient receives an antibiotic for suspected septic arthritis or an unrelated infection before the culture specimen is obtained, the culture may be inaccurately negative. In addition, a fastidious organism may not be detected by culturing. Arthroscopy can be a useful diagnostic and therapeutic modality for such a patient. Specimens can be obtained from multiple sites, and cultures from a synovial tissue biopsy obtained through the arthroscope may have a higher yield for fastidious organisms than joint fluid cultures.

Table 2

The Differential Diagnosis of Septic Arthritis

Ankylosing spondylitis

Chronic seronegative arthritis

Crystal-induced arthritis

Drug-induced arthritis

Gout

Infectious endocarditis

Inflammatory bowel disease–associated arthritis

Lyme disease

Mycobacterial, fungal, or viral arthritis

Pseudogout

Pseudoseptic arthritis

Psoriatic syndrome

Reiter syndrome

Rheumatoid arthritis

(Adapted with permission from Garcia-De La Torre I: Advances in the management of septic arthritis. *Rheum Dis Clin N Am* 2003;29:61-75.)

Table 3

Classification System for Septic Arthritis

Anatomic Type	Description
I	Periarticular soft-tissue infection without septic arthritis
II	Isolated septic arthritis
III	Septic arthritis with soft-tissue extension but without osteomyelitis
IV	Septic arthritis with contiguous osteomyelitis
Host Class	**Description**
A	Normal immune system
B	Compromise
B_L	Local tissue compromise
B_S	Systemic immune compromise
C	Aggressive treatment requires unwarranted risk
Clinical Setting	**Description**
1	Symptom duration less than 5 days; nonvirulent organism
2	Symptom duration 5 or more days; virulent organism

(Adapted with permission from Cierny G, Mader JT, Pennick JJ: A clinical staging system for adult osteomyelitis. *Contemp Orthop* 1985;10:17-37.)

Classification

The lack of a uniform classification system for septic joints has caused difficulty in reporting the outcomes of patients with septic arthritis. No existing system to describe osteomyelitis or infection surrounding a total joint is universally accepted. A modification of the Cierny-Mader classification of osteomyelitis[15] is recommended, as outlined in **Table 3**. This system serves as a reminder to consider multiple aspects of the infection, provides a framework for risk stratification, and allows for more informed treatment decision making.

The modified Cierny-Mader system stages the infection using three factors: the site and extent of tissue involvement (anatomic type), the patient's systemic and local physiologic status (host class), and the duration of symptoms and virulence of the organism (clinical setting). Anatomic type I, periarticular soft-tissue infection without septic arthritis, can occur in a postsurgical deep wound infection. Anatomic type II exists when the purulent material is confined within the capsule. Anatomic type III exists when both the joint and the surrounding soft tissue are infected, as in a deep wound infection or septic bursitis. There is no bony involvement in type III. Osteomyelitis contiguous with joint infection is classified as type IV.

A patient whose physiologic status is in host class A is metabolically and immunologically normal. A patient in class B has a local (B_L) or systemic (B_S) compromise. Local compromise can result from retained nonabsorbable suture or other biomaterial, irradiation, scarring from multiple procedures, or lymphedema. Systemic compromising factors include advanced age, a chronic disease, or any condition causing suppression of the immune system. For a patient in class C, the risks associated with aggressive treatment outweigh the negative consequences of the infection.

The two clinical-setting factors are the duration of symptoms and the aggressiveness of the organism. Patients in group 1 have symptoms of less than 5 days' duration and infection with a bacterial strain of relatively low virulence. Patients in group 2 have infection with a virulent organism or symptoms lasting for 5 or more days. The 5-day period was chosen because animal studies found that irreversible joint damage occurred when septic arthritis persisted beyond 5 days.[9] The prevalent virulent organisms vary by institution and geographic region, but usually they include methicillin-resistant *S aureus*, gram-negative bacilli, vancomycin-resistant *Enterococcus* species, and clostridia.

Treatment

Antibiotics

Prompt diagnosis of septic arthritis must be followed by joint decompression and an organism-specific antibiotic regimen to avoid disabling sequelae.[16,17] The selection of an antibiotic ideally is based on identification of the pathogen and its susceptibility profile. The organism sometimes cannot be isolated, and for these patients the probable infecting organism must be identified before determining an empiric treatment. The

Table 4

Guidelines for Choosing an Empiric Antibiotic to Treat Adult Septic Arthritis

Gram Stain Result or Clinical Condition	Probable Organisms	Preferred Antibiotics	Alternative Antibiotics
Gram-positive cocci	S aureus Streptococci	Nafcillin or cefazolin	Clindamycin Trimethoprim-sulfamethoxazole Vancomycin
Gram-negative cocci or negative stain Healthy, sexually active patient	N gonorrhoeae	Ceftriaxone	Doxycycline
Gram-negative bacilli	P aeruginosa Enterobacteriaceae	Piperacillin ± gentamicin	Third-generation cephalosporin
Gram-positive bacilli	P acnes	Penicillin G	Nafcillin Vancomycin
Intravenous drug abuse	S aureus P aeruginosa Serratia species	Cefazolin + gentamicin	Third-generation cephalosporin
Significant underlying disease Immunocompromise Nosocomial infection	S aureus Enterobacteriaceae P aeruginosa Streptococci	Cefazolin + gentamicin	Third-generation cephalosporin
Infected prosthesis	Staphylococcus epidermidis S aureus Enterobacteriaceae P aeruginosa	Vancomycin + gentamicin	Imipenem

(Adapted with permission from Hughes RA, Keat AC: Reiter syndrome and reactive arthritis: A current view. *Semin Arthritis Rheum* 1994;24:190-210.)

surgical options and overall disease treatment must also be considered in choosing an antibiotic agent.

The probable organisms vary with patient age and the presence of an underlying medical condition, such as rheumatoid arthritis, chronic illness, a history of intravenous drug abuse, a remote site of infection, or immunocompromise. Empiric antibiotic treatment can be initiated after a specimen is obtained for Gram staining, cultures, and sensitivity studies. A penicillinase-resistant antistaphylococcal drug is the usual initial choice for a typical gram-positive coccal infection. The first-generation cephalosporins have been favored in the United States because they are relatively nontoxic and inexpensive. A third-generation cephalosporin or vancomycin is chosen if the infecting organism is highly likely to be a gram-negative bacillus or methicillin-resistant staphylococcus, respectively.[6] An aminoglycoside should be added for coverage of *Pseudomonas aeruginosa* if the patient is receiving immunosuppressive agents or has a nosocomial infection. The initial antibiotics should cover both *S aureus* and *P aeruginosa* if the patient is an intravenous drug abuser. Gonococcal arthritis should be suspected in a young, sexually active patient for whom Gram staining was negative, and ceftriaxone should be used. Guidelines for initial empiric antibiotic therapy are summarized in Table 4.

When the microbiologic data become available, the spectrum of antibiotic coverage can be narrowed to maximize treatment efficacy and decrease the risk of systemic toxicity (Table 5). Consultation with an infectious disease specialist generally is recommended for full consideration of the characteristics of different pathogens, their institution-specific resistance profiles, and the continuing evolution of antimicrobial regimens.

The choice of oral or parenteral antibiotics is controversial. Several studies found that oral antibiotics were efficacious in treating osteomyelitis and septic arthritis in children.[18,19] However, the oral regimen was started only after intravenous treatment, most often of 3 to 7 days' duration. No well-designed, randomized, blinded, controlled study has determined whether oral antibiotics are as effective as parenteral antibiotics in treating septic arthritis. Thus, oral antimicrobial agents should be used only for an acute infection and after initial intravenous administration. In addition, the patient should have continuing clinical improvement including improved joint range of motion, decreased pain, and resolution of fever, as well as a normal WBC count and ESR.

The advantages of oral administration of antibiotics include lower cost, greater convenience, greater patient comfort, and decreased length of hospital stay. The patient should be evaluated before hospital discharge to

Table 5

Antibiotic Therapy for Specific Pathogens

Microorganism	Preferred Antibiotic (Duration of Therapy)	Alternative Antibiotic
Streptococcus species	Penicillin or ampicillin (2 to 3 weeks)	Clindamycin or first-generation cephalosporin Vancomycin
Methicillin-sensitive *S aureus*	Nafcillin or first-generation cephalosporin (4 to 6 weeks)	Vancomycin Linezolid Daptomycin
Methicillin-resistant *S aureus*	Vancomycin (4 to 6 weeks)	Linezolid Daptomycin Tigecycline
N gonorrhoeae	Ceftriaxone (7 to 10 days)	Fluoroquinolone
Gram-negative bacillus other than *P aeruginosa*	Third-generation cephalosporin (4 to 6 weeks)	Extended-spectrum penicillin Fluoroquinolone Trimethoprim-sulfamethoxazole
P aeruginosa	Piperacillin + aminoglycoside (4 to 6 weeks)	Cefepime + aminoglycosides Ciprofloxacin Levofloxacin

(Adapted with permission from Garcia-De La Torre I: Advances in the management of septic arthritis. *Rheum Dis Clin N Am* 2003;29:61-75.)

ensure that serum concentrations are adequate. Most clinicians arbitrarily require a serum bactericidal titer of at least 1:8; others recommend a 1:16 peak level and a 1:2 trough level. The risks associated with a postdischarge oral antibiotic regimen are that the patient may not follow instructions or may have difficulty in obtaining the medication. Thus, the importance of completing the full course of therapy must be stressed, and the patient must be carefully instructed as to the proper dosage and timing.

The duration of antibiotic therapy also is a subject of discussion. Guidelines have been established, although no controlled studies have determined the optimal length of treatment. The duration of the antibiotic regimen varies with the pathogen, the patient's underlying condition, and any adjuvant medical or surgical procedures. A course of 7 to 10 days generally is recommended for gonococcal septic arthritis. A 2- to 3-week course usually is adequate for septic arthritis caused by streptococci or a *Haemophilus* species. If a more virulent organism such as *S aureus* or a gram-negative bacillus is isolated, a 4- to 6-week course of an appropriate antibiotic is required. A patient who is immunocompromised or has a slow clinical response requires a full 6 weeks of treatment.

Nonsteroidal Anti-inflammatory Drugs
Bacterial products are not completely removed by sterilizing the joint with antibiotics and irrigation. These microbial fragments can persist in the joint for a prolonged period and can contribute to development of postinfectious inflammatory synovitis. Nonsteroidal anti-inflammatory drugs (NSAIDs) can be useful in

treating this inflammatory process. In addition, naproxen was found to decrease the amount of glycosaminoglycan and collagen when administered with antibiotics in an animal model.[16] This finding suggests that the addition of a NSAID to the antibiotic regimen can decrease the destruction of articular cartilage. However, NSAIDs should not be started early in the course of infection because their action can mask a poor clinical response to an antibiotic. The recommended timing is to begin administering a NSAID 4 to 5 days after antibiotic treatment is initiated.

Evacuation and Decompression
The treatment of septic arthritis includes sterilization and decompression of the joint, with removal of all inflammatory cells, lysosomal and proteolytic enzymes, and fibrinous materials. There are two different schools of thought as to the preferred method of joint decompression for an infection not related to surgery. One view is that treatment of septic arthritis requires only repeated needle aspiration[20] and appropriate antibiotics. The second view is that the best treatment of septic arthritis as well as osteomyelitis is surgical débridement.[21] Studies are available to support both beliefs.[22] Table 6 compares important aspects of the procedures.

Proponents of repeated arthrocentesis cite reasons for avoiding surgical intervention, including extended hospitalization, wound management complications, and risks associated with anesthesia. Several retrospective studies conducted during the 1970s and 1980s compared infected joints treated with needle aspiration and those treated with surgical drainage, concluding that septic joints can be medically managed with good results.[23]

Table 6

Comparison of Decompression Procedures for Septic Arthritis

Procedural Factor	Type of Procedure			
	Aspiration	Tidal Irrigation	Arthroscopy	Arthrotomy
Site	Bedside	Bedside	Operating room	Operating room
Anesthesia	Local	Local	Regional or general	Regional or general
Joint accessibility	All joints (Repeat aspiration limited to large, superficial joints)	Limited to large, superficial joints	Limited to large joints	All joints
Drainage accessibility	Modest	Modest	Excellent	Excellent
Adhesion lysis	No	No	Yes	Yes
Synovectomy	No	No	Yes	Yes
Morbidity	Minimal	Minimal	Moderate	Significant

Aspiration of an infected joint should be performed using a large-bore needle under sterile conditions. A long spinal needle may be necessary to penetrate the glenohumeral joint in an obese or muscular patient. It is essential to drain the joint completely, and aspiration should be done once or twice daily until the effusion ceases to recur.

Proponents of surgical drainage cite reasons for avoiding joint aspiration, including the technical difficulty of shoulder aspiration, inadequate needle evacuation of purulent material secondary to loculations and adhesions, pain associated with repeated arthrocentesis, and the risk of iatrogenic needle inoculation of subchondral bone. As with aspiration, only retrospective studies are available to support the preference for surgical treatment.[23]

Although the debate over medical and surgical drainage of joint infections is ongoing, evidence is accumulating to support the use of surgical arthroscopy. Arthroscopy has a diagnostic advantage because it allows direct viewing of the entire joint, which is essential for determining the extent of the disease. If the condition is atypical or otherwise challenging, a tissue biopsy can be obtained during arthroscopy. Arthroscopy also offers a therapeutic advantage, as the joint can be adequately drained, thoroughly débrided, and copiously irrigated. Arthroscopic irrigation and drainage can reduce hospital stay and allow early range-of-motion exercises, which may be helpful in preserving joint function. Arthroscopic or open surgical drainage should be preferred to repeated arthrocentesis under the conditions listed in Table 7.

Septic arthritis has been drained using percutaneous catheters placed under fluoroscopy, in combination with antibiotic therapy.[24] Experience with this technique is relatively limited, and its role in the treatment of joint infection has yet to be determined.

Rehabilitation should begin as soon as the joint

Table 7

Indications for Treating Adult Septic Arthritis With Arthroscopic or Open Surgical Drainage Rather Than Repeated Arthrocentesis

Symptom duration of at least 5 days before the initiation of treatment

Presence of an aggressive organism:

Methicillin-resistant *S aureus*

Gram-negative bacillus

Enterococcus

Clostridia

Glycocalyx-producing organisms

Age older than approximately 75 years

Patient immunocompromise:

Immunosuppressive therapy

Chronic debilitating illness

Malignancy

Acquired immunodeficiency syndrome

Malnutrition

Diagnostic dilemma requiring tissue biopsy

Related condition:

Rheumatoid arthritis

Osteoarthritis

Periarticular osteomyelitis

Postsurgical infection

Failure of repeated arthrocentesis:

No or little clinical improvement

Effusion persisting after 5 to 7 days of treatment

infection is diagnosed. The joint initially can be immobilized in a functional position. Because articular cartilage is nourished by being bathed in synovial fluid, it is important to begin active and passive range-of-motion exercises as soon as the acute symptoms subside or when drains are removed and drain sites are sealed.[25]

Summary

Septic arthritis is a medical and surgical emergency because it can lead to rapid destruction of the joint and irreversible loss of function. A variety of microorganisms can cause septic arthritis, although bacteria are the most common agents. Prompt clinical recognition with urgent diagnostic aspiration followed by appropriate antibiotic treatment and joint decompression are essential. Despite appropriate treatment, septic arthritis leads to loss of function in 25% to 50% of patients.

Annotated References

1. Goldenberg DL: Septic arthritis. *Lancet* 1998;351:197-202.

2. Ross JJ, Davidson L: Methicillin-resistant *Staphylococcus aureus* septic arthritis: An emerging clinical syndrome. *Rheumatology(Oxford)* 2005;44:1197-1198.

   This demographic and clinical study found a poorer outcome with methicillin-resistant *S aureus* septic arthritis than methicillin-sensitive *S aureus* septic arthritis. Patients with suspected septic arthritis, a history of infection or colonization with methicillin-resistant *S aureus*, and a recent hospitalization should receive an antibiotic regimen including vancomycin.

3. Al-Nammari SS, Bobak P, Venkatesh R: Methicillin-resistant Staphylococcus aureus versus methicillin-sensitive Staphylococcus aureus adult haematogenous septic arthritis. *Arch Orthop Trauma Surg* 2007;127:537-542.

   Patients with methicillin-resistant *S aureus* were older than patients with methicillin-sensitive S aureus (mean, 76 and 44 years, respectively [P < 0.05]), had more comorbidities (mean, 2.7 and 1.35, respectively [P < 0.05]), and had a poorer outcome.

4. Schelenz S, Bramham K, Goldsmith D: Septic arthritis due to extended spectrum beta lactamase producing Klebsiella pneumoniae. *Joint Bone Spine* 2007;74:275-278.

   Septic arthritis in patients who are immunocompromised may be caused by unusual organisms, including drug-resistant gram-negative bacteria. In hospitals where these organisms are prevalent, a broad-spectrum antibiotic such as meropenem (with or without amikacin) should be used empirically.

5. Rosenthal J, Giles G, Bole WDR: Acute nongonococcal infectious arthritis: Evaluation of risk factors, therapy, and outcome. *Arthritis Rheum* 1980;23:889-896.

6. Ross JJ: Septic arthritis. *Infect Dis Clin North Am* 2005;19:799-817.

   The pathogenesis, risk factors, clinical presentation, diagnosis, and treatment of septic arthritis are outlined.

7. Garcia-De La Torre I: Advances in the management of septic arthritis. *Rheum Dis Clin N Am* 2003;29:61-75.

   This review focuses on the pathogenesis, risk factors, and clinical manifestations of nongonococcal bacterial arthritis and other forms of infectious arthritis, including differential diagnosis and treatment.

8. Mehta P, Schnall SB, Zalavras CG: Septic arthritis of the shoulder, elbow, and wrist. *Clin Orthop Relat Res* 2006;451:42-45.

   Septic arthritis of the shoulder, elbow, and wrist is uncommon, but a high index of suspicion is necessary for patients with upper extremity joint symptoms. Joint aspirate with cell count and differentials may be helpful in the diagnosis. *S aureus* is the most common pathogen. Level of evidence: IV.

9. Riegels-Nielsen P, Frimodt-Moller N, Jensen J: Rabbit model of septic arthritis. *Acta Orthop Scand* 1987;58:14-19.

10. D'Angelo GL, Ogilvie-Harris DJ: Septic arthritis following arthroscopy with cost/benefit analysis of antibiotic prophylaxis. *Arthroscopy* 1988;4:10-14.

11. Armstrong R, Bolding F: Septic arthritis after arthroscopy: The contributing roles of intraarticular steroids and environmental factors. *Am J Infect Control* 1994;22:16-18.

12. Edwards CJ, Cooper C, Fisher D, Field M, van Staa TP, Arden NK: The importance of the disease process and disease-modifying anti-rheumatic drug treatment in the development of septic arthritis in patients with rheumatoid arthritis. *Arthritis Rheum* 2007;57:1151-1157.

    The incidence of septic arthritis was found to be increased 12.9 times in patients with rheumatoid arthritis. The higher risk was attributed to both the disease process and the use of disease-modifying antirheumatic drugs.

13. Masi AT, Eisenstein BI: Disseminated gonococcal infection and gonococcal arthritis (GCA): II. Clinical manifestations, diagnosis, complications, treatment and prevention. *Semin Arthritis Rheum* 1981;10:173.

14. Nade S: Septic arthritis. *Best Pract & Res Clin Rheumatol* 2003;17:183-200.

    Early diagnosis of septic arthritis and prompt medical and surgical intervention are essential if normal functioning of the infected joint is to be restored. The clinical features differ among neonates, children, and adults. Diagnosis may be aided by ultrasonography and arthrocentesis.

15. Cierny G, Mader JT, Pennick JJ: A clinical staging system for adult osteomyelitis. *Contemp Orthop* 1985;10: 17-37.

16. Smith JW, Chalupa P, Hasan MS: Infectious arthritis: Clinical features, laboratory findings and treatment. *Clin Microbiol Infect* 2006;12:309-314.

    This review of septic arthritis emphasizes the clinical features and treatment of bacterial, viral, and chronic monoarticular arthritis.

17. Weston V, Coakley G: Guideline for the management of the hot swollen joint in adults with a particular focus on septic arthritis. *J Antimicrob Chemotherap* 2006;58: 492-493.

    The British Society of Rheumatic Standards developed an evidence-based guideline for the management of hot, swollen joints, with an emphasis on septic joints.

18. Margaretten ME, Kohiwes J, Moore D, Bent S: Does this adult patient have septic arthritis? *JAMA* 2007;297: 1478-1488.

    The clinical diagnosis of septic arthritis may be characterized by suboptimal accuracy and precision. Meta-analysis of 14 studies involving 6,242 patients suggested that the synovial WBC count and the percentage of polymorphonuclear leukocytes are essential data for assessing the likelihood of septic arthritis before Gram staining and culture results are known.

19. Kocher MS, Madiga R, Murphy JM, et al: A clinical practice guideline for treatment of septic arthritis in children. *J Bone Joint Surg Am* 2003;85:994-999.

    A clinical practice guideline was developed by interdisciplinary experts using an evidence-based method of evaluating the outcome of septic arthritis of the hip in children. Process and efficacy of care were improved by using the clinical practice guidelines. Patients had less variation in care with no significant difference in outcome.

20. Goldenberg DL, Brandt KD, Cathcart ES: Treatment of septic arthritis. *Arthritis Rheum* 1975;18:83-90.

21. Leslie BM, Harris JM, Driscoll D: Septic arthritis of the shoulder in adults. *J Bone Joint Surg Am* 1989;71:1516-1522.

22. Mathews CJ, Kingsley G, Field M, et al: Management of septic arthritis: A systematic review. *Ann Rheum Dis* 2007;66:440-445.

    The overall impression of an experienced clinician is the gold standard for the diagnosis of septic arthritis. Demographic features can predict the likelihood of an atypical organism. The outcomes of medical and arthroscopic approaches to treatment are similar.

23. Esterhai JL, Gelg I: Adult septic arthritis. *Orthop Clin North Amer* 1991;22:503-514.

24. Renner JB, Agee MW: Treatment of suppurative arthritis by percutaneous catheter drainage. *Am J Rheumatol* 1990;154:135-138.

25. Salter RB: The biologic concept of continuous passive motion of synovial joints. *Clin Orthop Relat Res* 1989; 242:12-25.

4: Specific Situations

Chapter 14

Prosthetic Joint Infections

*Douglas R. Osmon, MD, MPH   Arlen Hanssen D., MD

4: Specific Situations

Introduction

Prosthetic joint infection is difficult and expensive to diagnose and treat effectively, and it often results in significant morbidity. Optimal treatment typically requires a multidisciplinary approach that includes an orthopaedic surgeon, an infectious disease physician, and, frequently, a plastic surgeon or internist. It is important to review current concepts in the prevention, diagnosis, and management of prosthetic joint infection.

Pathogenesis

Prosthetic joints are at risk for infection because they can be colonized by a small number of microorganisms that form an extracellular polysaccharide layer called a biofilm. The biofilm protects the bacteria against phagocytosis and antimicrobial agents. Infection can occur by contamination during surgery or the immediate postoperative period, hematogenous dissemination from an infection elsewhere in the body, or, rarely, contiguous spread from an adjacent soft-tissue infection. The microorganisms in a biofilm often have decreased in vitro susceptibility to antimicrobial agents. An infection also may persist on a prosthesis because of the presence of a small colony variant of a typical microorganism such as Staphylococcus. Small colony variants have a defect in the electron transport system that promotes resistance to host defense mechanisms. They can be extremely resistant to a variety of antimicrobial agents, and their slow growth makes them difficult to routinely identify in the microbiology laboratory. It has been suggested that the formation of small colony variants is promoted by the use of aminoglycoside-impregnated polymethylmethacrylate cement.[1]

Prevention

The risk of prosthetic joint infection following joint arthroplasty is approximately 1% to 2%, although the risk varies by institution. The risk is greater after total

knee arthroplasty (TKA) or revision arthroplasty than after total hip arthroplasty (THA).[2] The risk factors include revision arthroplasty; the development of a superficial surgical site infection; a National Nosocomial Infections Surveillance system risk index score of 1 or 2; and certain patient-specific conditions and characteristics, including a malignancy, rheumatoid arthritis, diabetes mellitus, steroid use, obesity, extreme old age, poor nutritional status, psoriasis, hemophilia, and sickle cell disease. A superficial surgical site infection during the early postoperative period often results from poor wound healing or hematoma formation. The risk of a hematogenous infection is increased after Staphylococcus aureus bacteremia; in two retrospective studies, the risk was reported to be approximately 34% to 42%.[3,4]

S aureus and coagulase-negative staphylococci together cause 50% to 60% of all prosthetic joint infections. Oxacillin resistance increasingly is found among staphylococci. Infections caused by a β-hemolytic Streptococcus, Enterococcus, gram-negative bacillus, or anaerobe are less common, as are polymicrobial infections. Prosthetic joint infections caused by mycobacteria, fungi, or other unusual organisms are relatively rare. An infection may not be identified on culture because antimicrobial agents were used before the culture specimens were obtained or because of the difficulty of growing biofilm organisms in the clinical microbiology laboratory.

The recommendations of the US Centers for Disease Control and Prevention for preventing surgical site infection should be followed whenever possible.[5] The strategies for preventing perioperative prosthetic joint infection center on minimizing the impact of preoperative comorbidities such as tobacco use and diabetes mellitus and providing appropriate perioperative antimicrobial prophylaxis at the optimal time relative to the incision or tourniquet inflation. Cefazolin or cefuroxime is the recommended agent, and it should be administered according to national guidelines. Vancomycin is an alternative for a patient with a type I hypersensitivity reaction to penicillin or cephalosporins; it should be considered for a patient who is known to be colonized with methicillin-resistant S aureus (MRSA). A preoperative evaluation by an allergist can prevent the suboptimal use of vancomycin. Although the use of laminar airflow and clean exhaust suits in the operating room remains controversial, they are used in many

*Douglas R. Osman, MD, MPH or the department with which he is affiliated has received research or institutional support from Cubist Pharmaceuticals.

Table 1

The Classification of Prosthetic Joint Infections as Related to Time Elapsed Since Implantation

Type	Time Elapsed Since Implantation	Therapeutic Strategy
Intraoperative	None (positive intra-operative culture)	Intravenous antimicrobial agents (4-6 weeks) *with or without* chronic oral suppression
Early	Less than 1 month	Débridement and prosthesis retention *plus* intravenous and oral antimicrobial agents (3-6 months) *with or without* chronic oral suppression
Acute or hematogenous	Months to years	Débridement and prosthesis retention *plus* intravenous and oral antimicrobial agents (3-6 months) *with* or *without* chronic oral suppression
Delayed or late (chronic)	Months to years	Two-stage revision *plus* intravenous antimicrobial agents (4-6 weeks)

institutions. The fixation of cemented implants with antimicrobial-impregnated cement also is controversial. Antimicrobial-impregnated cement is routinely used in Europe for primary arthroplasty procedures, however, and it is common in the United States if the patient is at high risk for infection.

Infection elsewhere in the body can lead to hematogenous seeding of the prosthesis, and preventing such infections therefore is a key to preventing hematogenous prosthetic joint infection. The patient and physician should take any necessary steps to minimize the risk of pneumonia, minimize lymphedema, avoid a urinary tract infection or cellulitis, avoid tobacco use, and make sure all appropriate vaccinations are up to date. Professional organizations including the American Academy of Orthopaedic Surgeons have published statements on antimicrobial prophylaxis for patients with a prosthetic joint (see appendix). The topic is controversial, and recommendations differ on the advisability of routine prophylaxis for various procedures. The clinician may prefer to administer prophylactic therapy before, for example, a clean dental procedure (although published data have not established that routine antimicrobial prophylaxis for a clean dental procedure can prevent hematogenous infection from an oral source).

Diagnosis

Prosthetic joint infections may be classified based on the timing and presumed mechanism of infection[6] (Table 1). Pain is the initial symptom in 90% of patients who develop a delayed infection (appearing several months to 2 years after implantation) or a chronic infection (appearing more than 2 years after implantation). The pain typically is accompanied by impaired function caused by loosening of the prosthesis. The presence of a sinus tract always should raise the suspicion of a deep infection. A delayed or chronic infection often is difficult to differentiate from aseptic loosening

or other mechanical causes of prosthesis dysfunction. The cause of a delayed or chronic infection typically is a relatively low-virulence pathogen such as a coagulase-negative staphylococcus, although sometimes *S aureus* or another organism is responsible. Most delayed and chronic infections are believed to be acquired during prosthesis implantation.

The initial symptoms of an acute hematogenous infection usually are rapid-onset erythema, swelling of the affected joint, pain, and fever and chills. Purulent drainage from the wound also may be present. Delayed wound healing or hematoma formation also can lead to deep infection during the immediate postoperative period. A history of superficial wound infection in a patient with a chronically painful prosthesis always should raise the suspicion of a deep periprosthetic infection. The most common causative organisms in early postoperative infections are *S aureus*, β-hemolytic streptococci, and aerobic gram-negative bacteria. Acute infections that occur more than 2 years after prosthesis implantation are believed to be caused by hematogenous seeding, most often by *S aureus* or a β-hemolytic *Streptococcus*.

Diagnosis of a prosthetic joint infection is relatively easy if a patient has a sinus tract or the typical signs of a wound infection. The diagnosis is more difficult if chronic pain is the only symptom. Information should be obtained from a patient with a suspected prosthetic joint infection about the type of prosthesis, the date of implantation, all other surgical procedures, the symptoms, any drug allergies or intolerances, any comorbidities, and past or current antimicrobial therapy (including local therapy).

The total white blood cell count and differential are not sensitive or specific for distinguishing chronic prosthetic joint infection from aseptic loosening. An elevated erythrocyte sedimentation rate (ESR) or C-reactive protein (CRP) level is a much better laboratory marker of the presence of infection, unless the patient has a condition such as rheumatoid arthritis that also can cause an elevation. Although both the ESR and CRP level may be elevated in the postoperative period, the CRP level usually returns to normal within 2 to 3 weeks. An elevated CRP level is more sensitive and specific than an elevated ESR. If both tests are normal, the likelihood of a prosthetic joint infection is very low. Interleukin-6 testing has promise for detecting prosthetic joint infection.[7,8]

Plain radiographs can reveal dislocation, lucency at the bone-cement interface, bony erosion, or new subperiosteal bone growth (**Figure 1**). These conditions are not sensitive or specific for the diagnosis of infection, but they are crucial for clinical decision making. CT and MRI are not commonly used in the diagnosis of prosthetic joint infection because of image distortion. Nuclear medicine tests occasionally are used, but they are relatively expensive. Technetium Tc 99m bone scanning is very sensitive but not specific for infection, and therefore a negative test can exclude infection with some certainty. However, a bone scan may have a false-positive result for many months after implantation. A combination of leukocyte imaging labeled for indium In 111 and marrow imaging with technetium Tc 99m bone scanning usually can differentiate an infection from aseptic loosening because neutrophils typically are present in prosthetic infection but absent in aseptic loosening. Fluorodeoxyglucose positron emission tomography detects increased glucose uptake, which is typical in infections; however, its reported reliability has been variable,[8,9] and it is not routinely used at most institutions. Ultrasonography may be useful in detecting periprosthetic fluid collections.

If at least one inflammatory marker is elevated, the clinician suspects infection, and there is no contraindication such as overlying cellulitis, synovial fluid should be submitted for white blood cell count and differential, Gram stain, and culture for aerobic and anaerobic organisms. An elevation in the number of neutrophils to 60% or 70% in the synovial fluid or a total leukocyte count of 1,100 to 1,700 is a sensitive and specific marker for prosthetic joint infection in a patient who had prosthesis implantation more than 6 months earlier and has no underlying inflammatory joint disease. The CRP level, ESR, and synovial fluid leukocyte count have the greatest value for diagnosing prosthetic joint infection when they are considered together.[10]

A pathology report on fresh-frozen periprosthetic tissue taken during revision surgery is a relatively sensitive and specific test for the diagnosis of a prosthetic joint infection. These reports can be difficult to interpret, however, because of the presence of acute inflammatory arthritis in some patients and the differing definitions of infection used by pathologists. As a result, many clinicians do not routinely use this test in diagnosis.

The pathogen can be identified through aerobic and anaerobic culturing of tissue or purulent fluid surrounding the prosthesis at the time of resection or revision. Pathogen identification is important so that the appropriate antimicrobial agents can be administered

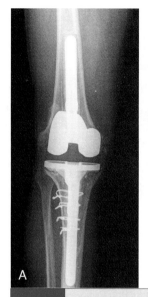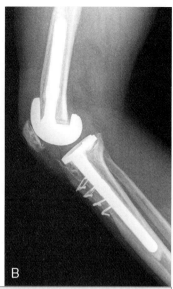

Figure 1 AP **(A)** and lateral **(B)** radiographs of a loose total knee prosthesis with a chronic coagulase-negative staphylococcal infection.

after surgery. Three to six intraoperative samples should be submitted to the laboratory to ensure optimal sensitivity and specificity. The sensitivity and specificity of the cultures can be improved by withholding antimicrobial agents for at least 2 weeks before the specimen collection. A positive Gram stain has a sensitivity of only 10% to 20%, given the low burden of organisms in infected periprosthetic tissue. However, a recent study found that a positive Gram stain with a high neutrophil count had greater sensitivity.[11]

Sonication dislodges bacteria from the surface of an explanted prosthesis into a liquid medium that is cultured for aerobic and anaerobic organisms. This process has greater sensitivity and specificity than culturing of periprosthetic tissue, particularly if antimicrobial agents were not withheld for at least 2 weeks before the surgery.[12] The validity of sonication has not been established for the recovery of fungi or mycobacteria, and periprosthetic tissue therefore should be submitted for culturing these unusual organisms. Polymerase chain reaction using sonicate fluid or tissue specimens can provide false-positive or false-negative results and is not currently used as a clinical microbiology test.

Treatment

The goal of treating a prosthetic joint infection is to achieve a painless, well-functioning joint. Often, but not always, the infection must be eradicated. The factors to be considered in surgical decision making include the possible loosening of the prosthesis, the patient's comorbidities, the virulence and antimicrobial susceptibility of the pathogen, and the status of the soft tissue and bone surrounding the prosthesis. With an

Table 2

Antimicrobial Therapy for Prosthetic Joint Infections as Related to Microorganism and Surgical Treatment

| Microorganism | Postoperative Antimicrobial Therapy* | |
	Two-Stage Revision *or* Resection Arthroplasty	Débridement and Prosthesis Retention *or* One-Stage Revision
Methicillin-susceptible *S aureus* Methicillin-susceptible coagulase-negative *Staphylococcus*	Nafcillin sodium *or* oxacillin sodium (1.5-2 g IV q 4 hr for 4-6 weeks) *or* cefazolin (1-2 g IV q 8 hr for 4-6 weeks)	Nafcillin sodium *or* oxacillin sodium (1.5-2 g IV q 4 hr for 2-6 weeks) *or* cefazolin (1-2 g IV q 8 hr for 2-6 weeks); *plus* rifampin (300-450 mg by mouth bid); *followed by* a quinolone, a first-generation cephalosporin, trimethoprim-sulfamethoxazole, *or* minocycline; *plus* rifampin for 6-10 weeks after THA, 20-24 weeks after TKA; *followed by* chronic oral suppression (a first-generation cephalosporin, an oral antistaphylococcal penicillin, trimethoprim-sulfamethoxazole, *or* minocycline)
MRSA Methicillin-resistant, coagulase-negative *Staphylococcus*	Vancomycin (15 mg/kg IV q 12 hr) *or* daptomycin (6 mg/kg IV q 24 hr) *or* linezolid (600 mg IV or oral q 12 hr for 4-6 weeks)	Vancomycin (15 mg/kg IV q 12 hr), daptomycin (6 mg/kg IV q 24 hr), *or* linezolid (600 mg IV or oral q 12 hr) for 2-6 weeks; *plus* rifampin (300-450 mg by mouth bid); *followed by* a quinolone, trimethoprim-sulfamethoxazole, *or* minocycline; *plus* rifampin for 6-8 weeks after THA, 20-22 weeks after TKA; *followed by* chronic oral suppression with trimethoprim-sulfamethoxazole *or* minocycline
β-hemolytic *Streptococcus*	Penicillin G (20 million units IV q 24 hr continuously or in 6 divided doses) *or* ceftriaxone (2 g IV q 24 hr) for 4-6 weeks	Penicillin G (20 million units IV q 24 hr continuously or in 6 divided doses) *or* ceftriaxone (2 g IV q 24 hr) for 4-6 weeks; *followed by* chronic oral suppression with penicillin VK, a first-generation cephalosporin, *or* an oral antistaphylococcal penicillin
Penicillin-susceptible, vancomycin-susceptible *Enterococcus*	Penicillin G (20 million units IV q 24 hr continuously or in 6 divided doses) *or* ampicillin sodium (12 g IV q 24 hr continuously or in 6 divided doses); *plus* aminoglycoside (optional) for 4-6 weeks	Penicillin G (20 million units IV q 24 hr continuously or in 6 divided doses) *or* ampicillin sodium (12 g IV q 24 hr continuously or in 6 divided doses); *plus* aminoglycoside (optional) for 4-6 weeks; *followed by* chronic oral suppression with penicillin VK
Penicillin-resistant *Enterococcus*	Vancomycin (15 mg/kg IV q 12 hr)	No nontoxic agent available for chronic suppression
Pseudomonas aeruginosa	Cefepime (2 g IV q 12 hr) *or* meropenem (1 g IV q 8 hr); *plus* aminoglycoside (optional). Double coverage can be considered.	Cefepime (2 g IV q 12 hr) *or* meropenem (1 g IV q 8 hr) *plus* aminoglycoside (optional). Double coverage can be considered. *Followed by* chronic oral suppression with ciprofloxacin.
Enterobacteriaceae	Cefepime (2 g IV q 12 hr) *or* meropenem (1 g IV q 8 hr)	Cefepime (2 g IV q 12 hr) *or* meropenem (1 g IV q 8 hr); *followed by* chronic oral suppression with trimethoprim-sulfamethoxazole *or* cephalosporin
Propionibacterium acnes	Penicillin G (20 million units IV q 24 hr continuously or in 6 divided doses) *or* ceftriaxone (2 g IV q 24 hr)	Penicillin G (20 million units IV q 24 hr continuously or in 6 divided doses) *or* ceftriaxone (2 g IV q 24 hr); *followed by* chronic oral suppression with penicillin VK *or* a first-generation cephalosporin *or* minocycline

Bid = twice daily, hr = hours; IV = intravenous, q = every.
*Assuming in vitro susceptibility, no contraindications, and no drug allergies. Dosage varies with creatinine clearance, hepatic function, drug intolerances, and drug interactions. Rifampin use is optional. Chronic suppression use varies with patient circumstances and clinician preference. *S aureus* usually is treated for 6 weeks.

early postoperative or hematogenous infection, the prosthesis typically is retained. A chronic infection accompanied by a loose prosthesis requires resection arthroplasty, with or without a staged reimplantation.

There are no prospective, controlled clinical studies comparing the different surgical modalities and evaluating the appropriate length of antimicrobial therapy

in patients with a prosthetic joint infection. The choice of antimicrobial treatment is based on the specific pathogen and the type of surgery (Table 2).

Débridement and Prosthesis Retention

Débridement with retention of the prosthesis is best used in patients who have a well-fixed prosthesis and

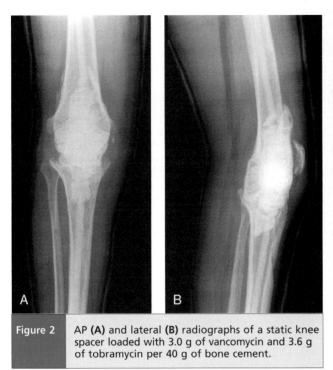

Figure 2   AP **(A)** and lateral **(B)** radiographs of a static knee spacer loaded with 3.0 g of vancomycin and 3.6 g of tobramycin per 40 g of bone cement.

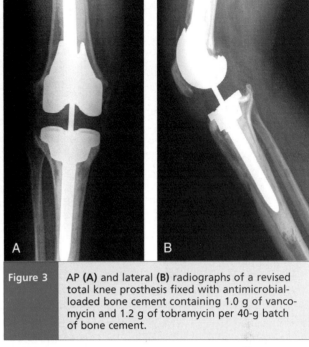

Figure 3   AP **(A)** and lateral **(B)** radiographs of a revised total knee prosthesis fixed with antimicrobial-loaded bone cement containing 1.0 g of vancomycin and 1.2 g of tobramycin per 40-g batch of bone cement.

an early postoperative infection or an acute hematogenous infection caused by a pathogen with relatively low virulence. A satisfactory outcome is more likely with a susceptible causative organism, a symptom duration of 1 to 3 weeks, and the absence of a sinus tract or prosthesis loosening. The polyethylene liner usually is exchanged during the débridement. Most available data on débridement and prosthesis retention relate to THA or TKA. There are fewer data comparing arthroscopic and open débridement, although recent studies suggest that arthroscopic débridement is less effective than open débridement.[13]

In an infection caused by *S aureus* or a coagulase-negative *Staphylococcus*, the risk of treatment failure is greater if the antimicrobial regimen does not include rifampin. Rifampin has excellent in vitro activity against staphylococci, including biofilm organisms. Rifampin should never be used alone because monotherapy commonly leads to the emergence of resistance. The quinolones usually are used in combination with rifampin after completion of a course of intravenous therapy combined with oral rifampin (Table 2). Less information is available on the use of other oral agents in combination with rifampin after intravenous therapy; these agents include fusidic acid (not available in the United States), the β-lactam antimicrobial agents, trimethoprim-sulfamethoxazole, and minocycline.

In a sentinel randomized, controlled clinical study, patients with an orthopaedic implant–related staphylococcal infection were treated with débridement and prosthesis retention followed by a combination of ciprofloxacin and either rifampin or a placebo.[14] All patients who received 3 to 6 months of treatment with ciprofloxacin and rifampin were cured; the rate was

58% among patients treated with ciprofloxacin and a placebo. The patients in both groups had received at least 2 weeks of intravenous antimicrobial therapy including rifampin before beginning the ciprofloxacin-rifampin or ciprofloxacin-placebo therapy. Because resistance to fluoroquinolone is increasing among the staphylococci, the use of combination drug regimens that do not include fluoroquinolone has become much more common in recent years. Recommendations vary as to the optimal length of rifampin-containing intravenous antimicrobial therapy, but a typical course is 2 to 6 weeks. After THA, this intravenous regimen is followed by 6 to 10 weeks of oral therapy (a total of 3 months of antimicrobial therapy); after TKA, the intravenous regimen is followed by 18 to 22 weeks of oral therapy (a total of 6 months of antimicrobial therapy). Chronic oral antimicrobial suppressive therapy may be used at the conclusion of the 3 to 6 months of combination rifampin therapy.

Two-Stage Revision

The first stage of a two-stage revision involves removal of the infected prosthesis, débridement of all infected tissue, and placement of an antimicrobial-impregnated spacer (Figure 2). Systemic antimicrobial therapy is subsequently administered. The second-stage procedure involves removal of the antimicrobial-impregnated spacer and implantation of a second prosthesis (Figure 3). Institutions and surgeons vary in preferred surgical technique, duration of antimicrobial therapy, type of antimicrobial spacer, and time to implantation of the new prosthesis. A two-stage revision usually is the procedure of choice in the United States for treating a chronic prosthetic joint infection or an infection associated with loosening of the prosthesis, particularly if a poor soft-tissue envelope or a sinus tract is present or if the infection is caused by a virulent pathogen. A review of multiple studies including 1,077 treated prosthetic joint infections found that the overall success rate was 87%.[15] Infections caused by methicillin-resistant staphylococci, enterococci, or *Candida* species also have been successfully treated with two-stage revision.[16] The guidelines for administering and monitoring outpatient intravenous antimicrobial therapy should be closely followed, and the patient should be closely monitored for the duration of the therapy.[17] Rifampin is not routinely recommended for the treatment of a methicillin-susceptible or methicillin-resistant staphylococcal infection after resection arthroplasty; existing data support its use only after prosthesis retention. A short course of systemic antimicrobial therapy recently was found to be adequate, although further data are needed before this approach can be recommended.[18]

The interval between the resection and reimplantation typically is 6 to 8 weeks for a TKA and 3 months for a THA. There is concern about treatment failure caused by infection after a two-stage revision; in addition, concern is increasing about mechanical failure and particularly the failure of a cemented component.[19] Cemented components historically were used to allow antibiotic-impregnated bone cement to be used for infection prophylaxis. Increasingly, cementless prostheses with local antimicrobial delivery are being used for reconstruction following infection. Research is needed to compare the prevention of infection and mechanical failure using a cemented prosthesis or a cementless prosthesis with local antimicrobial treatment.

One-Stage Revision
A one-stage revision is more common for a THA infection than a TKA infection, and it is more common in Europe than in the United States. The procedure involves removal of the infected prosthesis, débridement of the surrounding bone and soft tissue, and implantation of a new prosthesis, typically with antimicrobial-impregnated cement. Some clinicians use intravenous antimicrobial therapy for days to weeks after a one-stage revision, as well as chronic antimicrobial suppressive therapy.

The proposed criteria for the use of a one-stage revision include good patient health, a favorable soft-tissue envelope, preoperative identification of the causative pathogen, an antimicrobial-sensitive pathogen, and the expectation that the femoral osseous defect will be minimal after prosthesis removal.[20,21] The success rate of a one-stage revision for an infected THA is approximately 85%.

Permanent Resection Arthroplasty, Arthrodesis, and Amputation
The relative indications for permanent resection arthroplasty or arthrodesis include recurrent infection after a two-stage revision, infection in a patient who has severe immunodeficiency or is an active abuser of intravenous drugs, or infection in a patient who will not receive a functional benefit from revision arthroplasty. Treatment of a prosthetic joint infection with permanent resection arthroplasty usually is followed by 4 to 6 weeks of intravenous antimicrobial therapy. Permanent resection arthroplasty often has a poor functional outcome.

Arthrodesis for the treatment of TKA infection is done with an external fixation device or internal fixation using a plate or intramedullary nail. Bone grafting may be necessary. Like a two-stage revision, arthrodesis using an intramedullary rod usually is completed in staged fashion after antimicrobial therapy is administered for 4 to 6 weeks. The risk of infection following arthrodesis may be greater if internal fixation was used, but the risk of nonunion may be greater if external fixation was used.

The indications for amputation to treat prosthetic joint infection include uncontrollable pain, severe bone loss, and vascular insufficiency that precludes the use of other salvage procedures. If a residual bone infection is present above the level of amputation, the patient will require treatment of chronic osteomyelitis with 4 to 6 weeks of intravenous antimicrobial therapy; otherwise, it is reasonable to treat only the residual soft-tissue infection.

Chronic Oral Antimicrobial Suppression Therapy
Chronic oral antimicrobial suppression typically is used following débridement and prosthesis retention. Only limited data are available on the use of chronic oral suppression after a single-stage revision, after a two-stage revision in a patient who is at high risk of reinfection or relapse, or when surgery is not done. No prospective data are available on chronic oral suppression, and the retrospective information is limited to case series.[22] After débridement and component retention, 89% of 99 prosthetic joint infections were treated with a rifampin-free regimen for chronic suppression; at 2-year follow-up, 60% had survived free of treatment failure (range, 50%-71%; confidence interval, 95%).[22] The use of chronic antimicrobial suppression after débridement and prosthesis retention is controversial, particularly for a staphylococcal infection after a rifampin-based regimen was used. A first-generation cephalosporin, minocycline, or trimethoprim-sulfamethoxazole typically is used for chronic suppression of a staphylococcal infection, based on the results of in vitro susceptibility testing. The patient should be monitored for toxicity with routine laboratory testing while these long-term antimicrobial agents are being used.

Antimicrobial-Impregnated Cement and Spacers
Antimicrobial-impregnated polymethylmethacrylate cement is routinely used for prophylaxis and treatment of prosthetic joint infection.[23] The antimicrobial levels

that can be delivered locally usually are much higher than those achieved systemically. Six products have been approved by the US Food and Drug Administration for use in prosthesis fixation during revision arthroplasty after a resection for prosthetic joint infection. The commercially available products all contain a low dose of an aminoglycoside (gentamicin or tobramycin). Some data suggest that high-level resistance to both tobramycin and gentamicin is common among isolated staphylococci; 41% or 66% of staphylococcal isolates in one study were resistant to gentamicin or tobramycin, respectively.[24] The interpretation of these data is unclear, but they are nonetheless concerning. More information is needed on the predictive value of in vitro susceptibilities for the efficacy of local antimicrobial therapy. Although significant retrospective data support the use of antimicrobial-impregnated cement for prophylaxis against deep infection following primary THA,[25] its use for this purpose remains controversial in the United States because of the cost and the emergence of antimicrobial resistance. In addition, the increasing use of cementless prostheses means that the ability of the clinician to use antimicrobial-impregnated cement for primary or secondary prophylaxis is becoming more limited.

Antimicrobial-impregnated spacers are used in a two-stage revision, and they are considered by many to be the standard of care.[26] Antimicrobial-impregnated spacers deliver high local doses of antimicrobial agents and control dead space; in addition, they improve the patient's mobility before revision arthroplasty in a two-stage revision. The use of articulating spacers is becoming more common, and commercial devices are now available. Some articulating spacers have been approved by the Food and Drug Administration. Some investigators believe that an antimicrobial-impregnated spacer should not be used in patients infected with difficult-to-treat organisms such as methicillin-resistant staphylococci, enterococci, fungi, other multidrug-resistant bacteria, or small colony variants of a staphylococcus.[27] However, some data support the use of a spacer for a prosthetic joint infection caused by a methicillin-resistant *Staphylococcus*, an *Enterococcus*, or *Candida*, provided that active antimicrobial agents that will elute from the spacer are put into the spacer at the time of implantation.[16] The mechanical complications of using antimicrobial-impregnated spacers include pain, dislocation, and instability.

Summary

Prosthetic joint infection is uncommon, but it causes significant morbidity. It has a variable presentation and can be difficult to identify. Combined medical and surgical therapy often is the most effective treatment for a prosthetic joint infection.

Annotated References

1. Proctor RA, Kahl B, von Eiff C, Vaudaux PE, Lew DP, Peters G: Staphylococcal small colony variants have novel mechanisms for antibiotic resistance. *Clin Infect Dis* 1998;27(suppl 1):S68-S74.

2. Berbari EF, Hanssen AD, Duffy MC, et al: Risk factors for prosthetic joint infection: Case-control study. *Clin Infect Dis* 1998;27:1247-1254.

3. Chu VH, Crosslin DR, Friedman JY, et al: Staphylococcus aureus bacteremia in patients with prosthetic devices: Costs and outcomes. *Am J Med* 2005;118:1416.

   The risk of prosthetic joint infection following *S aureus* bacteremia is described.

4. Murdoch DR, Roberts SA, Fowler VG Jr, et al: Infection of orthopedic prostheses after Staphylococcus aureus bacteremia. *Clin Infect Dis* 2001;32:647-649.

5. Mangram AJ, Horan TC, Pearson ML, Silver LC, Jarvis WR: Guideline for Prevention of Surgical Site Infection: 1999: Centers for Disease Control and Prevention (CDC) Hospital Infection Control Practices Advisory Committee. *Am J Infect Control* 1999;27:97-132

6. Tsukayama D, Estrada R, Gustilo RB: Infection after total hip arthroplasty: A study of the treatment of one hundred and six infections. *J Bone Joint Surg Am* 1996;78:512-523.

7. Bottner F, Wegner A, Winkelmann W, Becker K, Erren M, Gotze C: Interleukin-6, procalcitonin and TNF-alpha: Markers of peri-prosthetic infection following total joint replacement. *J Bone Joint Surg Br* 2007;89:94-99.

   The utility of various laboratory tests in identifying prosthetic joint infection before revision arthroplasty was studied. The low sensitivity and specificity of the total leukocyte count and ESR were confirmed. CRP level is the most sensitive and specific widely available laboratory marker for detecting prosthetic joint infection; interleukin-6 testing had equal sensitivity but less specificity. Testing for procalcitonin and tumor necrosis factor–α was very specific but insensitive for diagnosing prosthetic joint infection.

8. Parvizi J, Ghanem E, Menashe S, Barrack RL, Bauer TW: Periprosthetic infection: What are the diagnostic challenges? *J Bone Joint Surg Am* 2006;88 (suppl 4):138-147.

   Issues in the tests used to diagnose prosthetic joint infection are reviewed.

9. Sampedro MF, Patel R: Infections associated with long-term prosthetic devices. *Infect Dis Clin North Am* 2007;21:785-819.

   The diagnosis and treatment of prosthetic joint infection are reviewed.

10. Ghanem E, Parvizi J, Burnett RS, et al: Cell count and differential of aspirated fluid in the diagnosis of infec-

4: Specific Situations

tion at the site of total knee arthroplasty. *J Bone Joint Surg Am* 2008;90:1637-1643.

The results of several preoperative tests, including synovial fluid tests, were combined to provide guidance for the clinical diagnosis of infection. Of 429 knees undergoing revision surgery, 161 had prosthetic joint infection. Combining serum inflammatory markers with the synovial fluid cell count and differential was found to be optimal for the diagnosis of prosthetic joint infection.

11. Ghanem E, Ketonis C, Restrepo C, Joshi A, Barrack R, Parvizi J: Periprosthetic infection: Where do we stand with regard to Gram stain? *Acta Orthop* 2009;80: 37-40.

This study describes the sensitivity of Gram staining in identifying prosthetic joint infection.

12. Trampuz A, Piper K, Jacobson M, et al: Sonication of removed hip and knee prostheses for diagnosis of infection. *N Engl J Med* 2007;357:654-663.

In a prospective study, culturing of fluid samples obtained by sonication of a resected hip or knee prosthesis was found to be significantly more sensitive than tissue culturing (78.5% compared to 60.8%), particularly in patients who had received antimicrobial therapy or for whom fewer than five tissue samples were submitted.

13. Byren I, Bejon P, Atkins BL, et al: One hundred and twelve infected arthroplasties treated with 'DAIR' (debridement, antibiotics and implant retention): Antibiotic duration and outcome. *J Antimicrob Chemother* 2009; 63:1264-1271.

A retrospective study identified 112 patients with prosthetic joint infection after treatment with débridement and retention followed by a mean 1.5-year course of antimicrobial therapy, including rifampin combinations for staphylococcal infection. At mean 2.3-year follow-up, treatment had failed in 18%. The risk factors included arthroscopic débridement, earlier revision surgery, and *S aureus* infection. Although patients who discontinued chronic oral antimicrobial suppression therapy were at higher risk, treatment did not fail in most such patients.

14. Zimmerli W, Widmer AF, Blatter M, Frei R, Ochsner PE: Role of rifampin for treatment of orthopedic implant-related staphylococcal infections: A randomized controlled trial. Foreign-Body Infection (FBI) Study Group. *JAMA* 1998;279:1537-1541.

15. Sia IG, Berbari EF, Karchmer AW: Prosthetic joint infections. *Infect Dis Clin North Am* 2005;19:885-914.

Outcome studies related to prosthetic joint infection are reviewed.

16. Mittal Y, Fehring TK, Hanssen A, Marculescu C, Odum SM, Osmon D: Two-stage reimplantation for periprosthetic knee infection involving resistant organisms. *J Bone Joint Surg Am* 2007;89:1227-1231.

This multicenter study analyzed the outcome of two-stage revision for TKA infection with MRSA or a methicillin-resistant, coagulase-negative *Staphylococcus*. Of 37 patients, 4 (11%) had reinfection with the same

microorganism and 5 (14%) had infection with a different organism. The authors concluded that two-stage revision is a reasonable procedure for patients with TKA infection caused by resistant staphylococci. Level of evidence: IV.

17. Tice AD, Rehm SJ, Dalovisio JR, et al: Practice guidelines for outpatient parenteral antimicrobial therapy: IDSA guidelines. *Clin Infect Dis* 2004;38:1651-1672.

Guidelines are provided on all aspects of outpatient administration of intravenous antimicrobial therapy, including patient selection and monitoring for toxicity.

18. Whittaker JP, Warren RE, Jones RS, Gregson PA: Is prolonged systemic antibiotic treatment essential in two-stage revision hip replacement for chronic Gram-positive infection? *J Bone Joint Surg Br* 2009;91:44-51.

In this retrospective case study, two-stage revision was required in 44 THAs because of aerobic gram-positive infection (63% caused by coagulase-negative staphylococci and 12% by *S aureus*). An antimicrobial-impregnated cement spacer was implanted during resection arthroplasty, followed by a 2-week course of intravenous vancomycin. At a median 49-month follow-up, there were only 6 treatment failures (18%), including three relapses of infection and three infections with a new microorganism. Several recent studies have questioned the optimal duration of intravenous antimicrobial therapy in patients treated with an antimicrobial-impregnated cement spacer during two-stage revision.

19. Sanchez-Sotelo J, Berry DJ, Hanssen AD, Cabanela ME: Midterm to long-term followup of staged reimplantation for infected hip arthroplasty. *Clin Orthop Relat Res* 2009;467:219-224.

A retrospective case study of 168 patients (169 hips) with prosthetic joint infection emphasized treatment failure caused by reinfection or mechanical failure. All hips were treated with two-stage reimplantation. In the second-stage surgery, 121 femoral components were fixed with antimicrobial-impregnated bone cement; all acetabular components were cementless. At a minimum 2-year follow-up, further surgery had been required because of infection in 12 hips (7.1%) or aseptic loosening or osteolysis in 13 hips (7.7%). At 10-year follow-up, 87.5% were infection free and 75.2% were free of mechanical failure. Although the study had low power for detecting differences between groups, the risk of infection or mechanical failure did not differ by type of femoral component fixation. Level of evidence: IV.

20. Jackson WO, Schmalzried TP: Limited role of direct exchange arthroplasty in the treatment of infected total hip replacements. *Clin Orthop Relat Res* 2000;381: 101-105.

21. Ure KJ, Amstutz HC, Nasser S, Schmalzried TP: Direct-exchange arthroplasty for the treatment of infection after total hip replacement: An average ten-year follow-up. *J Bone Joint Surg Am* 1998;80:961-968.

22. Marculescu CE, Berbari EF, Hanssen AD, et al: Outcome of prosthetic joint infections treated with debride-

ment and retention of components. *Clin Infect Dis* 2006;42:471-478.

A large retrospective study identified the success rates of débridement and retention for TKA and THA infection caused by a variety of microorganisms.

23. Jiranek WA, Hanssen AD, Greenwald AS: Antibiotic-loaded bone cement for infection prophylaxis in total joint replacement. *J Bone Joint Surg Am* 2006;88:2487-2500.

Published data are reviewed on antimicrobial-impregnated bone cement used for prophylaxis against prosthetic joint infection in total joint arthroplasty. The patterns of use, mechanical and elution properties, safety, cost, and advantages and disadvantages of different products are compared, with recommendations for the use of antimicrobial-loaded bone cement in primary and revision surgery and for secondary prophylaxis in revision surgery after resection arthroplasty for prosthetic joint infection.

24. Anguita-Alonso P, Hanssen AD, Osmon DR: High rate of aminoglycoside resistance among staphylococci causing prosthetic joint infection. *Clin Orthop Relat Res* 2005;439:43-47.

The in vitro susceptibilities of 93 staphylococcal isolates from patients with prosthetic joint infection were determined. Gentamicin or tobramycin susceptibility was found in 41% or 66% of the isolates, respectively. Methicillin-resistant isolates were more likely to be resistant to gentamicin and tobramycin than methicillin-susceptible isolates. Many microbiology laboratories do not routinely determine the susceptibility of staphylococci to these agents. Surveillance of aminoglycoside resistance in the staphylococci that cause orthopaedic device infections is warranted, as well as research to determine appropriate breakpoints for the local delivery of antimicrobial agents.

25. Parvizi J, Saleh KJ, Ragland PS, Pour AE, Mont MA: Efficacy of antibiotic-impregnated cement in total hip replacement. *Acta Orthop* 2008;79:335-341.

Strict inclusion criteria were used in a meta-analysis of the efficacy and safety of antimicrobial-impregnated cement for prophylaxis in primary and revision THA. The use of antimicrobial-impregnated cement was found to decrease the risk of prosthetic joint infection by approximately 50% in primary THA (from 2.3% to 1.2%). The data were insufficient to form a conclusion on the efficacy of antimicrobial-impregnated cement in preventing infection following revision THA for aseptic loosening.

26. Cui Q, Mihalko WM, Shields JS, Ries M, Saleh KJ: Antibiotic-impregnated cement spacers for the treatment of infection associated with total hip or knee arthroplasty. *J Bone Joint Surg Am* 2007;89:871-882.

This review article describes the classification, construction, efficacy, and safety of articulating and nonarticulating spacers in two-stage revision for THA or TKA infection. The rationale for local antimicrobial delivery, choice of antimicrobial agents, factors that affect elution from spacers, and hand mixing of antimicrobial-impregnated cement are discussed in detail.

27. Zimmerli W, Trampuz A, Ochsner PE: Prosthetic-joint infections. *N Engl J Med* 2004;351:1645-1654.

This excellent review describes the diagnosis and management of prosthetic joint infection from a European perspective.

Chapter 15

Bite Wounds and Infections

Stephen B. Schnall, MD   Jack L. LeFrock, MD

Introduction

An estimated 2 to 5 million people receive a bite wound in the United States each year. Although most such wounds are minor, some require medical treatment. Patients who have sustained a severe bite wound require appropriate acute and follow-up wound care, including antimicrobial therapy. Bite wounds account for approximately 1% of emergency department visits.[1] From 1% to 2% of these injuries are severe enough to require hospitalization.[2-5] The patients most often are male, and children are at particularly high risk.[6,7] Bite wound infections can cause extensive morbidity, including disability and cosmetic damage.

Patients who seek care within 8 hours of a dog bite have an estimated 20% to 30% risk of developing an infection.[8] Dog bites are responsible for 10 to 20 deaths annually, primarily among infants and small children.[4,9] A large percentage of severe dog bites in children are about the head and neck, reflecting the relative heights of the animal and the patient.

Microbiology and Clinical Syndromes

One important aspect of treating a bite wound is to identify the inoculated oropharyngeal flora. The microflora of a dog's mouth consist of more than 60 different bacterial species, many of which are known pathogens. Microflora from soil or excreta also may have been introduced into the wound. A combination of aerobic and anaerobic organisms usually is found in a dog or cat bite wound.[10] The organism most frequently responsible for an infection is *Pasteurella multocida*.[8,11] Other common infecting organisms include *Staphylococcus aureus*; α-, β-, and γ-hemolytic streptococci; some gram-negative bacilli; and a variety of anaerobic organisms, including *Bacteroides fragilis*.[12]

P multocida is found in the mouths of more than 50% of healthy dogs and is responsible for approximately 50% of infections from dog bites and as many as 90% of infections from cat bites.[1,8,13] *P multocida* also is responsible for a large percentage of infections following bites by other small domestic animals. It is occasionally identified in bite wounds caused by rats, mice, rabbits, cattle, opossums, sheep, swine, reindeer, horses, monkeys, wolves, lions, panthers, and lynx.

Pharyngeal cultures of asymptomatic animal handlers and veterinary students have revealed inoculation with this organism. *P multocida* can live as long as 3 weeks in water or soil, and infection therefore can develop in a contaminated skin abrasion, in the absence of a bite. A wound infection caused by *P multocida* is characterized by a rapidly developing, intense inflammatory reaction. Within 24 hours of the injury, local heat, redness, pain, and swelling develop, and in many patients purulent drainage, lymphnoditis, tender regional adenopathy, chills, and fever also develop. These symptoms may appear during administration of suboptimal antibiotic therapy. A review of the literature on disease caused by *P multocida* found that almost 40% of surveyed patients had significant complications resulting from the initial infection, including arthritis, osteomyelitis, tenosynovitis, and bacteremia.[14]

Four unclassified groups of the gram-negative *Capnocytophaga* bacteria (EF-H, M-5, IIj, and DF-2) are associated with dog bite infections.[15] These bacteria are frequently identified in the nasal and oral secretions and on the gingiva of healthy dogs. In a small group of dogs, approximately 10% yielded DF-2 from oropharyngeal washings, and 90% yielded IIj. These bacteria may appear alone or together in a bite wound. It has been suggested that IIj and DF-2 are species of *Flavobacterium* because of similarities in their fatty acid composition. IIj and DF-2 are slow growing and therefore may be missed in wound or blood cultures or incorrectly identified as *P multocida*. A DF-2 infection after a dog bite often leads to a fulminant septic disorder with disseminated intravascular coagulation, symmetric peripheral gangrene, renal cortical necrosis, and shock. Patients who are immunosuppressed or have had a splenectomy are at especially high risk of DF-2 sepsis.[15]

Blastomyces dermatitides may infect dogs living in endemic areas, and human cutaneous blastomycosis has been reported after inoculation via infected sputum from a dog bite. This form of primary cutaneous blastomycosis is manifested by a localized chronic ulcerated lesion with regional lymphadenopathy.[16] Erythema nodosum also may be present.

Approximately 40% of dog or cat bite wounds contain anaerobic organisms. The most commonly isolated anaerobes are *B fragilis, Fusobacterium, Peptococcus, Peptostreptococcus, Propionibacterium,* and *Veillonella*. Bites from chimpanzees, rats, horses, and squirrels also can introduce anaerobic organisms, including *Actinomyces*.[17] A human bite can introduce streptococci,

Table 1

Steps in the Evaluation of a Bite Wound

1. Take a complete patient history. Document the patient's allergies, medications, medical conditions, immunization status, and time of most recent meal.

2. Perform a complete physical examination, with attention to the number of wounds (especially critical for a small child); signs of wound infection such as fever, localized cellulitis, pain, and purulent discharge; signs of joint penetration such as a penetrating bite wound, pain, edema, or decreased range of motion near a joint; tendon exposure or injury; bone exposure; and the presence of foreign bodies.

3. Document any earlier care of the wound, such as cleansing or administration of antibiotic or tetanus prophylaxis.

4. Report the incident to law enforcement officials or animal control agents, as appropriate.

5. After a dog or cat bite, determine the ownership, current location, and rabies vaccination status of the responsible animal, whether the incident was provoked, and whether the animal had a history of biting humans.

Table 2

Steps in the Nonsurgical Treatment of a Bite Wound

1. Obtain specimens for culturing an infected wound before administering antibiotics. A fresh wound does not require culturing.

2. Order laboratory tests as indicated by the patient's condition. For example, a patient with sepsis requires a complete blood count and blood cultures; a patient with a snake bite requires coagulation studies.

3. For a patient with suspected *Capnocytophaga canimorsus* sepsis, examine the peripheral smear for the bacillus.

4. Obtain radiographic studies for every patient with a bite wound to identify any foreign bodies such as teeth, as well as fracture or osteomyelitis. A child with a head wound should be examined for bony penetration using plain radiography or CT. CT should be considered for a child or adult with a deep, penetrating bite wound. If the child was shaken, cervical spine evaluation should be considered.

5. Obtain a bone scan if osteomyelitis is suspected, even if radiographic findings are negative.

6. Administer rabies prophylaxis, if necessary.

7. Administer tetanus immunization, as appropriate.

8. Administer antimicrobial prophylaxis, as appropriate.

staphylococci, *Corynebacterium* species, *Haemophilus* species, and many anaerobic oropharyngeal organisms, including *B fragilis*.

Little is known about the presence of viral pathogens in soft-tissue infections, but the possibility of infection caused by hepatitis B or herpes simplex virus is a concern.[18,19] Human immunodeficiency virus is not commonly found in saliva, and the risk of transmission from a bite wound therefore is relatively low.[19,20] The risk of human bite transmission of the hepatitis C virus also is low.

General Treatment Recommendations

Tables 1 and 2 outline the evaluation and nonsurgical treatment of bite wounds. Table 3 summarizes the microbiology and empiric therapy of infections associated with bite wounds in adults. General principles of wound care should be followed when treating bite wounds. The wound first should be carefully inspected to identify deep injury and devitalized tissue. The area should be copiously irrigated with an isotonic sodium chloride solution, and necrotic tissue should be débrided. If a fracture is present, it should be stabilized

with appropriate coverage. Wounds with extensive crush injury and those requiring extensive débridement should not be closed primarily.

After a mammalian bite, rabies prophylaxis should be administered if the animal responsible for the bite has or is suspected to have rabies. A healthy-appearing animal should be observed for 10 days. Because of the devastating effects of rabies virus infection in humans, many physicians recommend that the patient be vaccinated if the animal is not available for observation. The rabies vaccine is administered as a 1-mL intramuscular injection in five doses (on days 0, 3, 7, 14, and 28). In addition, human rabies immune globulin is administered intramuscularly (30 IU/kg) in one dose on day 0; if anatomically possible, as much as half of this injection should be infiltrated around the wound.

The patient's tetanus immunization status should be determined, and the patient should be immunized as necessary. If the patient has completed primary tetanus immunization but has not received booster immunization within the past 5 years, tetanus-diphtheria toxin should be administered. If the patient's immune status is uncertain, 0.5 mL tetanus toxin and 250 IU tetanus immune globulin should be administered intramuscularly.

Table 3			

Microbiology and Empiric Drug Therapy for Common Bite-Associated Infections

Type of Bite	Common Organisms	Drug Treatments	Drug Treatments for a Penicillin-Allergic Patient
Cat	P multocida Streptococci Anaerobes	Amoxicillin-clavulanate 500 mg tid (oral) Ampicillin-sulbactam 3 g every 6 h (parenteral)	Levofloxacin 500 mg qd (oral) or gatifloxacin 400 mg qd (oral) plus Clindamycin 300 mg every 6 h or metronidazole 500 mg every 6 h (intravenous)
Dog	Streptococci S aureus Eikenella corrodens P multocida Anaerobes	Amoxicillin-clavulanate 500 mg tid, 875 mg bid (oral) Ampicillin-sulbactam 3 g every 6 h (parenteral)	Levofloxacin 500 mg qd (oral) or Gatifloxacin 400 mg qd (parenteral)
Human	S aureus E corrodens Haemophilus influenzae Anaerobes	Amoxicillin-clavulanate 500 mg tid Ampicillin-sulbactam 3 g every 6 h (parenteral) or cefoxitin 2 g every 8 h (parenteral)	Levofloxacin 500 mg qd (parenteral) or gatifloxacin 400 mg qd (IV) plus Clindamycin 900 mg every 8 h (parenteral) or metronidazole 500 mg every 6 h (IV)

Bid = twice daily, IV = intravenous, qd = daily, tid = three times daily.

Antimicrobial prophylaxis is controversial after mammalian bite wounds. However, antimicrobial prophylaxis definitely should be administered for a wound on the hand or near a joint prosthesis, a deep puncture wound, or a wound requiring surgical débridement. In addition, a patient who is older than 65 years or immunocompromised should receive antibiotic prophylaxis. The rate of infection after a cat bite is 56%;[6] therefore, antibiotic prophylaxis is recommended for every patient with a cat bite wound.

Antibiotics for prophylaxis or treatment are chosen based on the presumed oral microbiology of the responsible animal. For a dog, cat, or human bite, penicillin combined with a β-lactamase inhibitor is recommended if the patient has no history of penicillin allergy. The antibiotic choices are listed in Table 3.

Wounds Caused by Land Mammals

Most mammalian bites are inflicted by a dog (85%), cat (5% to 10%), rodent (2% to 3%), or human (2% to 3%). Bites by cats and humans are the most likely to become infected. Dog and cat bites are both responsible for substantial health care costs.[21]

Dogs

A dog bite is associated with a range of injuries from scratches and abrasions to deep open lacerations, puncture wounds, avulsions, and crush injuries.[3] In addition to local infections, depressed skull fractures and brain abscesses (caused by P multocida) have been reported. Dog bites to the head and neck primarily occur in children younger than 5 years. The animal responsible for the bite frequently is known to the person who was bitten.[22,23]

Dogs have relatively blunt teeth, and the wounds from a bite are related to tearing of flesh as well as direct puncture. Some dogs can exert an extremely strong biting force of as much as 450 lb per square inch.[1] A wound caused by a dog bite usually is open and visible, and it can be treated with irrigation, débridement, and appropriate antibiotic prophylaxis. As a result, only 15% to 20% of dog bites lead to an infection.[24] Open wound care can be used for a severely contaminated wound if the size and nature of the wound allow. Joints, tendons, nerves, and vessels must receive appropriate soft-tissue coverage, and wound closure can be considered after adequate débridement.

Cats

Domestic cats have sharp, pointed teeth that penetrate the skin and leave puncture wounds. These direct-inoculation wounds create an environment conducive to bacterial growth, and infection occurs in approximately half of all cat bites. Pasteurella is the most characteristic organism. Cat bites most frequently affect adult women. Most bites occur because the cat was provoked, and two thirds are received in an upper extremity.[1] Adequate surgical and antimicrobial treatment should be considered.

Cat-scratch disease can result from a scratch from a cat's claw or teeth, a cat bite, or, frequently, bites and scratches inflicted during the same incident.[3,25] The disease has recently been attributed to Bartonella henselae, a delicate-appearing pleomorphic, gram-negative organism that is found in lymph nodes, capillary walls in or near areas of follicular hyperplasia, and microabscesses.[3,25] The organism is best seen using Warthin-Starry silver impregnation stain. It is not known whether the organism is an obligate intracellular parasite with host specificity; its growth characteristics and antibiotic sensitivity patterns also are unknown. Cat-scratch disease develops clinically from a painless red papule at the injury site that undergoes pustulation and heals in 1 to 4 weeks. Subsequently, a sterile regional suppurative lymphadenitis develops, with fever, malaise, and weakness lasting as long as 3 months. Although the disease is usually benign and self-limited, it is occasionally associated with parotitis, pneumonitis, erythematic nodosum, thrombocytopenic purpura, or encephalitis. A patient who has severe disease or is immunocompromised can be treated with erythromycin or doxycycline.

Rodents

Rats are the rodents that most frequently bite a human. Children age 5 years or younger are most likely to be bitten. Most bites are to the face or hands and occur during the night.[26]

Rat bites are associated with two specific infecting organisms. *Streptobacillus moniliformis* causes rat bite fever; it is an aerobic, gram-negative organism commonly found in the nasopharynx of wild and laboratory rats.[3,4] *Spirillum minus* produces spirillary rat bite fever (sodoku).[3,4,9]

Humans

Human bite wounds are common. The injury can be devastating, especially if the wound becomes infected. The injury is most frequently at the metacarpophalangeal joint level; the joint is violated in almost 70% of such wounds, tendon injury occurs in almost 20%, and bone injury occurs in 17%.[27] Soft-tissue infection caused by a so-called love nip typically occurs in teenagers and adults in their 20s and can be found on any area of the body; occlusion bites usually involve the upper extremities, the breast in men, or the genitalia in women.

Almost 50 different aerobic and anaerobic organisms have been cultured from the human mouth, including *S aureus, E corrodens, H influenzae,* and the anaerobic bacterial strains that produce β-lactamase. *E corrodens,* a gram-negative facultative anaerobe, is common, and the appropriate cultures should be requested.[10,28-33] *E corrodens* is similar to *P multocida,* an organism common in cats and dogs, and it is sensitive to penicillin. Because *E corrodens* is resistant to first-generation cephalosporins, macrolides, clindamycin, and aminoglycosides, it should be treated with oral amoxicillin-clavulanic acid or with intravenous ampicillin-sulbactam or cefoxitin.

A recent human bite wound can be treated on an outpatient basis, but an infected wound usually requires hospitalization. A human bite wound should never receive primary suturing. Surgical exploration should be done with a sterile field, adequate exposure, and thorough débridement and lavage. It is important to remember that the extensor tendon has a more distal excursion when the hand is formed into a fist. The fingers are usually in extension during the surgical procedure, and a proximal extension of the wound is necessary to avoid overlooking a tendon injury.

Monkeys

Although monkey bites are rare, they carry a high risk of infection. A monkey bite can lead to infectious diseases including herpetic encephalitis, which is frequently fatal; monkeypox, an illness simulating mild variola; tuberculosis; hepatitis A; and Marburg disease, a rare and often-fatal hemorrhagic-uremic disorder characterized by thrombocytopenia, leucopenia encephalitis, and hepatocellular sepsis, frequently accompanied by shock and disseminated intravascular coagulation.

Wounds Caused by Other Animals

Marine Animals

Most wounds caused by marine animals are not bite wounds. Pain and tissue necrosis can result from a puncture wound or a sting, and toxins sometimes cause severe systemic symptoms and shock. Infections after these injuries are caused by organisms in seawater. Among the commonly responsible animals are sea urchins, jellyfish, catfish, stingrays, and coral. The spines of a sea urchin are composed of calcite covered with epithelium, which may contain venom. The calcium in a spine is initially visible on radiographs of the wound, although it is eventually absorbed. The tissue reaction is caused by the venom or foreign proteins present in the epithelium, and even nonvenomous spine penetration can be painful.[34] Jellyfish inject toxin via a nematocyst. Catfish and stingray spines cause severe pain; immersion of the affected extremity in hot water (104° to 115°F) and antibiotics to cover gram-negative organisms are used.

In addition to supportive care, pain control may be required, as when symptoms of significant envenomation occur. Wound care requires removal of any spines, débridement with thorough irrigation, and open treatment. Prophylactic antibiotics and tetanus prophylaxis should be administered after a marine sting, puncture, or bite.

Seal finger is an infection that can be caused by contact between the skin of a seal and a small skin break in a human finger. Alternatively, the infection can result from a direct bite by a seal. The responsible microbe is unknown;[35] none of the microorganisms usually associated with marine contact, such as *Erysipelothrix, Mycobacterium,* or even *Pasteurella,* have been identified. Infection can develop within 3 to 7 days. The patient has exquisite pain and swelling with erythema and possibly lymphangitis. Joint involvement leads to permanent arthritic damage. A throbbing, painful abscess appears at the site of infection. Progressive swelling and involvement of the entire hand sometimes occur without lymphangitis or fever. The natural course of the infection is slow resolution. The patient should be treated with tetracycline.[35]

Vibrio vulnificus can cause a rapidly progressing cellulitis. Typically, the infection occurs when contaminated seawater enters a wound incurred during shellfish harvesting or cleaning. The characteristic progressively necrotizing violet-colored lesion requires incision, drainage, débridement, and sometimes limb amputation.

Infection by *Mycobacterium marinum* has been reported after a dolphin bite, but it more commonly results from seawater contamination of an abrasion on an extremity. The infection is characterized by a small, tender papule. Progressive, persistent ulceration, a row of small papules, or proximally spreading papules sometimes follow. The normal course of the infection is indolent and slowly progressing. Like other mycobacteria (with the exception of *Mycobacterium tuberculosis*), *M marinum* should be cultured at 32°C in Löwenstein-Jensen medium.

Snakes

Approximately 10,000 poisonous snake bites occur in the United States each year. Most are inflicted by a rattlesnake or another member of the Crotalid family, such as the copperhead or cottonmouth (both of which belong to the *Agkistrodon* [moccasin] genus). Known as pit vipers because of the heat-sensing pits at the base of their snout, these snakes inject venom through hollow extensible fangs.

Pit viper venom contains a complex mixture of proteolytic enzymes. The hematologic consequences of a bite differ by species but often include coagulopathy.[36] Pit viper bites also can cause myonecrosis and neurologic symptoms. *Clostridium perfringens,* the most common anaerobic species in the oral flora of snakes, has been found in half of the cultures from fresh envenomated snake bite wounds, and *B fragilis* has been found in one third. Snake bites also can introduce enteric organisms such as *Salmonella* or *Shigella*. A broad-spectrum antibiotic covering aerobic coliform and anaerobic organisms should be considered.[37]

Before treating a snake bite, it is important to determine whether the bite was envenomated.[36,38] The size, age, and species of the snake should be ascertained, if possible. A relatively small, young poisonous snake may inject a smaller quantity of more lethal venom. The time of day the bite occurred and the type of attack can help in determining whether the snake was a pit viper (which strikes and then retreats) or a species such as a coral snake, which makes chewing motions.[39,40] Coral snake venom is a neurotoxin and does not cause the pain, swelling, and discoloration characteristic of pit viper venom. The immediate symptoms and signs as well as the rate of progression are paramount in evaluating a patient with a venomous snake bite.[38] Determining the severity of envenomation is important for

all aspects of snake bite treatment, including the need for administering an antivenin. The commercially available antivenins are CroFab (Savage Laboratories, Melville NY), which is an ovine Crotalidae polyvalent immune Fab; and Antivenin Crotalidae Polyvalent (Wyeth, Madison, NJ), an equine-derived product.[38]

Pain, swelling, erythema, and ecchymosis begin 30 minutes to 1 hour after a pit viper bite. The neurologic changes after a coral snake bite include tremors and altered sensorium.[36] In approximately 20% of bites from a poisonous snake, no venom is injected. No signs or symptoms appear after these dry bites, and only local wound care is necessary. A minimally envenomated pit viper bite produces local pain, swelling, and discoloration, but systemic signs are not present, and laboratory test results are unremarkable. Treatment with antivenin is not warranted. More extensive swelling appears after a moderate envenomation, with rapidly progressing symptoms. Coagulopathy can result, even though vital signs remain normal. Antivenin should be administered for moderate envenomation, especially if the patient is a child, is older than 65 years, or is immunocompromised. After severe envenomation, the patient has abnormal vital signs, perioral tingling, diaphoresis, diarrhea, and vomiting.[36] Antivenin should be administered. Serial examination is required, with particular attention to compartment syndrome, and compartment pressures should be noted if signs of compartment syndrome appear. A fasciotomy is performed if the examination reveals compartment syndrome or compartment pressures are elevated. Despite the marked swelling, compartment syndrome usually does not develop.[37]

The use of ice or tourniquets should be avoided in treating a snake bite. A complete laboratory panel should be ordered, including complete blood count, metabolic studies, and coagulation studies. Tetanus prophylaxis should be administered as necessary. Broad-spectrum antibiotics are used as prophylaxis for wounds created by the primary bite or subsequent surgical procedures. However, antibiotics may not be necessary for an envenomated but uninfected wound.[41]

Arachnids

Scorpions and spiders are responsible for most injuries caused by arachnids. *Centruroides* is the genus responsible for most scorpion stings in the United States and Mexico. Scorpion venom is injected via a telson and contains neurotoxins that block ion channels and cause profound acetylcholine and catecholamine release. The systemic symptoms, including severe pain and paresthesias, are rare in adults but more common in children and in adults older than 65 years. Supportive care is critical.[42,43]

The venom of a spider is intended to immobilize and liquefy its prey, as spiders do not have teeth. Most spider bites cause a local reaction. However, a bite from the brown recluse spider or its cousins in the *Loxosceles* genus causes significant tissue necrosis and some systemic signs. It is therefore important to identify the species of the spider responsible for the bite. A brown recluse spider bite is characterized by the so-called red, white, and blue phenomenon, which describes the bluish central necrotic area surrounded by an area of blanching and an outside erythematous circle. Differential diagnosis is important because early lesions can resemble those of Lyme disease,[3,42,43] and later lesions may simulate an oxacillin-resistant staphylococcal infection. True *Loxosceles* spiders have a distinct geographic distribution, primarily in the south central United States, and a bite that occurred elsewhere most likely was caused by another spider or an insect.[43]

A bite from a black widow spider (*Latrodectus mactans*) has significant systemic signs and symptoms, although there is little tissue injury. The venom is a rapidly acting neurotoxin that causes severe abdominal pain and cramping and can simulate peritonitis. Blood pressure elevation and diaphoresis occur. An antivenin is available but is used only for severe symptoms. Like some snake-bite antivenin, it is derived from horse serum, and the possibility of allergic reaction must be considered.

Local wound care is the preferred treatment of a spider bite. Antibiotics are used if infection is observed. Dapsone, glucocorticoids, hyperbaric oxygen, electric shock, excision and grafting, and antivenin have been used, although no benefit over local wound care has been proved.[44] Dapsone can be used to treat a documented *Loxosceles* bite, but its toxicity must be considered.[43]

Summary

Adequate patient history and evaluation are paramount for optimal treatment of bite wounds and infections. An epidermal-only wound not involving the hands or feet carries a low risk of infection, regardless of whether antibiotics are administered, if it is treated within 24 hours of injury. However, antibiotic prophylaxis is warranted for a wound with evidence of deeper penetration, especially a hand injury or a human, dog, or cat bite wound.[45] Prophylactic antibiotics also are recommended for any deep puncture wound in a patient who is older than 65 years or immunocompromised; or a wound near a prosthetic joint and or in an extremity with compromised venous or lymphatic drainage. *P multocida* should be suspected in a mammalian bite wound that becomes infected within 24 hours; pending culture results, coverage for aerobic and anaerobic organisms is prudent.[45] All patients with a cat bite wound should receive antibiotic prophylaxis.

Annotated References

1. Dire DJ: Emergency management of dog and cat bite wounds. *Emerg Med Clin North Am* 1992;10:719-736.

2. Brook I: Human and animal bite infections. *J Fam Pract* 1989;28:713-718.

3. Hodge D, Tecklenburg FW: Bites and stings. In Fleisher GR, Ludwig S, Henretig FM (eds): *Textbook of Pediatric Emergency Medicine*, ed 5. Philadelphia, PA, Williams and Wilkins, 2006, p 1045.

   This extensive review of animal bites and stings in children cites 103 references covering mammalian, insect, arachnid, and marine animal wounds.

4. Fleisher GR: The management of bite wounds. *N Engl J Med* 1999;340:138-140.

5. Talan DA, Citron DM, Abrahamian FM, et al: Bacteriologic analysis of dog and cat bites. *N Engl J Med* 1999;340:85-92.

6. Weiss HB, Friedman DI, Coben JH: Incidence of dog bite injuries treated in emergency departments. *JAMA* 1998;279:51-53.

7. Patrick GR, O'Rourke KM: Dog and cat bites: Epidemiologic analyses suggest different prevention strategies. *Public Health Rep* 1998;113:252-257.

8. Goldstein EJ: Bite wounds and infection. *Clin Infect Dis* 1992;14:633-638.

9. Ginsberg C: Animal and human bites, in Behrman RE, Kliegman RM, Jenson HB: *Nelson's Textbook of Pediatrics*, ed 17. Philadelphia, PA, WB Saunders, 2004, pp 2385-2387.

   The diagnosis and treatment of pediatric animal bite wounds are outlined.

10. Wiggins ME, Akelman E, Weiss APC: The management of dog bites and dog infections to the hand. *Orthopedics* 1994;17:617-623.

11. Arons MS, Fernando L, Polayes IM: Pasteurella multocida: The major cause of hand infections following domestic animal bites. *J Hand Surg Am* 1982;7:47-52.

12. Goldstein EJC, Citron DE, Finegold SM: Role of anaerobic bacteria in bite wound infections. *Rev Infect Dis* 1984;6(suppl 1):S177-S183.

13. Cummings P: Antibiotics to prevent infection in patients with dog bite wounds: A meta-analysis of randomized trials. *Ann Emerg Med* 1994;23:535-540.

14. Weber DJ, Wolfson JS, Swartz MN, Hooper DC: Pasteurella multocida infections: Report of 34 cases and review of the literature. *Medicine* 1984;63:133-157.

15. Kalb R, Kaplan MH, Tenenbaum MJ, et al: Cutaneous infection at dog bite wounds associated with fulminant DF-2 septicaemia. *Am J Med* 1985;78:687-690.

16. Gnann JW, Bressler GS, Bodet CA, Avent CK: Human blastomycosis after a dog bite. *Ann Intern Med* 1983;98:48-49.

17. Peel MM, Hornidge KA, Luppino M, Stacpoole AM, Weaver RE: *Actinobacillus* spp and related bacteria in infected wounds of humans bitten by horses and sheep. *J Clin Microbiol* 1991;29:2535-2538.

18. Muguti GI, Dixon MS: Tetanus following human bite. *Br J Plast Surg* 1992;45:614-615.

19. Richman KM, Rickman LS: The potential for transmission of human immunodeficiency virus through human bites. *J Acquir Immune Defic Syndr* 1993;6:402-406.

20. Havens PL: Postexposure prophylaxis in children and adolescents for nonoccupational exposure to human immunodeficiency virus. *Pediatrics* 2003;111:1475-1489.

    This clinical report reviews child and adolescent exposure to human immunodeficiency virus and specifically mentions the low risk of transmission from saliva in human bite wounds involving other children.

21. Benson LS, Edwards SL, Schiff AP, Williams CS, Visotsky JL: Dog and cat bites to the hand: Treatment and cost assessment. *J Hand Surg Am* 2006;31:468-473.

    This retrospective review found that after a dog or cat bite to the hand, almost two thirds of patients required hospitalization for intravenous administration of antibiotics or a surgical procedure. Thirteen of 111 patients incurred medical costs greater than $77,000.

22. Sutton LN, Alpert G: Brain abscess following cranial dog bite. *Clin Pediatr (Phila)* 1984;23:580.

23. Klein DM, Cohen ME: Pasteurella multocida brain abscess following perforating cranial dog bite. *J Pediatr* 1978;92:588-589.

24. Anderson CR: Animal bites. *Postgrad Med* 1992;92:134-146.

25. Leonard SN, Welch D: Bartonella species including cat scratch, in Mandell GL, Bennett JE, Dolin R: *Principles and Practice of Infectious Diseases*, ed 5. Philadelphia, PA, Churchill Livingstone, 2000, pp 2444-2453.

26. Byington CL, Basow RD: Rat-bite fever. In Feigin RD, Cherry JD (eds): *Textbook of Pediatric Infectious Diseases*. Philadelphia, PA, WB Saunders, 1998, pp 1529-1542.

27. Patzakis MJ, Wilkens J, Bassett RL: Surgical findings in clenched fist injuries. *Clin Orthop Relat Res* 1987;220:237-240.

28. Dreyfuss UY, Singer M: Human bites of the hand: A study of one hundred six patients. *J Hand Surg Am* 1985;10:884-889.

29. Goldstein EJC, Barones MF, Miller TA: Eikenella corrodens in hand infections. *J Hand Surg Am* 1983;8:563-567.

30. Shields C, Patzakis MJ, Meyers MH, Harvey JP Jr: Hand infections secondary to human bites. *J Trauma* 1975;15:235-236.

31. Goldstein EJC, Citron DM: Comparative susceptibilities of 173 aerobic and anaerobic bite wound isolates to sparfloxacin, temafloxacin, clarithromycin, and older agents. *Antimicrob Agents Chemother* 1993;37:1150-1153.

32. Rayan GM, Putnam JL, Cahill SL, et al: Eikenella corrodens in human mouth flora. *J Hand Surg Am* 1988;13:953-956.

33. Zubowicz VN, Gravier M: Management of early human bites of the hand: A prospective randomized study. *Plast Reconstr Surg* 1991;88:111-114.

34. Newmeyer WL III: Management of sea urchin spines in the hand. *J Hand Surg Am* 1988;13:455-457.

35. Mass DP, Newmeyer WL, Kilgore ES: Seal finger. *J Hand Surg Am* 1981;6:610-612.

36. Gold BS, Barish RA, Dart RC: North American snake envenomation: Diagnosis, treatment, and management. *Emerg Med Clin North Am* 2004;22:423-443.

    A bite from a venomous snake is a medical emergency, and treatment decisions must be based on close monitoring of the potentially erratic envenomation syndrome.

37. Rowland S, Pederson WC: The management of snake (pit viper) bites, in Green D, Hotchkiss R, Pederson W, Wolfe S (eds): *Green's Operative Hand Surgery*, ed 5. Philadelphia, PA, Churchill Livingstone, 2006, p 2013.

    This review of envenomation injuries caused by pit vipers is focused on acute treatment. Antibiotic recommendations and surgical treatment are included, with a synopsis of a treatment algorithm.

38. Kitchens CS: Snakebite. *Conn's Curr Ther* 2007;1338-1341.

    The diagnosis and treatment of snake bites are described, with an emphasis on distinguishing between the severity of evenomation and its role in treatment.

39. Seiler JG III, Sagerman SD, Geller RJ, Eldridge JC, Fleming LL: Venomous snake bite: Current concepts of treatment. *Orthopedics* 1994;17:707-714.

40. Snyder C: Animal bite infections. *Hand Clin* 1998;14:691-711.

41. LoVecchio F, Klemens J, Welch S, Rodriguez R: Antibiotics after rattlesnake envenomation. *J Emerg Med* 2002;23:327-328.

42. Saucier JR: Arachnid envenomation. *Emerg Med Clin North Am* 2004;22:405-422.

    This extensive review of arachnid bite wounds includes types, envenomation, and treatment options.

43. Swanson DL, Vetter RS: Bites of brown recluse spiders and suspected necrotic arachnidism. *N Engl J Med* 2005;352:700-707.

The geographic distribution of certain arachnids, the brown recluse spider bite, and the importance of correct diagnosis of an arachnid bite are discussed.

44. Phillips S, Kohn M, Baker D, et al: Therapy of brown spider envenomation: A controlled trial of hyperbaric oxygen, dapsone, and cyproheptadine. *Ann Emerg Med* 1995;25:363-368.

45. Nakamura Y, Daya M: Use of appropriate antimicrobials in wound management. *Emerg Med Clin North Am* 2007;25:159-176.

Most simple, uncomplicated wounds do not require systemic antibiotics but benefit from the use of topical antibiotics. Antibiotics cannot substitute for good local wound care.

Chapter 16

Hand Infections

Montri D. Wongworawat, MD   Stephen B. Schnall, MD

Introduction

Infection rates higher than 10% have been reported after open fractures of the hand.[1] Most hand infections are caused by *Staphylococcus* or *Streptococcus* species. If appropriate treatment of a hand infection is delayed, the risk of complications and the time required for resolution are likely to increase.[2]

Microbiology and Epidemiology

Resistance to antimicrobial treatment of infection increasingly is becoming a concern. During a 3-year period, 443 patients were surgically treated for hand and upper extremity infections at one institution. The reasons for patient admission included human bite (51%) as well as cellulitis, septic arthritis, abscess, gangrene, purulent flexor tenosynovitis, osteomyelitis, animal bite, web space infection, and paronychia.[3] Bacterial cultures were obtained for 395 patients, of which 247 were culture positive. A total of 719 organisms were isolated. Gram-positive aerobes accounted for almost two thirds of the organisms; 30% of these were *Streptococcus* species, 15% were *Staphylococcus aureus*, and 12% were coagulase-negative *Staphylococcus*. Bacteria that are resistant to first-line antibiotic therapy were found in 16% of the cultures, of which resistant *S aureus* was found in 20%. In addition, resistant strains of *Enterococcus* were found in 47%; *Enterobacter*, in 67%; *Acinetobacter*, in 92%; and *Pseudomonas*, in 100%.[3] Another study found a 34% rate of methicillin-resistant *S aureus* (MRSA) in surgically treated hand infections.[4] MRSA was the predominant single organism cultured from patients with a hand infection during a 2-year period at one institution.[5] The prevalence of community-acquired MRSA is increasing.

Evaluation and Treatment

A complete patient history and a thorough physical examination are important in assessing hand infections. Conditions that can mimic infection, such as gout, inflammatory arthritis, metastatic lesions, and factitious disorders, should be considered. The type of material expressed from the infected site should be noted because its consistency, odor, and color may be useful in choosing an empiric antibiotic. A purulent abscess with relatively thick material suggests a bacterial infection; vesicular watery fluid, a viral etiology; and material with the consistency of cottage cheese, a fungal etiology.

Cultures usually should be obtained before empiric antibiotic therapy is initiated. However, obtaining cultures may be unnecessary if the physician can identify the organism with a high degree of certainty.[6] Table 1 summarizes the recommended empiric antibiotic treatments. A greater-than-expected number of mixed flora infections, including anaerobic, mycobacterial, and fungal species, were found in cultures from patients who received antibiotics for a persistent infection.[7]

The surgical treatment of a hand infection should include incisions adequate for exposing the entire infected and draining area. The area must be irrigated and débrided to dilute the infection and remove necrotic debris. Most infected wounds should be left open after initial débridement. A secondary coverage procedure may be performed after the wound has developed a healthy granulation bed and the contamination is significantly reduced.

Immobilization initially may be necessary to maintain hand posture in the intrinsic-plus position (the wrist at 30° extension, metacarpophalangeal joints at 70° flexion, and interphalangeal joints at full extension). The timely initiation of motion exercises is crucial for maximum functional recovery; therefore, the patient's care must be coordinated with a hand therapist.[8]

Bacterial Infections

Felon

Pulp space infections often are caused by direct bacterial inoculation. The symptoms include severe pain, tenderness over the fingertip, and swelling. Osteomyelitis of the adjacent distal phalanx, septic arthritis, or purulent flexor tenosynovitis may develop if treatment is delayed.

Surgical decompression is the mainstay of treatment. A longitudinal incision is made on the midlateral aspect of the digit just below the nail or at the finger pulp.[9] A fishmouth incision should be avoided because it can lead to flap compromise and painful bulbous fingertip deformity.[9] Blunt disruption of all fibrous septae is

---

Table 1

Empiric Antibiotic Treatment of Common Hand Infections

Type of Infection	Organisms	Drugs
Abscess	S aureus MRSA Group A streptococci Anaerobes	First-generation cephalosporin Ertapenem Vancomycin (if MRSA is suspected)
Bite wound, cat	S aureus Pasturella multocida Anaerobes	Ertapenem Ampicillin + sulbactam (administered intravenously)
Bite wound, dog	S aureus P multocida Anaerobes	Penicillin Clindamycin + quinolone (if patient has penicillin allergy)
Bite wound, human	Streptococcus viridans S aureus Eikenella corrodens Anaerobes	Amoxicillin + clavulanate (administered orally)
Cellulitis	S aureus Group A streptococci	First-generation cephalosporin
Felon	S aureus Streptococci	First-generation cephalosporin
Gonorrhea, disseminated	Neisseria gonorrhoeae	Ceftriaxone
Mycobacterium marinum	M marinum	Clarithromycin Doxycycline Rifampin + ethambutol
Necrotizing fasciitis	S aureus Group A streptococci Enterobacteriaceae Anaerobes	Clindamycin + vancomycin (if atypical mycobacterium is suspected) + piperacillin + tazobactam
Osteomyelitis	S aureus Streptococci (Less common: Enterobacteriaceae, Pseudomonas aeruginosa, anaerobes)	Oxacillin or nafcillin First-generation cephalosporin Vancomycin (if MRSA is suspected)
Osteomyelitis, tuberculous	Mycobacterium tuberculosis	Isoniazid Rifampin + pyrazinamide + ethambutol
Paronychia	S aureus Group A streptococci	First-generation cephalosporin
Purulent flexor tenosynovitis	S aureus Group A streptococci	Ertapenem Ampicillin + sulbactam
Sporotrichosis	Sporothrix schenckii	Itraconazole
Whitlow	Herpes simplex virus 1 or 2	Acyclovir Valacyclovir Famciclovir

performed to decompress all compartments. Daily soaking in warm water should be initiated after surgery, and the wound is allowed to heal by secondary intention.

Paronychia

Infection around the nail bed often is caused by minor trauma such as from a hangnail, a poorly performed manicure, or nail biting. Patients with immunocompromised status are especially at risk of paronychia.[10] Acute infections usually are caused by *Staphylococcus* species, and gram-negative or fungal organisms may be found in chronic infections.

Incision and drainage of acute paronychia do not achieve better results than treatment with oral antibiotics.[11] Treatment can begin with warm soaking and oral antibiotics for *Staphylococcus* coverage. Surgical drainage is recommended if nonsurgical treatment does not eradicate the infection and fluctuance is observed. The incision over the fluctuance should be performed carefully, with or without partial nail excision, while avoiding injury to the nail matrix. Another method of providing drainage is marsupialization, in which a crescent of skin proximal to the eponychial fold is removed and healing is allowed by secondary intention.[12]

A recalcitrant infection may be an indication that the etiology is fungal or the patient is immunocompromised. A randomized, double-blinded, double-dummy study compared treatment of chronic paronychia using topical steroids or systemic antifungal therapy in 45 patients. Cure or improvement resulted from methylprednisolone treatment in 41 of 48 fingernails (85%); from terbinafine treatment, in 30 of 57 (53%); and from itraconazole treatment in only 29 of 64 (45%). This finding suggests that an environmental dermatitis was a more important cause than *Candida*.[13]

Human Bites

A human bite to the hand requires immediate attention. The deep structures of the hand often are injured, even in a wound that appears innocuous. A review of 194 skin lacerations in 191 patients found joint capsule violation in 132 (68%), tendon involvement in 39 (20%), articular-bone indentations in 33 (17%), and free articular cartilage fragments in 12 (6%).[14] The incisions should be made proximal and distal to the wound to allow adequate visualization and exploration of all possibly injured structures. Thorough débridement of the wound is necessary.

Patient compliance with postsurgical treatment was found to be poor. This finding may be related to the characteristics of the patients, most of whom were young adult men who received a clenched fist injury during an altercation.[14]

E corrodens was formerly believed to be the characteristic organism in a human bite to the hand, but recent studies suggest that *Streptococcus* species are more frequently responsible. A total of 380 organisms were isolated from specimens collected from 57 patients; *Streptococcus* species were the most common aerobic organisms, and *Prevotella* species were the most prevalent anaerobes.[15] In a multicenter prospective study of 50 patients treated in the emergency department, the median number of isolates per wound culture was four. *Streptococcus* species were isolated in 82% of the cultures; *E corrodens* was present in 30%.[16] This finding underscores the polymicrobial nature of human bite infections.

Purulent Flexor Tenosynovitis

The tendon sheath mechanism provides a gliding surface for the flexor tendons, and the thickened pulley system of the sheaths provides stability. As a result, the functioning of the mechanism resembles that of a fishing rod rather than a bow and arrow. The vascular supply to the tendons is complex.[17] There can be a clinically significant increase in digital tissue pressure in a patient with suppurative flexor tenosynovitis.[18,19]

The sheaths of the index, long, and ring fingers usually begin 1 cm proximal to the deep transverse metacarpal ligaments, although many variations exist. The sheaths of the thumb and little finger frequently are confluent to the radial or ulnar bursa, respectively. These bursae allow purulent material to easily track proximal to the wrist through one bursa and distal to the wrist through the other bursa, after traversing Parona's space, and thereby to create a so-called horseshoe abscess. Although hematogenous spread of infection can cause a horseshoe abscess, particularly with gonococcus,[20] the most common scenario involves a penetrating injury.

The clinical signs of purulent flexor tenosynovitis are a slight flexion posture of the finger, fusiform swelling, tenderness along the flexor sheath, and exquisite pain with passive extension of the digit.[21] Purulent flexor tenosynovitis is classified according to severity. In stage I, the sheath has serous exudate and congestion; in stage II, the sheath has murky or cloudy fluid, purulence, and synovial granulation; and in stage III, marked sheath or tendon necrosis is present.[22]

Surgical treatment is recommended. Continuous closed tendon sheath irrigation has been a standard method of surgical drainage for many years. A palmar incision can allow access to the sheath at the level of the A1 pulley, and a second incision in the digit distal to the A4 pulley can be used to irrigate the sheath. A transverse or short longitudinal incision is made in the palm (without extending beyond the proximal digital crease) to gain access to the fibroosseous tunnel proximally. A small Brunner or short midlateral incision allows distal access to the sheath. Irrigation is performed from proximal to distal using a small angiocatheter and is continued until the effluent is clear. The hand is placed in a bulky dressing with an indwelling catheter, and irrigation is continued with saline at approximately 25 mL/h for the next 24 to 48 hours. The catheter is then removed, the dressing is changed, and range-of-motion exercises are initiated. A 2000 study found that continuous postsurgical irrigation with an indwelling catheter may not be necessary.[23] Regardless of method, an early, aggressive range-of-motion program, under the direct supervision of a physician or therapist, is of paramount importance to maximize results.

A recent study identified several risk factors in patients with pyogenic flexor tenosynovitis.[24] Poor outcome was associated with the presence of subcutaneous purulence, digital ischemia, or polymicrobial infection; patient age greater than 43 years; and the presence of diabetes, peripheral vascular disease, or renal failure.

Palmar Space Infections

A diagnosis of a palmar space infection may be delayed because the affected spaces are deep to the soft-tissue structures of the palm. Swelling of the dorsum of the

4: Specific Situations

hand is often present, and the palmar contour is usually lost.

The thenar, hypothenar, and midpalmar spaces lie between the fascial planes of the hand.[25] The thenar space includes the thenar musculature and the first dorsal interosseous muscle and is separated from the midpalmar space by the septum arising from the third metacarpal. A straight dorsal incision over the first web space is used for surgical drainage and is combined with a volar incision in line with the thenar crease. Care should be taken to avoid the recurrent motor and palmar cutaneous branches of the median nerve.

The hypothenar space includes the hypothenar muscles and is separated from the midpalmar space by a fascial septum arising from the fifth metacarpal. Hypothenar space infections are rare. The space is drained through an incision placed on the radial aspect of the hypothenar eminence.

The midpalmar space lies between the thenar and hypothenar spaces, and it may be continuous with Parona's space in the distal forearm. Several palmar incisions, including longitudinal, transverse, oblique, or combined incisions, can be used for evacuation.

Web space infections are also referred to as collar button abscesses. An isolated collar button abscess does not involve the thenar, hypothenar, or midpalmar space and therefore is not a true deep space infection. There may be relatively little swelling in the palm but marked swelling on the dorsum of the web space. Combined incisions should be used because of dorsal-palmar communication. In designing palmar and web space incisions, it is important to avoid creating scar contractures. Oblique or zigzag palmar incisions are recommended; straight, longitudinal incisions are used on the dorsum.[8]

Bone and Joint Infections

Bone and joint infections most commonly occur after traumatic penetrating injury. The most common causative organisms are *S aureus* and *Streptococcus* species.[26] The patient may have a predisposing condition such as diabetes, vascular disease, sickle cell anemia, a connective tissue disorder, or intravenous drug use. A review of 700 patients with a hand infection found that 22% had vascular insufficiency or were immunocompromised. Patient history, physical examination, plain radiography, and biopsy or culture were the most useful factors in diagnosing the infection.[27]

Surgical débridement is the mainstay of treatment. If septic arthritis is present, the goal of surgical planning, including incision planning, should be to preserve the extensor mechanism and thereby prevent late deformities such as the septic boutonniere deformity. A metacarpophalangeal joint incision usually is performed on the dorsal aspect in a curvilinear, longitudinal fashion. The proximal interphalangeal joint is drained from a midlateral approach palmar to the lateral bands or in the plane between the lateral bands and central slip. Postsurgical mobilization is important for a good functional outcome.[28]

Several options are available for treating osteomyelitis, from simple curettage to staged reconstruction. Early treatment is important and should include débridement of necrotic bone and tissue.[29] The overall amputation rate for osteomyelitis of the hand is 39%. However, the amputation rate is 86% if treatment is delayed more than 6 months.[27]

Viral Infections

Superficial viral infections of the hand usually are herpetic in origin. The cause of herpetic whitlow in adolescents and adults is inoculation of herpes simplex virus type 2; in children, the cause usually is herpes simplex virus type 1.[30] The patient has vesicular lesions with clear or turbid fluid, not purulent material, and may have lymphadenopathy, lymphangitis, or fever. An infant or child may have oral lesions. The erythema and pain may be less severe than with a bacterial infection.[31] Viral infections present a risk to medical and health care personnel; cross contamination between patients and workers is well recognized. The risk of contracting herpetic whitlow is increased in a person who is immunocompromised.[32-34]

Viral infections should be observed; resolution usually requires approximately 2 weeks. Surgical treatment can lead to a secondary bacterial infection. Oral antiviral agents are not used unless the patient is immunocompromised or the infection is extremely extensive. Intravenous acyclovir has been used to treat severe viral infections.

Atypical Infections

Fungal Infections

Fungal or mycobacterial hand infections are often classified as atypical.[35] A person who is immunocompromised may be particularly susceptible to a fungal infection.[36] The pathogenesis of a fungal infection is indolent, and the diagnosis therefore is frequently delayed. Lack of appropriate biopsy specimens or inadequate instruction to the laboratory as to the suspected fungal pathology also can lead to a delayed diagnosis.

A fungal infection of the fingernail can be diagnosed using a wet potassium hydroxide technique with subsequent growth on Sabouraud culture medium. *Candida albicans*, *Trichophyton*, *Microsporum*, and *Epidermophyton* are the most common organisms.[37] Tinea manus caused by *Trichophyton* can be treated using a topical antifungal cream such as tolfinate or miconazole. If the infection cannot be controlled locally, a systemic agent such as oral griseofulvin or ketoconazole may be required.

S schenckii, a saprophyte found in soil and plant materials, can exist in virtually any climate. It is the cause of upper extremity lymphocutaneous sporotrichosis.[38] Inoculation can easily occur if the hand or finger is impaled by a sharp plant thorn.[38] This chronic granulomatous infection first appears in the form of ulcerations and subsequently spreads through the lymphatic system. The lymph nodes and subcutaneous nodules form violet-colored ulcerations that may drain fluid. Material should be cultured using modified Sabouraud medium at approximately 30°C; the temperature should not exceed 37°C because warmth can prevent or delay growth. In the past, lymphocutaneous sporotrichosis was treated with saturated potassium iodide administered orally. Antifungal drugs such as itraconazole have now become the treatment of choice.

Blastomycosis, coccidioidomycosis, histoplasmosis, mucormycosis, aspergillosis, and candidiasis are among the commonly seen fungal infections. Histoplasmosis is endemic to the Mississippi and Ohio River valleys. Coccidioidomycosis is most often seen in the southwestern United States, particularly the San Joaquin valley in California. These infections can cause tenosynovitis, and bone involvement is also common.[39] Synovectomy and débridement usually are sufficient surgical treatment. Pharmacologic treatment also is necessary, usually with amphotericin B. In disseminated fungal infections, the hand infection may not respond to routine débridement and drug therapy; amputation is sometimes necessary. Patients who are immunocompromised, including those with diabetes, are particularly at risk for a systemic fungal infection.

Mycobacterial Infections

A mycobacterial infection has an indolent, mildly painful course that can lead to a delay in the diagnosis. *M tuberculosis* affects as many as 10 million people worldwide. Approximately 20% of patients in whom the condition is newly diagnosed have involvement of sites other than the pulmonary system; in 2%, the elbow, wrist, or hand is affected.[40,41] The patient may have a so-called cold abscess, with swelling, mild pain, and only slightly increased warmth. The severe bone destruction usually associated with bacterial septic joints or osteomyelitis does not appear on radiographs. Lack of significant periosteal reaction or joint space narrowing may be subtle clues to the diagnosis. An open biopsy is suggested because an aspiration culture may be negative. The laboratory should be requested to obtain aerobic, anaerobic, fungal, and mycobacterial cultures from the biopsy specimen. Mycobacterial and fungal cultures require several weeks to grow, so the necessity for a biopsy specimen for histopathology cannot be overemphasized; it is also important to alert the laboratory to the type of cultures being sent. *M tuberculosis* will grow best on Löwenstein-Jensen medium at 37°C, which is a warmer temperature than is used for other mycobacteria. Aggressive débridement should be performed. Primary wound closure is acceptable for *M tuberculosis* infections, unlike many other infections. The use of appropriate antituberculosis drugs is of paramount importance to eradicating the infection.

The patient's occupational, recreational, and environmental history may suggest infection with a *Mycobacterium* other than *M tuberculosis* (a so-called MOTT infection). *M marinum* is associated with injury occurring in warm water, and *Mycobacterium terrae*, with injury occurring at a farm or other rural area. *Mycobacterium avium* usually is found in patients who are immunocompromised.[42,43] These organisms are cultured on Löwenstein-Jensen medium at 30°C to 32°C.

Necrotizing Infections

A necrotizing soft-tissue infection can appear as a clinical, microbiologic, or pathologic syndrome. The risk factors for a necrotizing infection include diabetes mellitus, intravenous drug use, age older than 50 years, hypertension, malnutrition, and obesity.[44] In one study, 32% of the patients were intravenous drug users and 62% had a premorbid condition.[45] The presence of three or more risk factors was found to predict a 50% mortality rate.[46] Age and positive blood cultures were also found to be related to mortality.[47] Evidence was found that patients with a greater propensity for producing inflammatory cytokines in response to streptococcal supra-antigens develop significantly more severe systemic manifestations than other patients.[48] One study found that increased mortality was associated only with delayed débridement.[49] Mortality was found to range from 6% to 76%.[50,51]

A necrotizing infection may initially appear as a tender localized abscess with erythema. Bluish patches, which are considered pathognomonic, do not appear until 2 or 3 days later.[52] The presence of edema extending beyond the erythema can help differentiate necrotizing fasciitis from cellulitis.[45] Numbness and bullae may be present in the affected area.[52] True purulence is not seen; a "dishwater fluid" exudate is more typical. The infection spreads rapidly via fascial planes, and a probe can be easily advanced superficial to the fascia.[53]

Routine radiographs infrequently reveal the presence of gas.[54] CT is not useful,[55] but MRI may be of value.[56] Although it is not routinely available, fluorescence in situ hybridization, targeted to ribosomal RNA, was reported to promise rapid identification of pathogens.[57] *Streptococcus* species have been designated as the primary culprits in this disease. However, polymicrobial findings are common.[58,59]

The treatment of a necrotizing infection is predicated on early recognition and aggressive débridement. It can be useful to obtain a frozen section during surgery to confirm that the margins are clear.[60] The wounds should be kept moist, and repeated examination is important. Irrigation with 5% mafenide acetate solution is valuable,[61] although saline also can be used to maintain a moist wound. There is evidence that hyperbaric oxygen is a useful adjunct in the treatment of necrotizing fasciitis, particularly if anaerobic organisms are present.[62-65]

Gas Gangrene

Gas gangrene is categorized either as caused by *Clostridium* species or as nonclostridial. Clostridial organisms are anaerobic gram-positive rods. Nonclostridial infections occur primarily in patients with diabetes; the mixture of aerobic and anaerobic organisms can be gram negative or positive. Crushed, devitalized tissue resulting from trauma is an excellent in vivo environment for a gas gangrene infection, although anaerobic organisms can flourish in any closed space. Immune system compromise, vascular injury, diabetes, or a malignancy can predispose a patient to a gas gangrene infection. The patient has short-onset, rapidly expanding edema, skin discoloration, and hemorrhagic bullae. Foul purulence can be observed. Usually the patient has tachycardia and severe pain. Muscle necrosis and renal failure ensue. Radiographs usually, but not always, reveal gas in the soft tissues, and clinical suspicion is therefore necessary.

Surgical débridement is the mainstay of treatment, and antibiotics including penicillin are used. The wounds initially should be left open. Hyperbaric oxygen therapy is considered a useful adjunct.[65]

Summary

Accurate diagnosis is the initial step in treating an infection of the hand. For the best outcome, the clinical examination, history, and cultures (aerobic, anaerobic, fungal, and mycobacterial, including biopsy specimens) should be completed before antibiotics are chosen or débridement is done.

Annotated References

1. McLain RF, Steyers C, Stoddard M: Infections in open fractures of the hand. *J Hand Surg Am* 1991;16: 108-112.

2. DeLong WG Jr, Born CT, Wei SY, Petrik ME, Ponzio R, Schwab CW: Aggressive treatment of 119 open fracture wounds. *J Trauma* 1999;46:1049-1054.

3. Weinzweig N, Gonzalez M: Surgical infections of the hand and upper extremity: A county hospital experience. *Ann Plast Surg* 2002;49:621-627.

4. Downs DJ, Wongworawat MD, Gregorius SF: Timeliness of appropriate antibiotics in hand infections. *Clin Orthop Relat Res* 2007;461:17-19.

   A retrospective review of 110 patients found MRSA infection in 34%. The patients had a substantial delay before receiving appropriate antibiotics. Level of evidence: III.

5. LeBlanc DM, Reece EM, Horton JB, Janis JE: Increasing incidence of methicillin-resistant Staphylococcus aureus in hand infections: A 3-year county hospital experience. *Plast Reconstr Surg* 2007;119:935-940.

This retrospective review of patients with a hand infection found that the incidence of community-acquired MRSA at a large county facility increased from 34% to 64% between 2001 and 2003.

6. Goldstein EJ: Bite wounds and infection. *Clin Infect Dis* 1992;14:633-638.

7. Bhatty MA, Turner DP, Chamberlain ST: Mycobacterium marinum hand infection: Case reports and review of literature. *Br J Plast Surg* 2000;53:161-165.

8. Wongworawat MD, Schnall SB: Hand Infections. *Current Treatment Options in Infectious Disease* 2002;4: 295-301.

9. Jebson PJ: Infections of the fingertip. Paronychias and felons. *Hand Clin* 1998;14:547-555.

10. Roberge RJ, Weinstein D, Thimons MM: Perionychial infections associated with sculptured nails. *Am J Emerg Med* 1999;17:581-582.

11. Shaw J, Body R: Best evidence topic report: Incision and drainage preferable to oral antibiotics in acute paronychial nail infection? *Emerg Med J* 2005;22:813-814.

    No relevant studies were found comparing incision and drainage to oral antibiotics in acute paronychial nail infection. The authors concluded that evidence is not available to support the use of one treatment over the other.

12. Bednar MS, Lane LB: Eponychial marsupialization and nail removal for surgical treatment of chronic paronychia. *J Hand Surg Am* 1991;16:314.

13. Tosti A, Piraccini BM, Ghetti E, Colombo MD: Topical steroids versus systemic antifungals in the treatment of chronic paronychia: An open, randomized double-blind and double dummy study. *J Am Acad Dermatol* 2002; 47:73-76.

14. Patzakis MJ, Wilkins J, Bassett RL: Surgical findings in clenched-fist injuries. *Clin Orthop Relat Res* 1987;220: 237-240.

15. Merriam CV, Fernandez HT, Citron DM, Tyrrell KL, Warren YA, Goldstein EJ: Bacteriology of human bite wound infections. *Anaerobe* 2003;9:83-86.

    Mixed organisms are common in human bite wound infection, with *Prevotella* species the most common anaerobes and streptococci the most prevalent aerobic organisms.

16. Talan DA, Abrahamian FM, Moran GJ, et al: Clinical presentation and bacteriologic analysis of infected human bites in patients presenting to emergency departments. *Clin Infect Dis* 2003;37:1481-1489.

    A prospective study of 50 patients with human bites found that 56% were clenched fist injuries and 44% were occlusional injuries. The median number of organisms isolated was four (three aerobes and one anaerobe). Ampicillin–clavulanic acid and moxifloxacin were useful antibiotics for these infections.

17. Lundborg G, Myrhage R, Rydevik B: The vascularization of human flexor tendons within the digital synovial sheath region: Structural and functional aspects. *J Hand Surg Am* 1977;2:417-427.

18. Schnall SB, Vu-Rose T, Holtom P, Doyle B, Stevanovic M: Tissue pressures in pyogenic flexor tenosynovitis of the finger. *J Bone Joint Surg Br* 1996;78:793-795.

19. Floyd WE III, Troun S, Frankle MA: Acute and chronic sepsis, in Peimer CA (ed): *Surgery of the Hand and Upper Extremity.* New York, NY, McGraw Hill, 1996.

20. Schaefer RA, Enzenauer RJ, Pruitt A, et al: Acute gonococcal flexor tenosynovitis in an adolescent male with pharyngitis. *Clin Orthop Relat Res* 1992;281:212-215.

21. Kanavel AB: *Infections of the Hand*, ed 7. Philadelphia, PA, Lea and Febiger, 1939, pp 453-469.

22. Juliano PJ, Eglseder WA: Limited open tendon sheath irrigation in the treatment of pyogenic flexor tenosynovitis. *Orthop Rev* 1991;20:1065-1069.

23. Lille S, Hayakawa MW, Neumeister MW, Brown RE, Zook EG, Murray K: Continuous post-operative catheter irrigation in not necessary for the treatment of suppurative flexor tenosynovitis. *J Hand Surg Br* 2000;25:304-307.

24. Pang HN, Teoh LC, Yam AK, Lee JY, Puhaindran ME, Tan AB: Factors affecting the prognosis of pyogenic flexor tenosynovitis. *J Bone Joint Surg Am* 2007;89:1742-1748.

    Five risk factors for a poor result were identified in 75 patients with pyogenic flexor tenosynovitis studied over 5 years. Clinical findings were used to classify the patients into three groups with prognostic value. Level of evidence: II.

25. Jebson PJ: Deep subfascial space infections. *Hand Clin* 1998;14:557-566.

26. Freeland AE, Senter BS: Septic arthritis and osteomyelitis. *Hand Clin* 1989;5:533-552.

27. Reilly KE, Linz JC, Stern PJ, Giza E, Wyrick JD: Osteomyelitis of the tubular bones of the hand. *J Hand Surg Am* 1997;22:644-649.

28. Boustred AM, Singer M, Hudson DA, et al: Septic arthritis of the metacarpophalangeal and interphalangeal joints of the hand. *Ann Plast Surg* 1999;42:623-628.

29. Barbieri RA, Freeland AE: Osteomyelitis of the hand. *Hand Clin* 1998;14:589-603.

30. Wu IB, Schwarts RA: Herpetic whitlow. *Cutis* 2007;79:193-196.

Herpetic whitlow usually is caused by herpes simplex virus 1 in children and herpes simplex 2 virus in adolescents and adults. Most instances can be attributed to autoinoculation.

31. Walker LG, Simmons BP, Lovallo JL: Pediatric herpetic hand infections. *J Hand Surg Am* 1990;15:176-180.

32. Bleicher JN, Blinn DL, Massop D: Hand infections in dental personnel. *Plast Reconstr Surg* 1987;80:420-422.

33. Hurst LC, Gluck R, Sampson SP, et al: Herpetic whitlow with bacterial abscess. *J Hand Surg Am* 1991;16:311-314.

34. Louis DS, Silva J: Herpetic whitlow: Herpetic infections of the digits. *J Hand Surg Am* 1979;4:90-93.

35. Hoyen HA, Lacey SH, Grahm TJ: Atypical hand infections. *Hand Clin* 1998;14:613-634.

36. Gonzalez MH, Bochar S, Novotny J, Brown A, Weinzweig N, Prieto J: Upper extremity infections in patients with diabetes mellitus. *J Hand Surg Am* 1999;24:682-686.

37. Patel MR: Chronic infections, in Green DP, Hotchkiss R, Pederson WC (eds): *Green's Operative Hand Surgery,* ed 4. New York, NY, Churchill Livingstone, 1999, pp 1048-1095.

38. Carr MM, Fielding JC, Sibbald G, et al: Sporotrichosis of the hand: An urban experience. *J Hand Surg Am* 1995;20:66-70.

39. Szabo RM, Lanzer WL, Gelberman RH, et al: Extensor tendon rupture due to Coccidioides immitis. *Clin Orthop Relat Res* 1985;194:176-180.

40. Bush DC, Schneider LH: Tuberculosis of the hand and wrist. *J Hand Surg Am* 1984;9:391-398.

41. Watts HG, Lifeso RM: Current concepts review: Tuberculosis of bones and joints. *J Bone Joint Surg Am* 1996;78:288-299.

42. Kozin SH, Bishop AT: Atypical mycobacterium infections of the upper extremity. *J Hand Surg Am* 1994;19:480-487.

43. Phillips SA, Marya SKS, Dryden MS, et al: *Mycobacterium marinum* infection of the finger. *J Hand Surg Br* 1995;20:801-802.

44. McHenry CR, Brandt CP, Piotrowski JJ, Jacobs DG, Malangoni MA: Idiopathic necrotizing fasciitis: Recognition, incidence, and outcome of therapy. *Am Surg* 1994;60:490-494.

45. Lille ST, Sato T, Engrav L, Foy H, Jurkovich GJ: Necrotizing soft tissue infections: Obstacles in diagnosis. *J Am Coll Surg* 1996;182:7-11.

46. Francis KR, Lamaute HR, Davis JM, Pizzi WE: Implications of risk factors of necrotizing fasciitis. *Am Surg* 1993;59:304-307.

47. Schnall SB: Necrotizing fasciitis: Clinical presentation, microbiology and determinants of mortality [letter]. *J Bone Joint Surg Am* 2004;86:869.

    In 99 patients with necrotizing fasciitis who were older than 40 years, a positive blood culture was a statistically significant predictor of mortality.

48. Norrby-Teglund A, Chatellier S, Low DE, McGeer A, Green K, Kotb M: Host variation in cytokine responses to superantigens determine the severity of invasive group A streptococcal infection. *Eur J Immunol* 2000; 30:3247-3255.

49. Wong CH, Chang HC, Pasupathy S., Khan LW, Tan JL, Low CO: Necrotizing fasciitis: Clinical presentation, microbiology, and determinants of mortality. *J Bone Joint Surg Am* 2003;85A:1454-1460.

    A retrospective review of 89 patients found that 53.9% had a polymicrobial infection. Mortality was related to a delay in surgery of more than 24 hours. Advanced age, two or more comorbidities, and delayed surgery led to a poorer outcome.

50. Sudarsky LA, Laschinger JC, Coppa GF: Improved results from a standardized approach in treating patients with necrotizing fasciitis. *Ann Surg* 1987;206:661-665.

51. Freischlag JA, Ajalat G, Busuittil RW: Treatment of necrotizing soft tissue infections: The new approach. *Am J Surg* 1985;149:751-755.

52. Janevicius RV, Hann SE, Batt MD: Necrotizing fasciitis. *Surg Gynecol Obstet* 1982;154:97-102.

53. Wall DB, de Virgilio C, Black S, Klein S: Objective criteria may assist in distinguishing necrotizing fasciitis from nonnecrotizing soft tissue infection. *Am J Surg* 2000;179:17-21.

54. Fisher JR, Conway MJ, Takeshita RT, Sandoval MR: Necrotizing fasciitis: Importance of roentgenographic studies for soft-tissue gas. *JAMA* 1979;241:803-806.

55. Rogers JM, Gibson JV, Farrar WE, Schabel SI: Usefulness of computerized tomography in evaluating necrotizing fasciitis. *South Med J* 1984;77:782-783.

56. Rahmouni A, Chosidow O, Amthieu D, et al: MR imaging in acute infectious cellulitis. *Radiology* 1994;192: 493-496.

57. Trebesius K, Leitritz L, Adler K: Culture independent and rapid identification of bacterial pathogens in necrotising fasciitis and streptococcal toxic shock syndrome by fluorescence in situ hybridization. *Med Microbiol Immunol* 2000;188:169-175.

58. Kilborn JA, Manz LA, O'Brien MO, et al: Necrotizing cellulitis caused by Legionella micdadei. *Am J Med* 1992;92:104-106.

59. Ou LF, Yeh FL, Fang RH, Yu KW: Bacteriology of necrotizing fasciitis: A review of 58 cases. *Zhonghua Yi Xue Za Zhi (Taipei)* 1993;51:271-275.

60. Stamenkovic I, Lew DP: Early recognition of potentially fatal necrotizing fasciitis: The use of frozen-section biopsy. *N Engl J Med* 1984;310:1689-1693.

61. Heinle EC, Dougherty WR, Garner WL, Reilly DA: The use of 5% mafenide acetate solution in the postgraft treatment of necrotizing fasciitis. *J Burn Care Rehabil* 2001;22:35-40.

62. Brown DR, Davis NC, Lepawski M, Cunningham J, Kortberk J: A multicenter review of the treatment of major truncal necrotizing infections with and without hyperbaric oxygen therapy. *Am J Surg* 1994;167: 485-489.

63. Kol S, Melamed Y: Hyperbaric oxygenation for necrotizing fasciitis . *Am J Obstet Gynecol* 1993;168;1336.

64. Monestersky JH, Myers RA: Hyperbaric oxygen treatment of necrotizing fasciitis. *Am J Surg* 1995;169: 187-188.

65. Tibbles PM, Edelsberg JS: Hyperbaric-oxygen therapy. *N Engl J Med* 1996;334:1642-1648.

Chapter 17

Spine Infections

Seth K. Williams, MD   Frank J. Eismont, MD

Introduction

A spine infection can result in significant disability and even death. Successful treatment depends on prompt, accurate diagnosis of the disease and initiation of appropriate antibiotics. Neurologic sequelae, including paralysis, are possible, and therefore a sense of urgency should accompany the diagnosis and treatment. Spine infections often are difficult to diagnose because of their deep anatomic location. Surgery is sometimes necessary to achieve pain relief, eradication of infection, maintenance or restoration of spine stability and alignment, and preservation of neurologic function. Residual spinal instability and deformity can cause chronic pain and disability after the infection is eradicated.

Several types of spine infections exist. They can be categorized anatomically, histologically, or etiologically. The infection may primarily involve the disk space, the vertebral body, or the epidural space, and these patterns of infection frequently coexist. The host response may be pyogenic, as it is with most bacterial infections; or granulomatous, as it is with *Mycobacterium tuberculosis*, *Brucella* species, fungal, and *Treponema pallidum* infections. The infection may involve direct inoculation, hematogenous spread, or local spread from adjacent structures. Spine infections have different characteristics in children and adults. The characteristics of infection also vary depending on whether the patient's immune system is normal or compromised.

General Considerations

Risk Factors and Causative Organisms

Smoking, obesity, malnutrition, diabetes, immunodeficiency, local radiation treatment, or the presence of a malignancy predisposes a patient to develop an infection in any part of the musculoskeletal system, including the spine. A transcolonic gunshot wound or other penetrating trauma also is known to lead to spine infection. Infections in another part of the body, such as the urinary tract, the heart, or an extremity, can lead to bacteremia and subsequently to remote spread to the spine.

Pyogenic infections are most commonly caused by *Staphylococcus aureus*, although *Staphylococcus epidermidis*, *Streptococcus* species, and *Escherichia coli*

also may be responsible. Granulomatous infections are usually caused by *M tuberculosis;* the responsible organism may also be another *Mycobacterium* species, a *Brucella* species, a fungus such as *Candida albicans* or *Coccidioides immitis*, or *T pallidum*.

Symptoms and Diagnosis

The lumbar spine is the most common site of infection. Pain in the back or neck usually is the first symptom of a spine infection, regardless of the causative organism, and radicular pain may be present. A neurologic deficit, such as sensory disturbance, motor weakness, gait abnormality, or sphincter dysfunction, is less common and usually results from neural compression rather than direct infection of the neural elements. The systemic manifestations of a spine infection can include fever, malaise, weight loss, altered mental status in a geriatric patient, or irritability in an infant.

The process of initial diagnosis does not vary with patient factors or the suspected offending organism. Laboratory tests, imaging studies, and acquisition of tissue for organism identification are typically included. The laboratory tests should include assessment of complete blood count with differential, erythrocyte sedimentation rate (ESR), and C-reactive protein (CRP) level, all of which are nonspecific and reflect the extent of systemic immune response. The ESR and the CRP level are almost always elevated in a patient with a spine infection, and therefore a patient with normal ESR and CRP values is highly unlikely to have a spine infection. CRP is an acute-phase protein that increases within 6 hours of the onset of infection, doubling every 8 hours and reaching its peak within 1 to 2 days of the onset of infection. The ESR begins to increase after several days, reaching its peak at 1 week after onset. When the infection is eradicated, the CRP level usually returns to normal within 10 days; the ESR returns to normal in approximately 3 weeks.[1-3] An elevated white blood cell (WBC) count is unreliable for confirming the presence of spine infection.

Blood cultures should be performed at the same time as the initial blood testing. However, several days usually are required for growing an organism, and the culture yields the causative organism only for approximately 50% of patients. A positive blood culture is particularly valuable because it allows biopsy to be avoided. If the organism is identified via blood culture, antibiotic treatment can be started immediately. Fastidious organisms such as *M tuberculosis* often require 6 or more weeks to culture. When the presence of such an organism is suspected, polymerase chain reaction testing should be performed, if it is available. The results often are available within several days.

Plain radiography of the spine should be ordered immediately, although bony changes usually cannot be detected until 10 or more days after symptom onset. Disk space narrowing, blurring of the vertebral end plates, and soft-tissue swelling are the first radiographic signs of infection. However, the disk space often is not affected by tuberculosis early in the disease process. Later findings include disk space collapse, vertebral body destruction or patchy sclerosis, and spinal deformity. The additional information gained from CT usually is insufficient to justify obtaining the studies.

MRI is the preferred imaging study for diagnosis because it is approximately 80% sensitive and specific for infection.[4,5] Inflammation in and about the vertebral bodies is seen as low-intensity bone marrow changes on T1-weighted MRI studies and high-intensity bone marrow changes on T2-weighted studies. Intravenous gadolinium is administered to optimize the evaluation of neural compression and to differentiate between purulence and granulation tissue. Although MRI is best at showing anatomic detail, radionuclide imaging techniques should be considered if MRI is contraindicated or multiple sites of infection are suspected. Gallium and technetium scans, especially when used in combination, are highly sensitive and specific and are excellent for localizing the site of infection. The entire skeleton can be studied, revealing other areas of osteomyelitis including the extremities or noncontiguous regions of the spine. Although radiolabeled leukocyte imaging is specific for spine infection, its sensitivity is low and therefore it has not been particularly useful in diagnosis.

Biopsy provides the most reliable means of isolating the causative organism and is indicated for all patients other than those with a positive blood culture. The treatment can be modified when biopsy culture and specificity results become available.[6] Image-guided percutaneous biopsy is generally reliable and safe, particularly if CT guidance is used. It is preferable to use a large-bore device, such as the Craig needle, to obtain relatively large amounts of solid tissue from the site of interest. The tissue should immediately be transported to the laboratory for Gram and acid-fast stains; anaerobic, aerobic, fungal, and *M tuberculosis* cultures; polymerase chain reaction, if tuberculosis is suspected; and routine histology. The culture yield can be improved by culturing the specimen for 10 days. In most institutions, aerobic and anaerobic bacteria cultures usually are considered final after 3 to 5 days, and a 10-day culture therefore must be specified in the microbiology laboratory orders. Skin flora and other slow-growing, low-virulence organisms are easily missed if the specimen is held for fewer than 10 days. If percutaneous biopsy is not feasible or does not yield sufficient tissue, open biopsy is usually indicated. When neurologic involvement necessitates urgent surgical decompression, as is common if an epidural abscess is present, an open biopsy is performed during the definitive surgical procedure.

Initial Treatment

Antibiotic Administration

Determining the causative organism and its sensitivity to specific antimicrobial treatment is of great importance. Blood specimens for culture are obtained at the first patient encounter, and biopsy is planned. Microbial isolation is dramatically hindered if antibiotics are administered before biopsy; therefore, all antibiotics should be withheld before the biopsy unless the patient is medically or neurologically unstable. In a patient with sepsis, empiric broad-spectrum antibiotics must be administered, with the hope that the blood culture or biopsy will be positive. The initial antimicrobial therapy for such a patient should be directed at gram-positive, gram-negative, and anaerobic species. Broad-spectrum intravenous antibiotics are subsequently used for the full treatment course, which usually is 6 weeks. A patient with sepsis generally does not require empiric treatment with antituberculous or antifungal agents because these types of infections are only rarely associated with acute medical instability.

Bracing

Immobilization with an orthotic device helps control the patient's pain and may prevent deformity and subsequent neurologic deterioration. The brace usually should be fitted after any early surgery to correct deformity. For a patient with thoracolumbar involvement, a custom-made rigid thoracolumbar orthosis is used. For a patient with cervical involvement, a rigid collar usually is appropriate. A cervicothoracic brace may be necessary for a patient with a lesion around the upper thoracic spine or cervicothoracic junction. Bracing should be continued for several months and gradually discontinued when the symptoms are resolved and the radiographic appearance is stable (**Figure 1**). Mobilization should begin as soon as the patient's pain level allows.

Pyogenic Vertebral Diskitis and Osteomyelitis

Adult Infections

Epidemiology and Etiology

Pyogenic vertebral diskitis and osteomyelitis can affect adults of any age, although geriatric patients are particularly susceptible. Men are more frequently affected than women. Patients who have diabetes, are intravenous drug abusers, or are immunocompromised also are predisposed to these infections. Any remote-site infection can lead to bacterial seeding; urinary tract infection and the transient bacteremia associated with genitourinary procedures are common sources.

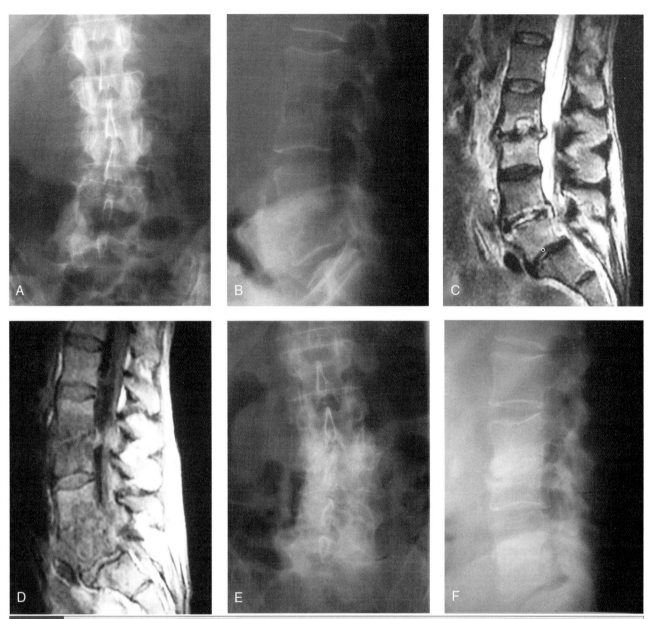

Figure 1 Diskitis and osteomyelitis were diagnosed at L2 through L5 in a 57-year-old man who was an intravenous drug abuser. The infection was successfully treated with bracing and a 6-week course of intravenous antibiotics, followed by a 10-week course of oral antibiotics. **A,** Initial AP radiograph of the lumbar spine, showing a slight deformity. **B,** Initial lateral radiograph of the lumbar spine, showing destructive changes in the vertebral bodies and an obscured vertebral body–disk border at L2-L3 and L4-L5. **C,** Initial T2-weighted MRI study, showing enhancement of the inferior portion of L2 and L4, all of L3 and L5, and the L4-5 disk space. An abscess in the L2-3 disk space also can be seen. **D,** Initial T1-weighted MRI study, showing decreased signal intensity in the regions enhanced on the T2-weighted study. These signal changes are characteristic of a pyogenic infection. AP **(E)** and lateral **(F)** radiographs of the lumbar spine 1 year after successful treatment, showing minimal progression of the deformity and spontaneous fusion across the L2-3 and L4-5 disk spaces.

Pathogenesis and Microbiology

The adult intervertebral disk is an avascular structure that depends on nutrient diffusion from adjacent vertebral body end plates. Hematogenous vertebral osteomyelitis is therefore believed to originate in the vertebral body. The rich end-arteriole vascular network in the vertebral metaphysis and end plates is the probable site of hematogenous seeding; retrograde flow through the Batson venous plexus is also possible. The bacterial infection spreads from the vertebral end plate to the adjacent disk space, which is a potent bacterial breeding ground because of its avascularity. The disk therefore bears the brunt of the infection early in the disease course. Disk space collapse soon follows. Isolated diskitis in adults is rare because of the anatomy of the blood supply to the vertebral column; however, it can occur with direct inoculation, as from a penetrating injury or iatrogenic access to the disk. Adult pyogenic vertebral diskitis and osteomyelitis usually are best considered as coexisting entities. Most spine infections involve these anterior spinal elements, although primary involvement of the posterior column sometimes occurs, usually after direct inoculation.

S aureus is responsible for the infection in approximately half of patients with adult pyogenic vertebral osteomyelitis and diskitis,[7,8] and *S epidermidis* is the next most common organism. Gram-negative organisms such as *E coli* and *Pseudomonas aeruginosa* are less common; they appear to be associated with genitourinary infections and procedures as well as intravenous drug use. Anaerobes are rarely involved. Multiple-organism infections are unusual. Although organisms of low virulence, such as skin flora, sometimes are found on culture, often they are disregarded as contaminants. However, these organisms are capable of causing vertebral osteomyelitis, and they should be dismissed as contaminants only after cautious thought and investigation.

Diagnosis

Adult pyogenic vertebral diskitis and osteomyelitis can be temporarily classified as acute, subacute, or chronic. The virulence of the organism and the patient's physiologic condition determine the clinical manifestations. Axial spine pain is the most common symptom; other manifestations include paraspinal muscle spasm, loss of range of motion, and, occasionally, neurologic deficit. The initial symptoms of subacute and chronic infections may be relatively vague, and delayed presentation and diagnosis are common. Laboratory and imaging studies are done, followed by biopsy.

Treatment

Antibiotics are the mainstay of successful treatment, and their use has resulted in a dramatic drop in the mortality rate from spine infection. There is a lack of controlled studies on which to base decisions as to the duration of antibiotic treatment and the route of administration. The standard treatment is a 6-week course of intravenous antibiotics, which may be followed by a course of oral antibiotics for a difficult-to-treat infection. The response to therapy is monitored by assessing the patient's symptoms as well as the ESR and CRP level. In particular, the CRP level appears to be reliably correlated with clinical symptoms.[9] The laboratory tests should be repeated 1 week after antibiotic therapy is discontinued and approximately 6 weeks later to ensure the infection has been completely eradicated. The patient should be followed clinically and radiographically after therapy is discontinued until full recovery is established.

Surgery is indicated if the infection is refractory to appropriate nonsurgical treatment (**Figure 2**). Spinal cord compression causing a neurologic deficit should be surgically treated as soon as possible, provided that an internal medicine physician determines that the patient can tolerate the surgery. Spinal cord compression must be distinguished from isolated nerve root compression. Isolated nerve root compression usually responds favorably to antibiotic therapy, if the infection can otherwise be treated nonsurgically. Abscesses are relatively well protected from antibiotic penetration and may need to be drained surgically, especially if the patient has clinical sepsis. Surgery may be required to correct a deformity, typically in the sagittal plane. Deformity is most likely to develop in the cervical spine and is more likely in the thoracic spine than in the lumbar spine. The deformity can be corrected during the active phase of infection if débridement or decompression is done. Otherwise, the deformity can be corrected when the infection is eradicated and the patient is better able to tolerate surgery.

Vertebral pyogenic osteomyelitis most commonly involves the vertebral body rather than the posterior elements, and an anterior surgical approach therefore is typically used. The involved vertebral bodies and disks should be thoroughly débrided. Autograft is preferred to allograft for reconstruction; structural iliac crest graft can be used to reconstruct a defect as much as 6 cm in length. Multiple structural rib grafts also can be used, but only if rigid instrumentation is added to provide adequate stability. For a defect longer than 6 cm, bone allograft or structural cages with morcellized autograft should be considered.[10] Bone morphogenetic protein was successfully used to augment fusion in a small number of patients, according to a recent report of this off-label use.[11] Anterior and posterior instrumentation can be safely used and do not appear to hinder the eradication of infection.[10-13]

A posterior approach is sometimes used alone, especially to achieve stability in the mid or low lumbar spine, if the patient's deformity is not significant and anterior débridement is unnecessary. Such a patient most commonly has persistent pain that prevents mobilization, with minimal vertebral body destruction. The posterior approach allows débridement and drainage of any associated epidural abscesses. Posterolateral fusion, with or without screws and rods, also can be performed. Laminectomy alone can result in instability because the anterior column is already compromised.

If infection recurs after nonsurgical treatment, it may be reasonable to administer another 6-week intravenous antibiotic regimen, followed by an oral regimen. The infection must be otherwise amenable to nonsurgical treatment. Surgical treatment is a reasonable option for a recurrent infection and is definitely indicated after a second recurrence of infection. If relapse occurs after surgical treatment, revision surgery may be necessary, with a second débridement.

Prognosis

The underlying physiologic condition of an adult patient with vertebral osteomyelitis is generally predictive of the final outcome. Regardless of whether surgical dé-

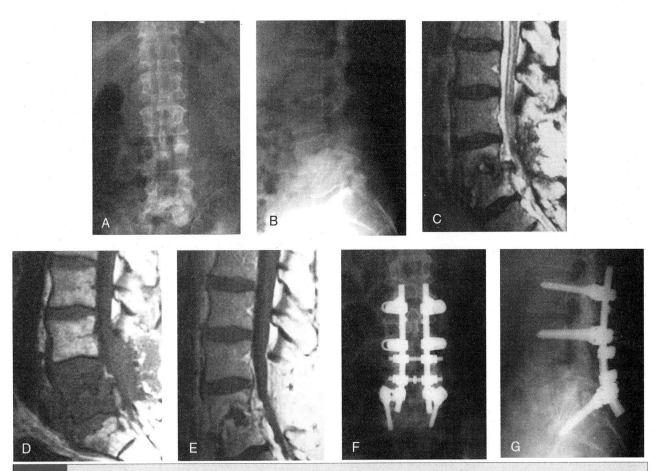

Figure 2 After unsuccessful treatment with intravenous antibiotics, a 66-year-old man with diskitis and osteomyelitis at L4-L5 underwent anterior débridement with corpectomies and fusion with rib autograft, followed by posterolateral instrumented fusion. The infection was eradicated. Initial AP **(A)** and lateral **(B)** radiographs of the lumbar spine, showing collapse of the L4-5 disk space and L4-L5 anterolisthesis. **C,** Initial T2-weighted MRI study, showing L4-5 disk space collapse with surrounding mild enhancement of the vertebral bodies. **D,** Initial T1-weighted MRI study, showing L4-5 disk space collapse and diffuse decreased signal intensity through the L4-L5 vertebral bodies. **E,** Initial T1-weighted MRI study with intravenous gadolinium contrast, showing sequestrum between and extending into the L4 and L5 vertebral bodies, with mild surrounding enhancement. Postsurgical AP **(F)** and lateral **(G)** radiographs of the lumbar spine, showing pedicle screw instrumentation and the rib graft extending from the inferior aspect of L4 to the superior aspect of the sacrum.

bridement is necessary, the factors specifically associated with a favorable outcome include age younger than 60 years and uncompromised immune status, as well as infection with *S aureus* and a rapidly decreasing ESR.[3] Relapse occurs in a relatively small number of patients, usually those who are older than 60 years or have an underlying comorbidity such as rheumatoid arthritis or diabetes. Patients with a neurologic deficit usually experience either a partial or full recovery, especially if the deficit is incomplete and involves caudal levels.[14] Diabetes mellitus, rheumatoid arthritis, age older than 60 years, and a more cephalad level of infection are associated with increased risk of paralysis.[14] Spontaneous interbody fusion is most likely to occur in patients with severe disk and end plate destruction. Patients who do not have spontaneous interbody fusion usually have a painless fibrous ankylosis.[15,16] Fusion occurs in approximately 96% of those treated surgically.[17]

Posterior instrumentation may help prevent progressive sagittal decompensation.[18] Residual deformity most frequently occurs in the thoracic spine, but it is not common and appears to depend on the extent of initial bone and disk destruction.[15]

Pediatric Infections

The disk vascular supply is more robust in young children than in adults. The arterioles penetrate the vertebral end plates and supply the nucleus pulposus, which is avascular in adults. Probably as a result of the ample vascular supply, most pediatric spine infections begin as isolated diskitis. As the infection spreads from the disk to the vertebral bodies, vertebral osteomyelitis results.[19]

The illness is systemic. A child who is old enough to communicate verbally may report back pain. Abdominal pain and refusal to ambulate are other common clinical manifestations. Fever is sometimes but not invariably present. The physical examination findings often are nonspecific and may include such subtle symptoms as local spine tenderness or refusal to assume a position that requires flexion of the spine. The ESR and the CRP level usually are elevated, although the WBC count may be normal. Blood cultures are positive in approximately half of the patients.

Initial radiographs usually appear normal; disk space narrowing and end plate erosion can be seen later. A bone scan is sensitive and reliable for diagnosis and treatment of the infection, and it allows evaluation of the entire skeletal system to detect any other areas of infection. MRI is best used when the area of involvement is known; it can determine whether an abscess is present if the infection is refractory to treatment.

S aureus is the most common offending organism. Blood cultures should be obtained immediately, and treatment with antistaphylococcal antibiotics should be initiated. If the child's condition does not rapidly improve or if the symptoms are atypical, disk space aspiration should be performed. A brace or cast is unnecessary for isolated diskitis because it rarely results in deformity. However, infants younger than 1 year often have an aggressive infection, and the threshold for applying a cast should be low.[20] Surgery is reserved for patients whose infection is refractory to nonsurgical treatment, patients requiring abscess débridement, and those with a neurologic deficit secondary to spinal cord compression. Most patients recover fully. The long-term prognosis is generally favorable if the choice and duration of antibiotic treatment are appropriate.[21-23]

Granulomatous Infections

Granulomatous spine infections are caused by fungi, a limited number of bacteria species, or spirochetes. These infections have similar symptoms, underlying pathology, and disease course.

Spinal Tuberculosis
Epidemiology and Etiology
Tuberculous spondylitis is more common in relatively undeveloped regions of the world than in developed regions. The patient risk factors include advanced human immunodeficiency virus (HIV) infection, immunosuppression, and alcohol or drug abuse.

Pathogenesis and Microbiology
Mycobacteria are acid-fast aerobic bacilli. The two organisms that cause tuberculosis are *M tuberculosis,* which is an airborne pathogen, and *Mycobacterium avium-intracellulare,* which is contracted by drinking contaminated milk. *M tuberculosis* is much more common. It initially infects the lungs, where a delayed hypersensitivity immune response usually eradicates the organism. The characteristic scar tissue in the lung parenchyma and hilar lymph nodes is called the Ghon complex. In some patients, the pulmonary infection

leads to secondary disseminated disease, which can affect any area of the body and become apparent in many ways. The typical histologic finding is a granuloma with central caseating necrosis. The body's delayed hypersensitivity reaction leads to progressive destruction of local tissues. The disease course is therefore insidious and not marked by sepsis. The spinal involvement usually is predominantly anterior and rarely is posterior alone. Unlike pyogenic infections, tuberculous spondylitis commonly spares the disks. Disk space infection does occur, however, and it is not unusual to see disk space collapse. Neurologic involvement typically results from spinal deformity that leads to secondary spinal cord compression, although it may be caused by epidural disease or, rarely, direct involvement of the neural elements.

Diagnosis
The symptoms of tuberculous spondylitis vary greatly, depending on the sites involved in the infection, the extent of disease, the duration of infection, and the patient's underlying physiologic condition. Insidious, nonspecific systemic manifestations are typical, including weight loss, fever, and malaise. The patient is not septic or otherwise critically ill unless another, superimposed bacterial infection is present. Back pain occurs most commonly in the thoracic spine, less commonly in the lumbar spine, and rarely in the cervical spine. A neurologic deficit may be present, especially with cervical or thoracic lesions; it usually has a slow onset. Kyphotic deformity secondary to collapse of the vertebral body and disk is common, especially in the thoracic spine (**Figure 3**).

The definitive diagnosis of tuberculous spondylitis is based on detection of the tubercle bacillus through vertebral biopsy. The tubercle bacillus grows very slowly, and 6 to 8 weeks are required for a positive culture to be identified. Polymerase chain reaction provides an immediate result and should be performed whenever possible. Other molecular detection techniques have recently been developed.[24,25] To determine which techniques are available and appropriate, an infectious disease specialist or pathologist can be consulted.

Laboratory studies often reveal a normal WBC count and elevated ESR and CRP level. The abnormalities often present on plain radiographs are not specific to tuberculosis infection. They include a variable amount of vertebral body destruction, disk space collapse, and kyphotic deformity. As the preferred method of imaging, MRI is often helpful in differentiating tuberculous spondylitis from pyogenic infection or tumor.[26] The disk spaces are for the most part spared, and this finding may suggest metastatic disease. However, other features usually are present to distinguish the two conditions. An anterior lesion spreading underneath the anterior longitudinal ligament is strongly associated with tuberculous infection. Tuberculous infection also is characterized by hyperemic granulation tissue throughout the involved area, as revealed by gadolin-

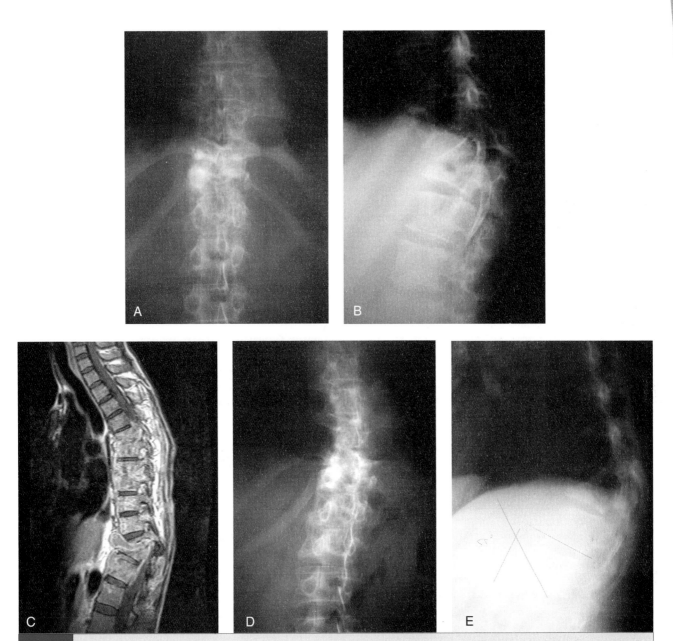

Figure 3 A 49-year-old woman with multilevel thoracic tuberculous spondylitis and focal thoracolumbar kyphosis refused surgical treatment. A prolonged multidrug oral antituberculous regimen and bracing led to resolution of the infection with residual deformity. **A,** Initial AP radiograph of the thoracic spine, showing sclerotic changes at the thoracolumbar junction; the deformity is not appreciable. **B,** Initial lateral radiograph of the thoracic spine, showing collapse of the vertebral bodies anteriorly with preservation of the posterior elements, resulting in focal kyphosis of approximately 50°. **C,** Initial MRI study, showing collapse of the two vertebral bodies, with a fluid collection that probably represents a tuberculous abscess. **D,** AP radiograph of the thoracic spine at 9-month follow-up. **E,** Lateral radiograph of the thoracic spine at 9-month follow-up, showing the residual deformity measured at 55° *(lines)* after healing of the infection.

ium enhancement. In contrast, pyogenic abscesses tend to be enhanced only on the periphery. Bone scans usually reveal the extent of tuberculous involvement, but they are not as helpful as MRI and are not routinely necessary. CT reveals the extent of bony involvement and may be helpful in surgical planning. However, CT adds little information to a good-quality MRI study.

Treatment

Tuberculous spondylitis should first be treated using antibiotics. A multidrug antimicrobial therapy regimen is necessary because of the high incidence of drug-resistant strains. The success of the initial drug regimen depends on the regional sensitivity patterns. Six to 8 weeks are required for sensitivities to be determined, and the drug regimen is then modified if necessary.

Consultation with an infectious disease specialist is recommended before beginning therapy. The duration of treatment is at least 6 to 9 months. Bed rest does not affect the extent of final deformity and therefore is not necessary. Bracing may help to prevent progressive deformity.

Surgery is used after unsuccessful treatment with antibiotics or if the patient has a neurologic deficit, significant initial or progressive later kyphotic deformity, or disease recurrence. Studies of tuberculous spondylitis in developing regions of the world have found that recovery from neurologic deficit is possible with antibiotic treatment alone. However, surgical treatment appears to increase the likelihood of neurologic recovery and is therefore recommended under these circumstances.[27,28] Because the extent of neurologic recovery is related to the duration of the deficit, early surgery is usually preferred to delayed surgery. In addition, surgery is technically easier during the early, active phase, before the formation of scar tissue that characterizes medically treated disease. If possible, the patient should be treated with antituberculous medication for several days before surgery. The purpose of this treatment is to decrease the likelihood that the operating room staff will become infected, as tuberculous organisms can be aerosolized during surgery.

Anterior débridement and strut grafting is the preferred surgical technique for direct access to vertebral body involvement. Débridement should be performed until bleeding healthy bone surfaces are exposed. Instrumentation is placed anteriorly, posteriorly, or circumferentially.[29] A posterior approach is rarely used alone and only for isolated posterior disease. In general, posterior decompression and fusion cannot control progressive deformity unless anterior débridement and reconstruction also are performed. Anterior débridement with anterior instrumented fusion (using a newer screw-and-rod or screw-and-plate instrumentation system) may be sufficient to maintain sagittal alignment, provided that screw purchase is robust in the uninfected adjacent vertebral bodies; supplementary posterior instrumentation is not required.[30]

Instrumentation has been used for many years to treat tuberculous spondylitis and does not hinder disease eradication when properly applied. Appropriate antibiotics must be administered for surgery to be successful. The graft for anterior reconstruction is chosen based on the extent of the reconstruction and the availability of graft material. Autograft is preferable, although a rib graft can fracture and should be used only with instrumentation. For a very large anterior defect, the use of allograft or a cage with morcellized autograft is acceptable.

Prognosis
The patient's general health status and age as well as the duration and extent of neurologic involvement determine the prognosis. A neurologic deficit often improves, especially if the deficit is incomplete and of short duration, although a complete deficit of longer duration also may improve. Surgery should therefore be strongly considered, even if the neurologic deficit is complete. Successful treatment depends on the correct selection of antibiotics and surgery as well as the patient's compliance with the antibiotic regimen. Fusion occurs in more than 90% of patients who undergo surgery, and spontaneous fusion usually occurs in nonsurgically treated patients.[27,28] The final deformity tends to be less severe in surgically treated patients than in nonsurgically treated patients, provided the initial deformity is corrected during surgery.[27,28,30] The extent of the initial deformity can be used to predict the final deformity in nonsurgically treated patients. Recurrent infection is rare after completion of appropriate treatment. Late-onset paraplegia can occur in patients with residual deformity after successful nonsurgical treatment. Fortunately, subsequent surgical treatment of these patients is usually successful.

Other Granulomatous Infections
Other granulomatous infections are relatively rare. They have an insidious onset with variable spinal deformity. A variety of organisms can be responsible; their common characteristic is a granulomatous histologic response. The diagnosis is established through biopsy. The typical laboratory studies (ESR, CRP level, complete blood count, and blood cultures) and imaging studies (plain radiography and MRI) should be obtained. Appropriate antimicrobial therapy is the mainstay of treatment, and surgery is done only after unsuccessful nonsurgical treatment or for a patient with a significant initial or progressive later deformity or with neurologic involvement.

Actinomyces israelii, a gram-positive bacterium found in human oral flora, is known for causing chronically draining sinuses. Spine infection with *A israelii* can occur after penetrating trauma or surgery, or through spread from an adjacent wound infection originally caused by a different organism. *Nocardia asteroides,* a weakly gram-positive bacterium found in the soil, can cause infection through the respiratory tract, usually in an individual who is immunocompromised. Suppurative abscesses may result, in addition to granuloma formation. A variety of *Brucella* species, a gram-negative coccobacillus found in domestic animals, can cause brucellosis. The spirochete *T pallidum* causes syphilis, a sexually transmitted disease.

Fungal infections usually are found in a patient who is immunocompromised or otherwise medically frail. Fungal stains should be ordered in addition to cultures whenever a fungal infection is suspected. *C immitis,* found in the desert soil of the southwestern United States, Central America, and South America, can cause infection through spore inhalation. Serum immunoglobulin tests and skin tests can help establish the diagnosis. *Blastomyces dermatitidis,* found in areas with warm, moist soil, also causes infection through inhalation. An enzyme-linked immunosorbent assay is often used for disease screening when infection is suspected. *Cryptococcus neoformans* resembles yeast and is found in pigeon feces and soil throughout the world; infection occurs via inhalation. A latex agglutination test is available to detect antigen in the serum. The opportunistic candidiasis infection is caused by the normal human flora *Candida* yeast species. *Aspergillus* species, a ubiquitous mold, causes aspergillosis, another opportunistic infection, after spore inhalation. Fungal infections often are treated using intravenous amphotericin, which has numerous adverse effects and a high rate of failure.[31] Recent evidence suggests that oral fluconazole may be a better choice than amphotericin because it has superior disk penetration.[32]

Epidural Abscess

Epidural abscesses occur much more frequently in adults than in children. Usually they are associated with vertebral osteomyelitis and diskitis, but they also can result from hematogenous spread from a remote infected site or as a complication of surgery or another intervention, such as injection or biopsy. The offending organisms are similar to those of vertebral osteomyelitis. Mass effect from the abscess may cause neurologic compromise. In rare patients, the infection penetrates the dura and causes meningitis. If the infection is associated with vertebral osteomyelitis, the abscess usually is anterior to the dural tube. Otherwise, the abscess usually is posterior to the dura, as more epidural space is available posteriorly than anteriorly. Patients with diabetes, a history of intravenous drug abuse, or multiple comorbidities are most commonly affected. Patients typically have some combination of back pain, fever or malaise, neurologic deficit, and paraspinal tenderness. The diagnosis is usually made through gadolinium-enhanced MRI. The course may be acute, subacute, or chronic. Paralysis is to be expected if the abscess is not treated.

The treatment is usually surgical, and it is often considered an emergency because of the risk of rapid, progressive neurologic deterioration. The surgical approach depends on the location of the abscess. Laminectomy is the procedure of choice if the abscess is isolated and can be safely reached posteriorly. If possible, antibiotics should be withheld until intrasurgical cultures are obtained. Broad-spectrum antibiotics are then administered until adjustments can be made based on sensitivities. The appropriate duration of antibiotic therapy has not been well studied, but a 2- to 4-week course is recommended if the abscess is not associated with osteomyelitis. The recurrence rate is minimal.

Nonsurgical treatment can be considered for a few patients, including those who have a small abscess without neurologic involvement (particularly in the lumbar spine), medically frail patients for whom surgery would impose a high risk, patients whose abscess extends over multiple segments without neurologic deficit, and patients who have had complete paralysis for many days.[33] Nonsurgical treatment must be conducted with great caution and close observation.

Surgery for a patient with an epidural abscess and a significant neurologic deficit generally should proceed as soon as possible. There is an even greater sense of urgency if the neurologic deficit is progressive. Early intervention in patients who have a neurologic deficit has been shown to improve neurologic outcomes. The allowable time from symptom onset to surgical decompression is debatable. Some studies have found that patients who undergo surgery within 24 hours of neurologic symptom onset have a better outcome than those treated later.[34,35] It is unclear what the outcomes are when patients are treated at different times within the initial 24 hours. Patients with a complete deficit for more than 48 hours should not be expected to have any meaningful neurologic recovery.

HIV Infection

Untreated HIV infection leads to progressive destruction of the immune system. As the CD4 cell count drops, indicating disease progression, the risk of developing a spine infection increases. Diagnosis and treatment proceed as for a patient who is immunocompetent. Treatment is often successful, particularly if the patient's CD4 cell count is higher than 200. A patient with a CD4 cell count lower than 200 is more likely to develop tuberculosis or another opportunistic infection and is more likely to die from any cause than a patient with a normal immune system.[36] An infectious disease specialist should be consulted for evaluation of the immune status and viral burden and assistance in managing the antiretroviral medications of a patient with HIV infection.

Postsurgical Spine Infection

A postsurgical spine infection can appear as a superficial (above the fascia) or deep (below the fascia) wound infection, diskitis, an epidural abscess, a paraspinal abscess, or meningitis. Each of these conditions may be associated with or lead to vertebral osteomyelitis. A wound infection is the most common form of postsurgical infection. The source of infection usually is intrasurgical seeding or hematogenous spread. A postsurgical spine infection may be classified as early, delayed, or late. Manifestations of a high-virulence organism tend to appear soon after surgery; a late infection is often caused by a low-virulence organism. The likelihood of postsurgical spine infection depends on the extent and type of the surgical procedure and certain patient characteristics (immunocompromise, rheumatoid arthritis, diabetes, age older than 60 years, chronic corticosteroid use, excessive alcohol use, obesity, malnutrition, and smoking). The risk of infection probably is greater after an instrumented procedure than a noninstrumented procedure and when a posterior rather than an anterior approach is used.[37]

Diagnosis

The patient history, clinical examination, laboratory studies, and imaging studies are used in diagnosing the infection. The patient often has greater-than-expected postsurgical pain, sometimes with systemic manifestations. Wound drainage is sometimes but not always present. Neurologic changes are not typical unless there is an associated epidural abscess.

The ESR and CRP level normally increase and then gradually decrease after surgery. The WBC count is less likely to be elevated. Usually, the ESR peaks approximately 4 days after surgery and returns to normal within 2 to 3 weeks. The CRP level peaks at approximately 3 days and returns to normal within 10 to 14 days.[1,3,38] This expected postsurgical elevation of the ESR and the CRP level must be distinguished from elevation associated with infection. The ESR and the CRP level are perhaps the most helpful laboratory measures for diagnosing a postsurgical infection; an upward trend continuing beyond 4 or 5 days after surgery usually indicates an infection. Plain radiographs may reveal evidence of osteomyelitis, although such changes require at least 10 to 14 days to develop. Contrast-enhanced CT or MRI may reveal fluid collection; however, an early soft-tissue abscess can be difficult to distinguish from a sterile seroma or hematoma. MRI is particularly helpful in detecting an epidural abscess, diskitis, osteomyelitis, or a paraspinal infection such as a psoas abscess. The imaging findings are similar to those seen in a primary spine infection, and normal postsurgical changes may be difficult to differentiate from those caused by infection (Figure 4).

Bacteriology and Antibiotic Regimen

S aureus is the pathogen most commonly responsible for postsurgical infections. The incidence of methicillin-resistant S aureus is increasing. Specimens taken from a draining wound are likely to be contaminated, and therefore wound aspiration is a more useful method of obtaining a specimen. If the patient does not have sepsis and surgery is imminent, antibiotics should be withheld, if possible, until intrasurgical cultures can be obtained. Broad-spectrum antibiotics should be administered immediately thereafter; vancomycin, gram-negative coverage, and anaerobic coverage should be included. It is usually unnecessary to empirically treat the patient with antifungal agents, unless a coexisting fungal infection elsewhere in the body is believed to be the source of the spine infection. The antibiotic regimen is adjusted based on the culture results. If the cultures do not yield an organism, then a decision must be made as to continuing broad-spectrum coverage or directing the regimen toward the most common Staphylococcus species to minimize adverse effects and the risk of complications from the antibiotics.

The optimal duration of antibiotic administration has not been determined. After final débridement is performed and only viable tissue remains, a 2-week course of parenteral antibiotics is commonly administered to eradicate an isolated superficial wound infection. A 6-week course of parenteral antibiotics is required for all other postsurgical infections. Oral antibiotics may then be administered. The duration of treatment is determined by the patient's overall medical condition, the nature of the infection, and the trend in the ESR, CRP level, and WBC count. For a late infection occurring after fusion has been achieved, the evidence suggests that removal of instrumentation with débridement, primary wound closure, and a short course of oral antibiotics are sufficient to achieve a cure, provided the infection is detected soon after onset.[39]

For some patients, lifetime administration of suppressive oral antibiotics may be necessary. If the oral suppression regimen can be tolerated, this treatment can be considered a first-line option for a frail patient with multiple comorbidities or spinal metastases. For such patients, a relapse can be catastrophic. Lifetime administration of suppressive antibiotics also may be necessary if a relapse occurs after appropriate initial treatment. However, treatment with suppressive antibiotics sometimes can be concluded after a solid fusion is achieved, the hardware is removed, and no evidence of residual infection remains.

Types of Postsurgical Infections

A superficial wound infection generally occurs soon after the surgical procedure, and the diagnosis usually can be made from the clinical examination. A deep wound infection may appear somewhat later, during the subacute postsurgical phase. A deep wound infection usually requires débridement followed by a course of antibiotics.

An epidural abscess has the potential to cause rapid neurologic deterioration from mass effect and is a surgical emergency. MRI is the preferred imaging modality, although it can be difficult to distinguish a hematoma from an abscess in the spinal canal on MRI studies. The diagnosis and treatment of postsurgical and primary epidural abscesses are similar.

Meningitis is a rare postsurgical complication manifested by fever, altered mental status, headaches, and nuchal rigidity. The risk factors include a durotomy or inadvertent dural tear, especially one that cannot be repaired primarily. Meningitis is treated with antibiotics, which should be instituted immediately because of the devastating consequences of unchecked infection. Cerebrospinal fluid analysis, including culture, cell count, and protein and glucose levels, should be performed. A persistent leak of cerebrospinal fluid may require surgical repair or insertion of a drain.

Isolated postsurgical diskitis is a specific clinical entity associated with disk surgery. A variable period of pain relief, which is expected after disk surgery, is fol-

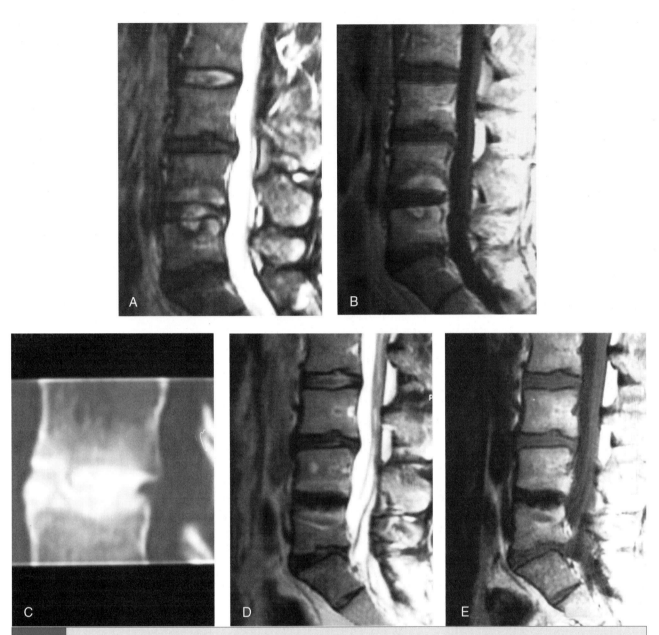

Figure 4   A 32-year-old man developed chronic fungal osteomyelitis at L4-L5 after lumbar laminectomy and diskectomy. *C albicans* was isolated. After unsuccessful treatment with amphotericin, the infection was eradicated through anterior lumbar débridement and interbody fusion. **A,** Initial T2-weighted MRI study, showing asymmetric enhancement of the L4-5 disc space. **B,** Initial T1-weighted MRI study, showing enhancement in the vertebral body end plates adjacent to the L4-5 disk. **C,** CT scan at 1-year follow-up, showing sclerosis consistent with fusion across the L4-5 disc space. T2-weighted **(D)** and T1-weighted **(E)** MRI studies at 1-year follow-up confirm resolution of the infection, although minimal residual enhancement can be seen around the L4-5 disk space.

lowed by worsening axial pain. During physical examination, the pain may appear to be greater than warranted. The wound usually has a benign appearance. Diskitis associated with a wound infection is not considered to be isolated diskitis. Neurologic deficit should not occur unless there is profound collapse of the disk space or an associated epidural abscess. The diagnosis is based on the typical pattern of abnormal laboratory and imaging study findings. T1-weighted MRI studies usually reveal disk hypointensity, and T2-weighted

studies reveal hyperintensity. The usual distinctive border between the disk and the vertebral bodies may appear to be lost. Percutaneous biopsy is performed, and antibiotics are administered. If an associated epidural abscess, sepsis, or a neurologic deficit is present, or if nonsurgical treatment has been unsuccessful, surgery is usually necessary. Parenteral antibiotics are usually administered for 6 weeks. However, the optimal duration of antibiotic therapy has not been clearly defined; clinical judgment and laboratory value trends are the basis

4: Specific Situations

of the decision, as for a primary spine infection. Because relevant imaging findings usually can be seen later than clinical findings, repeat MRI is not indicated unless the patient's clinical condition does not improve. Plain radiography is useful in detecting progressive involvement of the vertebral bodies.

Instrumentation and Bone Grafts

It is difficult or impossible to eradicate an infection in the spine or anywhere else in the skeletal system if mechanical instability is present. For an early infection after instrumented surgery, a thorough débridement should be performed and the instrumentation left in place. Antibiotics should be administered, with repeated débridement if necessary. Instrumentation that is not producing stability is serving only as a nidus for infection; it must be removed and usually is replaced. Instrumentation also should be removed if a late infection occurs after a solid fusion has been achieved; it need not be replaced. Braided cables should be removed if postsurgical infection occurs, and another means of fixation should be substituted. Postsurgical infection frequently recurs if the cables are left in place, presumably because of glycocalyx formation and poor antibiotic penetration into the cable.

If a postsurgical infection develops after bone grafting, the surgeon must decide during débridement whether the graft should be retained. Irrigation over an autogenous bone graft is recommended, with removal only of any dislodged graft material. Allograft bone and synthetic bone products usually are removed and can be replaced with autogenous bone graft, if necessary.

Emerging Treatment Strategies

Antibiotic-Impregnated Cement

The use of antibiotic-impregnated cement in the spine continues to be investigated. Antibiotic-impregnated polymethylmethacrylate beads can be placed in an infected wound bed to fill dead space and locally elute antibiotics. The benefit of this technique in the spine has not been proved.

Flap Coverage and Vacuum-Assisted Wound Closure

Débridement of a posterior postsurgical wound infection can create dead space, and sometimes it is difficult or impossible to adequately close the wound. Soft tissue can be successfully covered using various types of muscle flaps.[40] Latissimus dorsi muscle flaps are used for coverage in the thoracic and lumbar regions, and trapezius muscle flaps are used in the cervical region. Gluteal flaps are the primary option in the sacral region. Local paraspinal muscle advancement is a relatively straightforward technique if the area to be covered is small.

A vacuum-assisted wound closure device uses negative-pressure suction to drain and shrink the wound and sometimes can obviate the need for flap coverage. The application of the device is discussed in chapter 8. Although vacuum-assisted wound closure has been successfully used to treat spine wounds, including those with exposed instrumentation,[41] serious complications have been reported, including death from exsanguination.[42] Persistent bleeding is of particular concern when negative-pressure drainage is applied. To prevent this complication, the wound first should be serially débrided until it is stable, with clean granulation tissue and minimal bleeding potential. The device should not be applied directly over the dural tube or neural elements. The appropriate use of vacuum-assisted wound closure for spine infections has not been fully clarified, and the device should be used with caution.

Summary

A spine infection typically occurs in a patient with a compromised immune system, although it also can occur in a patient who is immunologically normal. Intravenous antibiotics usually lead to a cure. It is important to determine the causative organism before initiating antibiotic therapy. Some infections are refractory to antibiotic treatment. Surgery often is necessary for these infections and typically is successful in eradicating the infection. Neurologic deficit and significant deformity are relative indications for surgical intervention. Recurrent infection is rare after appropriate treatment is completed.

Annotated References

1. Khan IA, Vaccaro AR, Zlotolow DA: Management of vertebral diskitis and osteomyelitis. *Orthopedics* 1999; 22:758-765.

2. Rezai AR, Woo HH, Errico TJ, Cooper PR: Contemporary management of spinal osteomyelitis. *Neurosurgery* 1999;44:1018-1025.

3. Carragee EJ: Pyogenic vertebral osteomyelitis. *J Bone Joint Surg Am* 1997;79:874-880.

4. Carragee EJ: The clinical use of magnetic resonance imaging in pyogenic vertebral osteomyelitis. *Spine* 1997; 22:780-785.

5. Varma R, Lander P, Assaf A: Imaging of pyogenic infectious spondylodiskitis. *Radiol Clin North Am* 2001;39: 203-213.

6. Rankine JJ, Barron DA, Robinson P, Millner PA, Dickson RA: Therapeutic impact of percutaneous spinal biopsy in spinal infection. *Postgrad Med J* 2004;80: 607-609.

   Treatment for spine infection was changed in 35% of patients when biopsy results became available. If antibiotics were withheld before biopsy, cultures were positive in 50% of patients. If antibiotics were administered before biopsy, cultures were positive in 25%.

7. Butler JS, Shelly MJ, Timlin M, Powderly WG, O'Byrne JM: Nontuberculous pyogenic spinal infection in adults: A 12-year experience from a tertiary referral center. *Spine* 2006;31:2695-2700.

   Pyogenic vertebral osteomyelitis was reviewed in 48 patients. *S aureus* was responsible in 48%. Most patients were successfully treated nonsurgically with antibiotics and bracing.

8. Sapico FL, Montgomerie JZ: Pyogenic vertebral osteomyelitis: Report of nine cases and review of the literature. *Rev Infect Dis* 1979;1:754-776.

9. Chelsom J, Solberg CO: Vertebral osteomyelitis at a Norwegian university hospital 1987-97: Clinical features, laboratory findings and outcomes. *Scand J Infect Dis* 1998;30:147-151.

10. Ruf M, Stoltze D, Merk HR, Ames M, Harms J: Treatment of vertebral osteomyelitis by radical debridement and stabilization using titanium mesh cages. *Spine* 2007;32:E275-E280.

    Eighty-eight patients with vertebral diskitis and osteomyelitis were treated using antibiotics, anterior débridement, and a structural titanium cage with morcellized autograft, usually followed by posterior instrumented arthrodesis. All infections were eradicated, settling was not a problem, and fusion occurred in all patients.

11. Aryan HE, Lu DC, Acosta FL, Ames CP: Corpectomy followed by the placement of instrumentation with titanium cages and recombinant human bone morphogenetic protein-2 for vertebral osteomyelitis. *J Neurosurg Spine* 2007;6:23-30.

    Fifteen patients with vertebral osteomyelitis were treated using corpectomy and reconstruction with a titanium mesh cage, with bone morphogenetic protein and morcellized autograft or allograft. All infections were eradicated, the fusion rate was 100%, and no complications occurred.

12. Carragee EJ: Instrumentation of the infected and unstable spine: A review of 17 cases from the thoracic and lumbar spine with pyogenic infections. *J Spinal Disord* 1997;10:317-324.

13. Dimar JR, Carreon LY, Glassman SD, Campbell MJ, Hartman MJ, Johnson JR: Treatment of pyogenic vertebral osteomyelitis with anterior debridement and fusion followed by delayed posterior spinal fusion. *Spine* 2004;29:326-332.

    Anterior débridement and fusion, followed by posterior instrumentation, was found to be safe and effective in the treatment of medically refractory pyogenic vertebral osteomyelitis.

14. Eismont FJ, Bohlman HH, Soni PL, Goldberg VM, Freehafer AA: Pyogenic and fungal vertebral osteomyelitis with paralysis. *J Bone Joint Surg Am* 1983;65:19-29.

15. Garcia A Jr, Grantham SA: Hematogenous pyogenic vertebral osteomyelitis. *J Bone Joint Surg Am* 1960;42:429-436.

16. Frederickson B, Yuan H, Olans R: Management and outcome of pyogenic vertebral osteomyelitis. *Clin Orthop Relat Res* 1978;131:160-167.

17. Emery SE, Chan DP, Woodward HR: Treatment of hematogenous pyogenic vertebral osteomyelitis with anterior debridement and primary bone grafting. *Spine* 1989;14:284-291.

18. Klöckner C, Valencia R: Sagittal alignment after anterior debridement and fusion with or without additional posterior instrumentation in the treatment of pyogenic and tuberculous spondylodiscitis. *Spine* 2003;28:1036-1042.

    The effects of posterior instrumentation in preventing kyphotic decompensation were examined after anterior débridement and fusion. Posterior instrumentation appeared to effectively prevent sagittal deformity.

19. Song KS, Ogden JA, Ganey T, Guidera KJ: Contiguous discitis and osteomyelitis in children. *J Pediatr Orthop* 1997;17:470-477.

20. Eismont FJ, Bohlman HH, Soni PL, Goldberg VM, Freehafer AA: Vertebral osteomyelitis in infants. *J Bone Joint Surg Br* 1982;64:32-35.

21. Kayser R, Mahlfeld K, Greulich M, Grasshoff H: Spondylodiscitis in childhood: Results of a long-term study. *Spine* 2005;30:318-323.

    Twenty patients with pediatric spondylodiskitis were followed for a minimum of 10 years. A delayed diagnosis was common. Approximately half of the patients had isolated diskitis, and the other half also had osteomyelitis. Eighty percent fully recovered without sequelae, although 20% had focal kyphosis and some limitation in spine range of motion on radiographs. There were no neurologic deficits.

22. Brown R, Hussain M, McHugh K, Novelli V, Jones D: Discitis in young children. *J Bone Joint Surg Br* 2001;83:106-111.

23. Ventura N, Gonzalez E, Terricabras L, Salvador A, Cabrera M: Intervertebral discitis in children: A review of 12 cases. *Int Orthop* 1996;20:32-34.

24. Huggett JF, McHugh TD, Zumla A: Tuberculosis: Amplification-based clinical diagnostic techniques. *Int J Biochem Cell Biol* 2003;35:1407-1412.

    This review describes the molecular assays available for relatively rapid detection of the *M tuberculosis* organism.

25. Albay A, Kisa O, Baylan O, Doganci L: The evaluation of FASTPlaqueTB test for the rapid diagnosis of tuberculosis. *Diagn Microbiol Infect Dis* 2003;46:211-215.

4: Specific Situations

A new test was found to have potential for the rapid diagnosis of *M tuberculosis* in a comparison with three other methods.

26. Jung NY, Jee WH, Ha KY, Park CK, Byun JY: Discrimination of tuberculous spondylitis from pyogenic spondylitis on MRI. *AJR Am J Roentgenol* 2004;182: 1405-1410.

MRI was shown to be accurate in differentiating tuberculous spondylitis from pyogenic osteomyelitis. The characteristic findings of both conditions are discussed.

27. Tuli SM: Results of treatment of spinal tuberculosis by "middle-path" regime. *J Bone Joint Surg Br* 1975;57: 13-23.

28. Medical Research Council: A 15-year assessment of controlled trials of the management of tuberculosis of the spine in Korea and Hong Kong: Thirteenth Report of the Medical Research Council Working Party on Tuberculosis of the Spine. *J Bone Joint Surg Br* 1998;80: 456-462.

29. Kim DJ, Yun YH, Moon SH, Riew KD: Posterior instrumentation using laminar hooks and anterior interbody arthrodesis for the treatment of tuberculosis of the lower lumbar spine. *Spine* 2004;29:E275-E279.

Short-segment circumferential instrumentation was successfully used to treat tuberculous vertebral osteomyelitis.

30. Dai LY, Jiang LS, Wang W, Cui YM: Single-stage anterior autogenous bone grafting and instrumentation in the surgical management of spinal tuberculosis. *Spine* 2005;30:2342-2349.

Favorable outcomes were reported after single-stage anterior débridement and instrumented fusion, with maintenance of sagittal alignment.

31. Frazier DD, Campbell DR, Garvey TA, Wiesel S, Bohlman HH, Eismont FJ: Fungal infections of the spine: Report of eleven patients with long-term follow-up. *J Bone Joint Surg Am* 2001;83:560-565.

32. Conaughty JM, Khurana S, Banovac K, Martinez OV, Eismont FJ: Antifungal penetration into normal rabbit nucleus pulposus. *Spine* 2004;29:E289-E293.

In this study of the penetration of amphotericin and fluconazole into the normal rabbit nucleus pulposus, amphotericin reached therapeutic levels in none of 12 rabbits, whereas fluconazole reached therapeutic levels in five of seven rabbits. Level of evidence: II.

33. Sørensen P: Spinal epidural abscesses: Conservative treatment for selected subgroups of patients. *Br J Neurosurg* 2003;17:513-518.

Eight neurologically intact patients with an epidural abscess were successfully treated nonsurgically with appropriate antibiotic therapy. Other indications for nonsurgical treatment are reviewed.

34. Gleave JR, Macfarlane R: Cauda equina syndrome: What is the relationship between timing of surgery and outcome? *Br J Neurosurg* 2002;16:325-328.

35. Reihsaus E, Waldbaur H, Seeling W: Spinal epidural abscess: A meta-analysis of 915 patients. *Neurosurg Rev* 2000;23:175-204.

36. Weinstein MA, Eismont FJ: Infections of the spine in patients with human immunodeficiency virus. *J Bone Joint Surg Am* 2005;87:604-609.

All patients admitted with a spine infection were reviewed over a 6-year period. The prevalence of spine infection was significantly higher in HIV-positive than in HIV-negative patients ($P = 0.001$). The patient's CD4 cell count was predictive of clinical course. Epidural abscess and death most often occurred in patients with severe immunocompromise.

37. Fang A, Hu SS, Endres N, Bradford DS: Risk factors for infection after spinal surgery. *Spine* 2005;30:1460-1465.

Forty-eight postsurgical infections were retrospectively reviewed. The identified presurgical risk factors were age older than 60 years, smoking, diabetes, previous surgical infection, obesity, and excessive alcohol use. Staged anterior and posterior spinal fusion (performed under separate anesthesia) was the procedure most likely to be complicated by postsurgical infection.

38. Carragee EJ, Kim D, van der Vlugt T, Vittum D: The clinical use of erythrocyte sedimentation rate in pyogenic vertebral osteomyelitis. *Spine* 1997;22:2089-2093.

39. Clark CE, Shufflebarger HL: Late-developing infection in instrumented idiopathic scoliosis. *Spine* 1999;24: 1909-1912.

40. Dumanian GA, Ondra SL, Liu J, Schafer MF, Chao JD: Muscle flap salvage of spine wounds with soft tissue defects or infection. *Spine* 2003;28:1203-1211.

The authors describe their experience and generally successful outcomes in using muscle flaps in the treatment of spine infections.

41. Mehbod AA, Ogilvie JW, Pinto MR, et al: Postoperative deep wound infections in adults after spinal fusion: Management with vacuum-assisted wound closure. *J Spinal Disord Tech* 2005;18:14-17.

Twenty deep infections after spine fusion were treated with serial débridement followed by application of a wound VAC device and intravenous antibiotics. Instrumentation was retained, and wounds were closed an average of 7 days after the initial VAC device application. All infections were eradicated.

42. Jones GA, Butler J, Lieberman I, Schlenk R: Negative-pressure wound therapy in the treatment of complex postoperative spinal wound infections: Complications and lessons learned using vacuum-assisted closure. *J Neurosurg Spine* 2007;6:407-411.

The complications and limitations of wound VAC devices used in 13 patients were reviewed retrospectively. One patient died of exsanguination partly related to the use of wound VAC. Two patients had persistent infection, and one patient required a skin graft.

Chapter 18

Musculoskeletal Infections Caused by Mycobacterial, Fungal, and Atypical Microorganisms

Camelia E. Marculescu, MD, MSCR   J. Robert Cantey, MD

Introduction

Microorganisms such as *Staphylococcus epidermidis*, *Staphylococcus aureus,* and β-hemolytic streptococci have a well-recognized association with osteomyelitis, septic arthritis, and prosthetic joint infection. These microorganisms usually can be easily isolated by culturing using conventional media. However, some mycobacterial, fungal, and unusual or atypical microorganisms also can cause bone and joint infections. *Mycobacterium tuberculosis* is by far the most common worldwide cause of mycobacterial osteomyelitis and arthritis.[1] Fungal osteomyelitis and arthritis are uncommon diseases that often have an indolent course. Nontuberculous mycobacterial disease, once a rarity, has dramatically increased in incidence during the acquired immunodeficiency syndrome (AIDS) epidemic. Other microorganisms that can cause bone and joint infections can be difficult to culture or are not typically associated with osteomyelitis or septic arthritis.

It is important for the physician to recognize bone and joint disease caused by a mycobacterial, fungal, or atypical microorganism because these microorganisms usually are not susceptible to the antimicrobials used to treat other bacterial diseases. A high index of suspicion for such organisms should be maintained based on epidemiologic clues, geographic distribution, and patient history. Specialized diagnostic tests may be required.

Mycobacterium Tuberculosis Infections

Bony tuberculosis is found in the spine in approximately 40% of patients with tuberculosis. Some recent studies found spinal tuberculosis in 50% of patients, although the apparent increase may be attributable to the demographic characteristics of the study populations.[2,3] The disease also occurs in weight-bearing joints, especially the hip or knee, and occasionally in other joints.[4] Extraspinal musculoskeletal tuberculosis accounts for only 1% to 2% of all instances of tuberculosis.[5] The

risk of developing a tuberculous infection is greatest in a person who has a chronic debilitating condition; is older than approximately 65 years; is immunocompromised as a result of human immunodeficiency virus (HIV) infection, organ transplantation, or another cause; is a substance abuser; or has lived in a geographic region with a high incidence of tuberculosis.[6] The risk of developing tuberculous osteomyelitis or arthritis is increased in a person who is older than 65 years, is female, or has lived in a region where tuberculosis is prevalent.[7] In a large study conducted in the United States, foreign birth was not a significant risk factor for developing bone and joint tuberculosis.[7] This finding may be attributable to the prevalence among US-born patients of AIDS, which is associated with an increased incidence of extrapulmonary tuberculosis. The spine is affected in 60% of patients with tuberculosis who are HIV positive and only 1% of patients who are HIV negative.[6] Patients who are HIV positive have a 170-fold increase in the risk of reactivation of dormant earlier tuberculosis.

A musculoskeletal tuberculosis lesion usually results from either hematogenous dissemination of mycobacteria from a primary focus in the lung or genitourinary tract or lymphogenous dissemination from a primary or reactivated infected focus. In rare instances, mycobacterial disease results from direct inoculation. Although a pulmonary focus is often presumed, fewer than 50% of patients have active, intercurrent pulmonary tuberculosis.[8] Joint space involvement can result from hematogenous dissemination through the subsynovial vessels or from erosion of a epiphyseal lesion (usually in an adult) or a metaphyseal lesion (usually in a child) into the joint space.[9]

Spinal tuberculosis most commonly affects the thoracolumbar spine and less commonly the thoracic or lumbar spine (**Figure 1**). The cervical spine is affected only rarely, and the sacral region even more rarely.[6,10] Typically, the anterior part of the vertebra is initially destroyed. Bacilli then spread beneath the anterior spinal ligament and involve the anterosuperior aspect of the adjacent inferior vertebra, giving rise to the typical

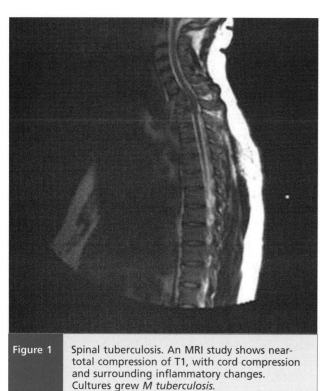

Figure 1 Spinal tuberculosis. An MRI study shows near-total compression of T1, with cord compression and surrounding inflammatory changes. Cultures grew *M tuberculosis.*

wedge-shaped deformity. Tuberculous arthritis usually is monoarticular, but multiple joints are involved in approximately 10% of patients.[8] The hip or knee is the most commonly affected joint, followed by the sacroiliac joint, shoulder, elbow, and ankle.[8]

Tuberculous osteomyelitis is less common than tuberculous arthritis. Although tuberculous osteomyelitis usually is multifocal and disseminated, the incidence of solitary lesions is increasing.[9] The disease most commonly occurs in the bones of the extremities.[8] Primary tuberculous tenosynovitis and tuberculous involvement of the muscle and fascia are uncommon. Tuberculous tenosynovitis involves the flexor tendon sheaths of the dominant hand.[8] Although secondary tuberculous involvement of the synovial bursa membranes is well known, primary bursitis is rarely reported. The trochanteric, subacromial, subgluteal, and radioulnar wrist bursae are most frequently affected. Tuberculous infection of a prosthetic joint is rare, accounting for 0.3% of prosthetic joint infections.[11] A hip or knee prosthesis is most commonly affected. Tuberculous prosthetic joint infection results from local reactivation or, less commonly, hematogenous spread. *M tuberculosis* infection of a prosthetic joint has been reported in patients with no history of tuberculosis.[11]

The nonspecific symptoms of tuberculous bone and joint infection and its indolent clinical course often lead to a delayed diagnosis. Pain and swelling are the most common complaints.[4] Chest radiographs suggest the presence of tuberculous infection in only 50% of patients. Abscesses, cutaneous fistulae, or joint deformities appear when the disease has been active for

months. Spinal disease may be associated with a neurologic deficit caused by impingement of the spinal cord, nerves, or nerve roots. Patients with thoracic spinal tuberculosis are at particular risk of paraplegia or paraparesis.

Tuberculin skin testing can be used if tuberculosis is suspected, and it is nearly 90% sensitive for bone and joint tuberculosis in patients who are immunocompetent.[12] However, the sensitivity decreases substantially in patients who are immunocompromised. A positive result neither confirms nor excludes the presence of tuberculosis, and mycobacterial culturing of bone biopsy or surgical specimens is essential to determine the antibiotic susceptibilities of the organism and guide subsequent therapy. Drainage fluid cannot be cultured with reliable results because the presence of colonizing bacteria or fungi can obscure the diagnosis.[4] Acid-fast smears are positive in some patients. The reported sensitivity of synovial tissue culturing is 94%, and that of synovial fluid culturing is 79%.[13] For a patient with suspected extrapulmonary tuberculosis, the diagnostic usefulness of molecular testing after a smear-negative or culture-negative result is unclear. Experience is limited in the use of polymerase chain reaction for detection of *M tuberculosis* in synovial fluid. Studies suggest a sensitivity of 57.7% in synovial fluid, which is lower than the sensitivity in the sputum or pleural fluid, and false-positive results can occur.[14]

Histologic evidence of mycobacterial infection has been reported in 94% of synovial biopsy specimens.[13] The presence of granulomatous inflammation is not specific for mycobacterial infection.[4] Cell counts and fluid biochemistry from tuberculous joint fluid also are not specific for mycobacterial infection.[4] A moderately elevated leukocyte count with a neutrophilic predominance, low glucose, and increased proteins is typical.[13]

Radiologic imaging can suggest the diagnosis and can be useful in obtaining culture material via directed biopsy. The findings of spinal MRI may favor tuberculosis over other causes of bone destruction such as a malignancy. MRI is the most sensitive radiologic method for diagnosing tuberculous spondylitis.[10] Typically, the infection starts at the anteroinferior aspect of the vertebral body and spreads to contiguous vertebrae along the anterior longitudinal ligament of the spine. The infection also can course down the posterior aspect of the spine, possibly leaving some vertebrae unaffected. The disks and posterior elements usually are spared early in the disease process.[4] The radiographic features of tuberculous arthritis include joint effusion, cortical irregularity, lytic lesions, joint space narrowing, and periosteal new bone formation.[8] The Phemister triad, which includes periarticular osteoporosis, peripheral osseous erosion, and gradual narrowing of the joint space, suggests the presence of tuberculosis. Focal areas of cartilaginous destruction may be present on MRI, interspersed with chondral elements that appear relatively normal. Bone marrow changes may reflect either osteomyelitis or bone marrow edema. Sinus tracts may have marginal tram-track enhancement on a gadolinium-enhanced MRI study. The MRI findings for tuberculous arthritis are nonspecific.[8] Tuberculous sequestration and sclerosis are uncommon on MRI and less extensive in extra-axial tuberculous osteomyelitis than in pyogenic osteomyelitis. MRI may reveal intraosseous involvement earlier than other imaging modalities. Ultrasonography is ideal for initial imaging of suspected tuberculous tenosynovitis, although MRI also is useful in detecting three forms of tuberculous tenosynovitis: hygromatous, serofibrinous, and fungoid.[8]

The medical treatment of patients with bone and joint tuberculosis is similar to that of patients with other forms of tuberculosis. The American Thoracic Society recommends a 6- to 9-month course of therapy for patients with drug-susceptible tuberculosis. A longer course may be required for a patient who does not respond during the first 6 to 9 months. The principles of treating drug-resistant bone and joint tuberculosis are the same as those for treating drug-resistant tuberculosis of other sites.[15] The optimal medical and surgical therapy for *M tuberculosis* prosthetic joint infection is unknown. Patients with *M tuberculosis* septic arthritis discovered incidentally during implantation surgery or the early postsurgical period were successfully treated using a nonrifampin antituberculosis drug combination for 12 to 18 months.[11] The use of corticosteroids is not recommended for treating tuberculous arthritis or osteomyelitis.

Surgery is used for draining abscesses and decompressing vital structures. A significantly damaged joint may require débridement and possibly fusion or replacement.[4] The possibility of an earlier *M tuberculosis* infection should be determined before a patient undergoes total joint arthroplasty; for a patient with such a history, mycobacterial culture specimens should be obtained during the arthroplasty.[11] When quiescent *M tuberculosis* septic arthritis necessitates total joint arthroplasty, the risk of *M tuberculosis* reactivation is higher for a patient receiving a prosthetic knee than a prosthetic hip (27% compared with 6%).[11] Late-onset *M tuberculosis* prosthetic joint infection has been treated using a two-stage exchange, a partial one-stage exchange, débridement with retention of the prosthesis, or medical treatment alone. Medical treatment usually is unsuccessful when used alone, and removal of the prosthesis is often required. Débridement with prosthesis retention was unsuccessful in three of six patients (50%).[11]

Spinal tuberculosis can be cured using medical treatment. Because of the close proximity of the spine to other vital structures, some researchers believe that aggressive surgical therapy is necessary to stabilize the spine and prevent kyphosis, unless the disease is very mild.[16] Radical débridement and bone grafting may be superior to simple débridement for improving kyphosis and preventing later spinal deterioration.[17-19]

Fungal Infections

Fungal arthritis and osteomyelitis are uncommon, and often they are indolent. The most important predisposing factors for fungal infection are alteration of human microbial flora, disruption of mucocutaneous membranes, impairment of immune function,[20] and prolonged antimicrobial therapy. Fungal osteomyelitis can occur as an isolated disease or as part of a multisystem process. The clinical appearance and outcome vary depending on the specific fungal pathogen and patient-specific factors.[21] The patient typically has localized pain affecting weight-bearing joints. Cold soft-tissue abscesses and sinus tracts may form in a chronic infection.[21] The slow progression of the disease and failure to recognize that a fungus may be responsible can lead to a delay in diagnosis.

Candida

Candida species are the fungi most commonly associated with an opportunistic infection. Bone and joint infections caused by *Candida* species commonly occur as disseminated disease but also can result from direct inoculation during trauma or surgery or as a direct extension from a joint infection or contiguous focus of infection.[20] A *Candida* bone infection can occur at the same time as an episode of fungemia or several months later, despite adequate therapy for the fungemia.[22] The vertebrae are most commonly affected. When the sternum is affected, draining sinus tracts often are present.[20] Hematogenous dissemination of *Candida* species often leads to monoarticular arthritis affecting a normal joint. The association of *Candida* arthritis with the intra-articular administration of steroids highlights the ability of cortisone to impair local defenses as well as the importance of aseptic technique.[23,24]

Candida typically affects a large weight-bearing joint. Knee involvement is most frequently reported, and hip, shoulder, ankle, cuneiform bone, and costochondral joint involvement also has been described. In contrast to bacterial arthritis, *Candida* arthritis begins as a synovitis, eventually involving adjacent bone and resulting in osteomyelitis.[20] Although fungal prosthetic joint infection is rare, *Candida* species are the most common pathogens; the percentage of all prosthetic joint infections caused by *Candida* species is estimated to be 1%.[25] A *Candida* prosthetic joint infection most often appears as a chronic infection during the late postsurgical period. The patient usually has pain and swelling or drainage. *Candida albicans* is the most frequently isolated species, and *Candida parapsilosis*, *Candida glabrata*, and *Candida tropicalis* also have been reported.[11,25-30] A *Candida* prosthetic joint infection can affect a hip, knee, or shoulder arthroplasty.

Candida osteomyelitis or arthritis can be difficult to diagnose. A high index of suspicion must be maintained in a patient with specific risk factors or with a joint infection that is unresponsive to antibiotic therapy. Blood cultures often are negative. The

4: Specific Situations

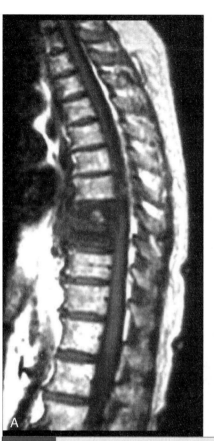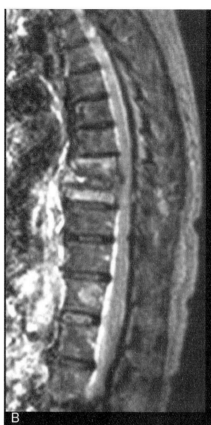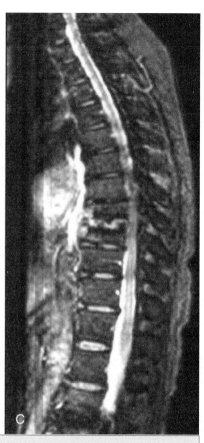

Figure 2   *Candida* spondylodiskitis. **A,** A T1-weighted sagittal MRI study of the thoracic spine reveals decreased or hypointense signal within the T8-9 disk and associated destruction of vertebral bodies and compromise of the spinal cord. **B,** A T2-weighted sagittal MRI study reveals a somewhat hyperintense marrow signal. **C,** A field echo MRI study reveals disk destruction and sclerosis of the adjoining end plates with a prevertebral and paravertebral soft-tissue mass. (Adapted with permission from Torres-Ramos FM, Botwin KP, Shah CP: Candida spondylodiscitis: An unusual case of thoracolumbar pain with review of imaging findings and description of the clinical condition. *Pain Physician* 2004;7:257-260.)

radiographic findings associated with *Candida* vertebral osteomyelitis are indistinguishable from those associated with bacterial infection; they include destruction of the superior end plate of a vertebral body and the inferior end plate of the adjoining body, accompanied by a decrease in disk space height.[6] MRI and CT are valuable in determining the presence and extent of cord compression, paraspinal abscess, and disk space or vertebral body involvement[26,31] (**Figure 2**). Disease activity and response to treatment can be reliably monitored through a gallium-enhanced bone scan.[32] Demineralization and a mottled trabecular pattern can be seen on plain radiographs in osteomyelitis of the long bones.[22] In *Candida* arthritis, synovial effusion may be present on plain radiographs, and purulence of the synovial fluid often allows *Candida* arthritis to be distinguished from arthritis caused by other fungi. In *Candida* arthritis, the synovial fluid white blood cell count ranges from 15,000 to 100,000 cells (primarily polymorphonuclear neutrophils); the glucose level may be low or normal, and the protein concentration typically is high.[20] Gram staining is positive in only 20% of patients; better results can be obtained by culturing the

synovial fluid or tissue.[21] The presence of *Candida* species in the synovial fluid should not be assumed to represent contamination. Histologic evidence of invasive *Candida* prosthetic joint infection is rare, and the diagnosis therefore is usually made through positive cultures from multiple periprosthetic specimens or multiple joint aspirates.[29] *Candida* prosthetic joint infection was diagnosed either by *Candida* isolation from at least two joint aspirates or from purulence in one joint aspirate combined with *Candida* identification on serial serologic tests, intrasurgical tissue culturing, or (rarely) histopathologic examination.[29] Joint aspiration was reported to yield hemorrhagic fluid in several patients.[28,33] Measurement of the serum level of β-D-glucan, a constituent of fungi, can be used for early diagnosis of a *Candida* bone infection,[34] although the results do not distinguish between types of fungi. The drug susceptibilities of C albicans and other *Candida* species vary, and the increasing incidence of species other than C albicans requires that the involved species be identified before the therapy is determined.

The treatment of *Candida* bone and joint infections is not well established. Antifungal therapy is typical, often in conjunction with surgical débridement. Several months of antifungal treatment may be required for eradication of *Candida* species.[20] Amphotericin B (0.5 mg/kg/day) is the most commonly recommended antifungal agent for initial treatment of osteoarticular infection.[20] Liposomal amphotericin B was found to be less nephrotoxic and as effective as conventional amphotericin B.[35] No evidence exists that amphotericin B with flucytosine is more efficacious than amphotericin B alone.[36] Azoles such fluconazole, itraconazole, voriconazole, and posaconazole are less toxic alternatives to amphotericin B. If standard therapy using amphotericin B is not feasible or is unsuccessful, an azole should be chosen based on the results of susceptibility testing, although clinical correlation data are lacking.[20] Limited data are available on the use of the echinocandins (caspofungin, micafungin, and anidulafungin) to treat *Candida* arthritis and osteomyelitis. Intra-articular amphotericin B is controversial when used as an adjunct to intravenous antifungal therapy in an infection limited to the joint capsule.[24] Vertebral osteomyelitis may require surgical stabilization and decompression, but medical treatment alone has been successful in patients without neurologic compromise.[22]

Successful treatment of *Candida* prosthetic joint infection often requires removal of the prosthesis followed by appropriate antifungal therapy.[11,28] Two-stage exchange offers the best functional outcome, but many investigators have been reluctant to perform delayed reimplantation because of the perceived high risk of relapse. However, the recurrence rate for *Candida* prosthetic joint infection after a two-stage exchange was estimated to be only 20%; the duration of antifungal therapy ranged from 6 weeks to 9 months for all patients.[29] The optimal interval before reimplantation has not been determined, although an infection-free interval of 3 months has been suggested.[30] The Infectious Diseases Society of America guideline suggests that reimplantation can be performed after eradication of the infection, which is defined as the absence of recurrent symptoms after antifungal therapy and a negative pre-reimplantation synovial fluid culture.[37]

After treatment, clinical symptoms and radiologic evaluation are used to evaluate the status of a *Candida* bone and joint infection. Eradication of *Candida* vertebral osteomyelitis is best confirmed with a posttreatment biopsy.[38]

Aspergillus

Aspergillus is a mold with septate hyphae. The common *Aspergillus* species grow on dead leaves, stored grain, compost piles, hay, and other decaying vegetation.[6] Like other fungal bone and joint infections, *Aspergillus* infection can occur in isolation or in association with invasive disease.[20] *Aspergillus* musculoskeletal disease is rare, although dissemination from a primary pulmonary focus can occur through hematogenous spread. Most instances of bone and joint aspergillosis occur in patients who are immunocompromised, have

chronic granulomatous disease, or have had trauma or surgery.[39,40] In patients who are immunocompetent, the disease has been reported as the cause of sternal osteomyelitis after trauma or surgery[4] or septic arthritis after intra-articular corticosteroid injection.[40]

Bone and joint aspergillosis is diagnosed through bone, soft-tissue, or synovial fluid culturing. *Aspergillus* isolated from the synovial fluid should not be dismissed as a contaminant.[41] The diagnosis of *Aspergillus* spondylitis can be difficult because the condition results in extensive destruction of the disk and vertebral bodies. Needle biopsy does not always provide a definitive diagnosis,[6] but radiologic evidence of bone and joint destruction often can be seen.

Aspergillus bone and joint infections often require both medical and surgical therapy. Surgical débridement and a course of amphotericin B followed by itraconazole have led to successful outcomes. Amphotericin B is the traditional drug of choice. However, the newer azoles, including voriconazole and posaconazole, are being used because they have excellent in vitro activity against *Aspergillus*, allow good bone penetration, and are less toxic than amphotericin B.[35,40,42] Itraconazole does not penetrate the central nervous system well and should not be used if there is evidence of central nervous system involvement. Caspofungin has been used in patients who do not respond to other antifungal agents, but its role in treating osteoarticular infection has not been determined. Medical therapy has been used alone or in combination with surgery to treat an *Aspergillus* spine infection. Surgical treatment is often initiated because medical treatment has had an unsatisfactory result or neurologic complications are present.[6]

Coccidioides Immitis

Coccidioides immitis is endemic in the southwestern United States. The primary infection is silent in 60% of infected individuals who are immunocompetent. Fewer than 1% of primary pulmonary *C immitis* infections progress to disseminated disease, and approximately 20% of disseminated infections involve the bone and joints.[20] Disseminated disease is more likely to occur among Hispanics and African Americans.[43] Reactivation of a preexisting infection can occur in a person who is immunocompromised.

Primary pulmonary coccidioidomycosis sometimes is associated with a sterile arthritis. Bone and joint infection can occur in isolation or in disseminated disease, most commonly involving large joints. The patient may have fever, joint pain, restricted range of motion, warmth, or joint effusion.[20] The radiologic findings can include cysts, cartilage erosion, or lytic lesions (in advanced stages of the disease). In coccidioidal spondylitis, most of the bony lesions are lytic and involve both anterior and posterior bony elements of the vertebrae. Paraspinal masses with contiguous rib involvement can be seen. The disk space is relatively uninvolved.[6]

The diagnosis of a *C immitis* infection relies on serology. Serum complement fixation titers of more

4: Specific Situations

than 1:32 indicate the presence of disseminated disease.[44] Peripheral eosinophilia may be present. The diagnosis is confirmed through synovial fluid culturing or tissue biopsy. On biopsy, spherules are the hallmark for diagnosis. Specimens should be handled with extreme care to prevent infection of laboratory personnel.[6]

C immitis infection is treated with débridement and a prolonged course of amphotericin B. *C immitis* can be very difficult to eradicate from bone and joints if the infection is chronic. Patients with coccidioidal spondylitis often require surgical decompression of the neural element, with radical excision of the infectious process and stabilization of the spine with instrumentation to prevent deformity.[6] Amphotericin B typically is administered for 2 to 3 months, followed by an azole such as fluconazole (400 to 600 mg per day for 12 months). To prevent a relapse, itraconazole (200 mg twice daily) can be used for long-term suppression, which may be required for years.[6] Posaconazole also may have a role in treatment.[31]

Histoplasma Capsulatum

Histoplasma capsulatum is a dimorphic fungus that is found worldwide but is endemic in the midwestern United States. Primary pulmonary, chronic pulmonary, and disseminated disease can occur. Bone and joint infections caused by *H capsulatum* are rare. Infectious arthritis can occur either with disseminated histoplasmosis or as a solitary monoarthritis[20] and sometimes is associated with immune-complex arthritis appearing as a symmetric arthritis.[21]

The radiographic findings may be normal in bone and joint histoplasmosis. The diagnosis relies on isolation of *H capsulatum* from synovial fluid or surgical tissue.[20] Caseating or noncaseating granulomas may be present.[44,45] Bone and joint histoplasmosis is treated with surgical débridement followed by amphotericin B or an oral azole (itraconazole). *H capsulatum* prosthetic joint infection was successfully treated using débridement and lifelong suppression with itraconazole.[46]

Blastomyces Dermatitidis

Blastomyces dermatitidis is found in soil in its mycelial form and in host tissue in its yeast form. It is endemic in the south central, southeastern, and midwestern United States, as well as Canada.

Infection caused by *B dermatitidis* has a predilection for the lungs, skin, soft tissue, and bone. The bone disease appears with pain and swelling in the affected area, sometimes accompanied by ulcerative or nodular skin lesions.[44] Joint involvement typically is monoarticular and is the result of spreading from an osteomyelitic focus.[20] The spine, particularly the lumbar or thoracic region, is the most common site of skeletal involvement; the skull, ribs, tibia, and bones of the foot and wrist are less frequently affected.[6] The radiologic findings include osteolytic lesions and synovial effusions.[44] *Blastomyces* spondylitis commonly affects the posterior elements of the vertebral body; the disk space

may be involved. Paraspinal soft-tissue abscesses and ulcerations are common.[6] A definitive diagnosis is made through histologic examination of synovial or bone tissue or culturing of the joint fluid or tissue. The characteristic round, broad-based budding yeast of *B dermatitidis* can be identified.[47] The synovial fluid is often purulent.

Treatment with itraconazole (200 to 400 mg per day for 1 year) has been recommended for osteomyelitis secondary to blastomycosis. Life-threatening disease requires treatment with amphotericin B.[20] In spondylitis caused by *B dermatitidis*, the absolute indications for surgery are progressive deformity and spinal canal compromise with neurocompression.[6]

Cryptococcus Neoformans

Cryptococcus neoformans is an encapsulated budding yeast that occurs widely and is found in large numbers in pigeon roosts. Patients who use corticosteroids or have a hematologic malignancy, diabetes, sarcoidosis, tuberculosis, or AIDS are especially susceptible to cryptococcosis. The bones become involved through hematogenous spread in 10% of patients with cryptococcosis.[20] Spinal involvement usually is a manifestation of disseminated cryptococcosis and occurs in 5% to 10% of patients with cryptococcosis.[48] Cryptococcal vertebral osteomyelitis has been reported in otherwise healthy patients.[20] Cryptococcal arthritis often is the result of local extension from an infected bone into the adjacent synovial space;[49] it most frequently is found in the knee but also can affect the elbow, ankle, wrist, sacroiliac, sternoclavicular, or metacarpophalangeal joint.[20]

The radiographic appearance of spinal cryptococcosis is variable and nonspecific. Lytic lesions may appear within a vertebral body, resembling the cystic form of tuberculosis with discrete margins and surrounding sclerosis. The infection may involve a single vertebral body and lead to collapse. Paravertebral soft-tissue masses suggestive of spinal tuberculosis can be seen in the later stages of the disease.[6] As in tuberculosis, posterior spinal elements usually are spared.[50] In arthritis, the radiographic findings include soft-tissue swelling, synovial effusion, and lytic lesions of contiguous bone.[20]

Cryptococcosis typically has a subacute onset characterized by swelling and pain. Serum or cerebrospinal fluid cryptococcal antigen testing may be helpful in the diagnosis, although a negative antigen does not completely rule out the presence of bone or joint cryptococcosis.[20] The diagnosis is confirmed by a positive culture of synovial fluid, tissue, or sinus tract drainage.[51] Multinucleate giant cells and granuloma formation can be seen on surgical biopsy specimens. Periodic acid–Schiff or methenamine silver staining may reveal the characteristic budding cryptococci.[20]

The treatment of cryptococcosis involves surgical drainage and antifungal therapy. Current data suggest that in a patient who is immunocompromised, cryptococcal joint or spinal infection is best treated using amphotericin B and 5-fluorocytosine followed by fluconazole.[6,20]

Sporothrix Schenckii

Sporothrix schenckii is a dimorphic fungus commonly found in soil or on animals or vegetation. The fungus enters the host through a minor wound or less commonly through the respiratory tract. Lymphocutaneous sporotrichosis, manifested as skin ulcerations or subcutaneous nodules, is the most common form of the disease. Alcoholism and myeloproliferative disorders have been associated with sporotrichosis.

The extracutaneous form of sporotrichosis is rare and can cause pneumonitis, arthritis, or osteomyelitis.[20] Extracutaneous sporotrichosis is osteoarticular in approximately 80% of patients. The disease typically involves the knee, although other joints also can be affected.[20] The estimated incidence of knee sporotrichoid arthritis ranges from 0.03% to 0.04%.[52] The symptoms are chronic and progressive and commonly include pain, swelling, and decreased range of motion in the affected joint.[20] Constitutional symptoms are uncommon. Chronic indolent *S schenckii* infection of a total knee prosthesis occurred in one patient.[53] The radiographic findings include joint space narrowing, erosion of the articular surfaces, joint effusions, soft-tissue swelling, and periarticular osteopenia.[20] Untreated sporotrichoid arthritis can lead to soft-tissue abscesses, cutaneous fistulae, or draining sinus tracts.[20]

Sporotrichosis can be difficult to diagnose, and a high level of suspicion is required. The role of serology has not been well studied;[54] synovial fluid may reveal moderate leukocytosis (8,000 to 23,600 cells) with neutrophilic and lymphocytic predominance.[20] Mycologic culturing of surgical specimens usually is required to establish the diagnosis. The diagnostic yield of synovial tissue cultures is higher than that of synovial fluid cultures;[52,54] the organisms are difficult to visualize using fungal stains.[55] Granulomatous inflammation and caseating or noncaseating granulomas may be seen.[52]

The Infectious Diseases Society of America guideline recommends that itraconazole be used for the initial treatment of osteoarticular sporotrichosis in most patients; the success rate is 60% to 80%.[56] Amphotericin B can be used for a patient with extensive involvement or after unsuccessful treatment with itraconazole. Fluconazole and ketoconazole have a minimal role in treating osteoarticular sporotrichosis.[56] In a patient who developed chronic indolent sporotrichosis after total knee arthroplasty, a periprosthetic cystic mass was débrided, and culturing yielded *S schenckii*. Treatment with amphotericin B to a cumulative dose of 2.4 g was followed by 2 years of treatment with oral itraconazole, leading to full suppression of the infection.[53]

Unusual or Atypical Infections

Nontuberculous Mycobacteria

Nontuberculous mycobacteria are ubiquitous and have been isolated from water and soil.[4] The incidence of infection with nontuberculous mycobacteria increased dramatically during the 1980s and 1990s, parallel with the AIDS epidemic. Most patients have pulmonary or disseminated disease. In patients who are immunocompetent, nontuberculous osteomyelitis and arthritis occur secondary to direct inoculation during trauma or surgery rather than through hematogenous dissemination.[4] In patients who are immunocompromised, hematogenous dissemination can lead to multifocal disease including the bone and joints.[4] Chronic granulomatous infection of the bone is rare and typically occurs as a result of direct inoculation of nontuberculous mycobacteria through trauma, surgical incision, puncture wound, or injection.[57] Nontuberculous mycobacteria have a tendency to cause infections associated with foreign bodies such as a prosthetic joint. The clinical appearance of nontuberculous mycobacterial bone and joint disease is similar to that of tuberculosis.

Rapidly Growing Mycobacteria

Prosthetic joint infection can be caused by rapidly growing mycobacteria such as *Mycobacterium fortuitum*, *Mycobacterium chelonae*, *Mycobacterium abscessus*, and *Mycobacterium smegmatis*.[11,58] Most prosthetic joint infections caused by *M fortuitum* occur in the early postsurgical period, and *M chelonae* usually causes a late infection.[11] The infection is diagnosed from pus, bone, synovial fluid, or abscess; on subculturing, the bacteria grow within 7 days.[2]

In the absence of randomized studies to determine the optimal treatment of rapidly growing nontuberculous mycobacterial bone and joint infections, a combination of surgery and antibiotics usually is recommended. For prosthetic joint infection caused by a rapidly growing mycobacterium, the desirable therapeutic approach is effective antibiotic therapy followed by a staged reimplantation.[58] The choice of antibiotic therapy should be guided by antimicrobial susceptibility testing because of interspecies and intraspecies variability in antimicrobial susceptibility patterns.[59] The first-line agents for *M tuberculosis* infection, such as isoniazid, ethambutol, and rifampin, are not active against rapidly growing mycobacteria and should not be used. For a bone, joint, or other infection caused by rapidly growing mycobacteria, the agents that should be tested against clinically important isolates are amikacin, cefoxitin, ciprofloxacin, clarithromycin, doxycycline, imipenem, sulfamethoxazole, tobramycin (for *M chelonae* only), and linezolid.[11] The number of agents required for effective treatment is not known, although a three-drug regimen often is used.[4] The optimal duration of antibiotic therapy also is unresolved; a course of 6 to 12 months generally is used. The duration of therapy is influenced by the type of surgical treatment and by resection or retention of an infected prosthesis. The duration of therapy sometimes is determined by the species of rapidly growing mycobacterium recovered; infection with some species (such as M abscessus) is more difficult to treat than infection with other species (such as M fortuitum).[58]

Patients with a nontuberculous mycobacterial bone infection must be followed closely because of the potential for drug toxicity over the extended duration of therapy. The patient's history and physical findings are likely to be the most relevant factors in assessing the response to therapy. The extent of clinical and radiologic improvement can suggest the required frequency of follow-up and intervention.[4]

Mycobacterium Avium-Intracellulare Complex

Disseminated infection caused by the Mycobacterium avium-intracellulare complex is found in patients with AIDS. In addition, the M avium-intracellulare complex causes pulmonary disease in patients who have preexisting lung disease, an underlying malignancy, or collagen vascular disease, as well as patients who are receiving corticosteroids or have received an organ transplant.[60,61] Extrapulmonary M avium-intracellulare complex infection is rare. However, cellulitis, tenosynovitis, septic arthritis, osteomyelitis, epidural abscess, spinal osteomyelitis, and prosthetic joint infection have been reported, primarily in patients who are immunocompromised.[11,27,60-66] Rare instances of septic arthritis or osteomyelitis have been reported in patients who are immunocompetent.[67,68]

The diagnosis of M avium-intracellulare complex infection usually is established by isolating the organism from a culture of blood, synovial fluid, or biopsy material. If synovial aspirate cultures are negative, synovial biopsy can be helpful in identifying the organism responsible for septic arthritis.[60] The infection has no typical histopathology; chronic osteomyelitis histology, with or without granulomas, does not exclude M avium-intracellulare complex infection.[67]

The M avium-intracellulare complex is highly resistant to standard antituberculous agents. The susceptibility testing is difficult and controversial compared to that of M tuberculosis. Only an in vitro susceptibility to macrolides (clarithromycin and azithromycin) was found to be correlated with the in vivo response.[69] The Clinical and Laboratory Standards Institute therefore suggests that macrolide susceptibility testing be performed for all clinically important isolates.[70] Multiple drug therapy that includes a macrolide as well as ethambutol and either rifampin or rifabutin is recommended for treating pulmonary or disseminated disease.[59,69] The duration of therapy is prolonged (more than 1 year) and may be lifelong in a patient with AIDS.[65] Adequate surgical débridement is critical to the outcome of an M avium-intracellulare complex infection and typically is followed by antimycobacterial

therapy.[61] For a prosthetic joint infection, a prolonged course has been suggested, using at least four antimycobacterial agents active against the M avium-intracellulare complex, with resection of the prosthesis. M avium-intracellulare complex prosthetic joint infection is believed to be associated with substantial risk of relapse after reimplantation.[66]

Mycoplasma and Ureaplasma

Mycoplasma septic arthritis and osteomyelitis have been reported in patients with hypogammaglobulinemia after organ transplantation, urethritis, cervicitis, or bronchitis.[71,72] True septic arthritis is rarely caused by Mycoplasma or Ureaplasma species.[72] Two patients who had rheumatoid arthritis with no genitourinary involvement developed a Mycoplasma hominis prosthetic joint infection with acute fever and joint pain.[11] M hominis prosthetic joint infection should be suspected in a patient who has a clinically infected joint with purulent aspirate, a negative Gram stain, and negative standard bacterial cultures; the microbiology laboratory should be instructed to specifically look for M hominis.[11]

Diagnosis of M hominis infection depends on polymerase chain reaction, if available, or cultivation on special media. Susceptibility testing of M hominis has not been standardized, and the results are not correlated with the clinical outcome. Many strains have in vitro susceptibility to clindamycin and are moderately susceptible to chloramphenicol and rifampin. Increased M hominis resistance to tetracycline has been documented.[73] Although fluoroquinolones usually are active in vitro against M hominis, in vitro resistance can be induced by exposing the microorganism to increasing concentrations of fluoroquinolones.[11]

Good outcomes have been reported after treatment using a combination of doxycycline and fluoroquinolones over several weeks or months.[72] One patient with a prosthetic joint infection required multiple joint aspirations and 6 months of doxycycline therapy. The patient developed gastrointestinal side effects that led to discontinuation of doxycycline and a relapse of the infection. The patient was then treated using ciprofloxacin for 2 weeks, with a good result.[74] The condition of a second patient improved after repeated aspiration and 1 month of clindamycin therapy.[75]

Whipple Disease

Whipple disease is a multisystem disorder caused by the fastidious actinomycete Tropheryma whippelii. The gastrointestinal manifestations of the disease often are preceded by a migratory, nondestructive peripheral arthritis. In one patient, Whipple disease was completely cured using trimethoprim-sulfamethoxazole for 20 months, but 2 years later the patient developed a prosthetic joint infection caused by T whippelii after total knee arthroplasty.[76] The symptoms were low-grade fever, joint pain, swelling, and tenderness.

A positive polymerase chain reaction of small bowel tissue may support a diagnosis of *T whippelii* joint infection. Polymerase chain reaction of the synovial fluid also can be useful.[77] Attempts to culture the causative organism often are unsuccessful. Microscopic examination of the infected tissue with periodic acid–Schiff stain reveals infiltration by large macrophages with diastase-resistant inclusions.[78]

A 2-week initial course of parenteral ceftriaxone is recommended, followed by oral trimethoprim-sulfamethoxazole for a period of at least 1 year.[72] A patient with a prosthetic joint infection was treated using débridement with retention of the prosthesis followed by chronic oral antimicrobial suppression (initially with trimethoprim-sulfamethoxazole and later with pristinamycin). At 1-year follow-up, the infection was controlled.[76]

Echinococcus

Echinococcus species are endemic in some sheep-raising areas of Asia, the Middle East, South America, Iceland, and northern Canada. Bone involvement is found in 0.5% to 2% of patients with echinococcosis, usually involving the pelvis, spine, humerus, or tibia.[79] Cysts grow slowly in the bones, and many years may pass before clinical manifestations appear. A combination of cysts and reactive sclerosis is most commonly observed. In a patient with rheumatoid arthritis, cysts were found during total hip arthroplasty, and the serology was positive for *Echinococcus*. Seven days after surgery, the patient developed a prosthetic joint infection, which was manifested by acute signs of local inflammation followed by sinus tract formation with local cystic and sclerotic changes.[80]

Although serologic tests can confirm a suspected diagnosis of echinococcosis, a negative serologic test does not rule out its presence. Immunoglobulin G enzyme-linked immunosorbent assay was found to be the most sensitive (84% to 94%) and specific (99%) test for most cyst locations.[81] Direct histopathologic inspection of the infected material is required for laboratory detection of *Echinococcus* species.

The treatment of bony echinococcal disease requires a complete resection of the involved area. Hemipelvectomy and hindquarter amputation have been recommended for complete eradication of the disease,[82] but the results have been discouraging. Adjunctive chemotherapy administered before and after surgery appears to reduce the risk of recurrence.[83] A patient with prosthetic joint infection caused by *Echinococcus multilocularis* after total hip arthroplasty had a favorable outcome 36 months after complete surgical removal of the cysts and prolonged treatment with albendazole.[79] Prosthesis removal and prolonged treatment with albendazole is required if complete cyst removal is not technically feasible.

Summary

The musculoskeletal infections caused by some microorganisms, such as *S epidermidis*, *S aureus,* and β-hemolytic streptococci, have been recognized for many years. Other, rare musculoskeletal infections can be caused by microorganisms including mycobacteria, fungi, and other atypical or unusual microorganisms. Prompt recognition and treatment of these infections crucially affects the prognosis and outcome. The epidemiology and risk factors associated with infection caused by a mycobacterial, fungal, or other unusual or atypical microorganism also must be considered.

Annotated References

1. Good RC, Snider DE Jr: Isolation of nontuberculous mycobacteria in the United States, 1980. *J Infect Dis* 1982;146:829-833.

2. Houshian S, Poulsen S, Riegels-Nielsen P: Bone and joint tuberculosis in Denmark: Increase due to immigration. *Acta Orthop Scand* 2000;71:312-315.

3. Jutte PC, van Loenhout-Rooyackers JH, Borgdorff MW, van Horn JR: Increase of bone and joint tuberculosis in the Netherlands. *J Bone Joint Surg Br* 2004;86:901-904.

   Of 12,447 patients in the Netherlands Tuberculosis Register from 1993 to 2000, 532 had bone and joint tuberculosis (of whom 56% had localization in the spine). Immigrants, particularly those from Somalia, were most likely to have bone and joint tuberculosis; the incidence also was related to female gender and increasing age.

4. Gardam M, Lim S: Mycobacterial osteomyelitis and arthritis. *Infect Dis Clin North Am* 2005;19:819-830.

   The incidence of mycobacterial bone and joint disease is expected to increase in North America because of increased travel, immigration, and the use of immunosuppressive medications. Treatment requires prolonged antibiotic therapy, often in conjunction with surgical intervention.

5. Hugosson C, Nyman RS, Brismar J, Larsson SG, Lindahl S, Lundstedt C: Imaging of tuberculosis: V. Peripheral osteoarticular and soft-tissue tuberculosis. *Acta Radiol* 1996;37:512-516.

6. Hadjipavlou AG, Tzermiadianos MN, Gaitanis I, Necessary J: Granulomatous infections of the spine, in Calhoun J, Mader JT (eds): *Musculoskeletal Infections.* New York, NY, Marcel Dekker, 2003, pp 421-471.

   The diagnosis and treatment of granulomatous spinal infections are reviewed.

7. Rieder HL, Snider DE Jr, Cauthen GM: Extrapulmonary tuberculosis in the United States. *Am Rev Respir Dis* 1990;141:347-351.

8. De Backer AI, Mortele KJ, Vanhoenacker FM, Parizel PM: Imaging of extraspinal musculoskeletal tuberculosis. *Eur J Radiol* 2006;57:119-130.

   Tuberculous spondylitis is the most common form of musculoskeletal tuberculosis; extraspinal musculoskeletal tuberculosis is among the least common manifestations. Radiologic assessment often is the key to adequate diagnosis and early treatment. The MRI characteristics of musculoskeletal tuberculosis are described.

9. Teo HE, Peh WC: Skeletal tuberculosis in children. *Pediatr Radiol* 2004;34:853-860.

   Skeletal tuberculosis in children most commonly is manifested as spondylitis, arthritis, or osteomyelitis. These conditions are described, with imaging techniques.

10. Wellons JC, Zomorodi AR, Villaviciencio AT, Woods CW, Lawson WT, Eastwood JD: Sacral tuberculosis: A case report and review of the literature. *Surg Neurol* 2004;61:136-139.

    Although sacral tuberculosis is an extremely rare cause of lower back pain, it should always be considered in the differential diagnosis of isolated sacral masses.

11. Marculescu CE, Berbari EF, Cockerill FR III, Osmon DR: Fungi, mycobacteria, zoonotic and other organisms in prosthetic joint infection. *Clin Orthop Relat Res* 2006;451:64-72.

    The current literature reporting prosthetic joint infection caused by zoonotic microorganisms, fungi, mycobacteria and other unusual microorganisms is reviewed. A high index of suspicion in diagnosis and the appropriate laboratory tests at surgical débridement are crucial for determining the microbiologic etiology of these infections.

12. Berney S, Goldstein M, Bishko F: Clinical and diagnostic features of tuberculous arthritis. *Am J Med* 1972;53:36-42.

13. Wallace R, Cohen AS: Tuberculous arthritis: A report of two cases with review of biopsy and synovial fluid findings. *Am J Med* 1976;61:277-282.

14. Titov AG, Vyshnevskaya EB, Mazurenko SI, Santavirta S, Konttinen YT: Use of polymerase chain reaction to diagnose tuberculous arthritis from joint tissues and synovial fluid. *Arch Pathol Lab Med* 2004;128:205-209.

    Compared with polymerase chain reaction, conventional bacteriologic methods for detection of *M tuberculosis* in samples obtained at arthroscopy are not sensitive and can be time consuming.

15. Blumberg HM, Burman WJ, Chaisson RE, Daley CL, Etkind SC, Friedman LN: American Thoracic Society/Centers for Disease Control and Prevention/Infectious Diseases Society of America: Treatment of tuberculosis. *Am J Respir Crit Care Med* 2003;167:603-662.

    The current guidelines emphasize concepts in tuberculosis treatment.

16. Leong JC: Tuberculosis of the spine. *J Bone Joint Surg Br* 1993;75:173-175.

17. Upadhyay SS, Saji MJ, Sell P, Sell B, Hsu LC: Spinal deformity after childhood surgery for tuberculosis of the spine: A comparison of radical surgery and debridement. *J Bone Joint Surg Br* 1994;76:91-98.

18. Upadhyay SS, Saji MJ, Sell P, Sell B, Yau AC: Longitudinal changes in spinal deformity after anterior spinal surgery for tuberculosis of the spine in adults: A comparative analysis between radical and debridement surgery. *Spine* 1994;19:542-549.

19. Upadhyay SS, Sell P, Saji MJ, Sell B, Hsu LC: Surgical management of spinal tuberculosis in adults: Hong Kong operation compared with debridement surgery for short and long term outcome of deformity. *Clin Orthop Relat Res* 1994;302:173-182.

20. Kohli R, Hadley S: Fungal arthritis and osteomyelitis. *Infect Dis Clin North Am* 2005;19:831-851.

    Fungal arthritis and osteomyelitis are uncommon, although their incidence is increasing with the prevalence of central venous catheters, broad spectrum antibiotics, immunocompromise, and abdominal surgery. The treatment is not well defined, but the use of azole antifungal agents is promising.

21. Kemper CA, Deresinski SC: Fungal disease of the bone and joint, in Kibler CC, Mackenzie DWR, Odds FC (eds): *Principles and Practice of Clinical Mycology.* Chichester, England, John Wiley, 1996, pp 49-68.

22. Gathe JC Jr, Harris RL, Garland B, Bradshaw MW, Williams TW Jr: Candida osteomyelitis: Report of five cases and review of the literature. *Am J Med* 1987;82:927-937.

23. Katzenstein D: Isolated Candida arthritis: Report of a case and definition of a distinct clinical syndrome. *Arthritis Rheum* 1985;28:1421-1424.

24. Silveira LH, Cuellar ML, Citera G, Cabrera GE, Scopelitis E, Espinoza LR: Candida arthritis. *Rheum Dis Clin North Am* 1993;19:427-437.

25. Darouiche RO, Hamill RJ, Musher DM, Young EJ, Harris RL: Periprosthetic candidal infections following arthroplasty. *Rev Infect Dis* 1989;11:89-96.

26. Bureau NJ, Ali SS, Chhem RK, Cardinal E: Ultrasound of musculoskeletal infections. *Semin Musculoskelet Radiol* 1998;2:299-306.

27. Evans RP, Nelson CL: Staged reimplantation of a total hip prosthesis after infection with Candida albicans: A report of two cases. *J Bone Joint Surg Am* 1990;72:1551-1553.

28. Lichtman EA: Candida infection of a prosthetic shoulder joint. *Skeletal Radiol* 1983;10:176-177.

29. Phelan DM, Osmon DR, Keating MR, Hanssen AD: Delayed reimplantation arthroplasty for candidal prosthetic joint infection: A report of 4 cases and review of the literature. *Clin Infect Dis* 2002;34:930-938.

30. Yang SH, Pao JL, Hang YS: Staged reimplantation of total knee arthroplasty after Candida infection. *J Arthroplasty* 2001;16:529-532.

31. Blair JE, Douglas DD: Coccidioidomycosis in liver transplant recipients relocating to an endemic area. *Dig Dis Sci* 2004;49:1981-1985.

    None of 41 liver transplant recipients who resided in and underwent transplantation in an area of low coccidioidal endemicity received antifungal prophylaxis. The incidence of new coccidioidal infection was 2.7% (one patient) at a minimum 1-year follow-up. Coccidioidomycosis was infrequent in liver transplant recipients from areas of low endemicity who relocated to a highly endemic area.

32. Lisbona R, Derbekyan V, Novales-Diaz J, Veksler A: Gallium-67 scintigraphy in tuberculous and nontuberculous infectious spondylitis. *J Nucl Med* 1993;34: 853-859.

33. Lambertus M, Thordarson D, Goetz MB: Fungal prosthetic arthritis: Presentation of two cases and review of the literature. *Rev Infect Dis* 1988;10:1038-1043.

34. Kawanabe K, Hayashi H, Miyamoto M, Tamura J, Shimizu M, Nakamura T: Candida septic arthritis of the hip in a young patient without predisposing factors. *J Bone Joint Surg Br* 2003;85:734-735.

    A 24-year-old woman had septic arthritis of the hip caused by *C albicans;* she underwent a two-stage total hip arthroplasty 3 years after infection onset. *Candida* was suggested by an elevated plasma level of β-D-glucan; the diagnosis could have been made earlier using this test. This is the first such report in a patient with no predisposing factors.

35. Maschmeyer G, Ruhnke M: Update on antifungal treatment of invasive Candida and Aspergillus infections. *Mycoses* 2004;47:263-276.

    New treatments for invasive *Candida* and *Aspergillus* infections are reviewed.

36. Arias F, Matta-Essayag S, Landaeta ME, et al: Candida albicans osteomyelitis: Case report and literature review. *Int J Infect Dis* 2004;8:307-314.

    This is the first instance of candidal foot osteomyelitis reported in Venezuela and only the second in the international literature.

37. Rex JH, Walsh TJ, Sobel JD, et al: Practice guidelines for the treatment of candidiasis: Infectious Diseases Society of America. *Clin Infect Dis* 2000;30:662-678.

38. Friedman BC, Simon GL: Candida vertebral osteomyelitis: Report of three cases and a review of the literature. *Diagn Microbiol Infect Dis* 1987;8:31-36.

39. Gunsilius E, Lass-Florl C, Mur E, Gabl C, Gastl G, Petzer AL: Aspergillus osteoarthritis in acute lymphoblastic leukemia. *Ann Hematol* 1999;78:529-530.

40. Sohail MR, Smilack JD: Aspergillus fumigatus septic arthritis complicating intra-articular corticosteroid injection [letter]. *Mayo Clin Proc* 2004;79:578-579.

    A letter to the editor describes a rare occurrence of *Aspergillus* septic arthritis after an intra-articular corticosteroid injection in an 88-year-old man who was immunocompetent.

41. Steinfeld S, Durez P, Hauzeur JP, Motte S, Appelboom T: Articular aspergillosis: Two case reports and review of the literature. *Br J Rheumatol* 1997;36:1331-1334.

42. Lodge BA, Ashley ED, Steele MP, Perfect JR: Aspergillus fumigatus empyema, arthritis, and calcaneal osteomyelitis in a lung transplant patient successfully treated with posaconazole. *J Clin Microbiol* 2004;42:1376-1378.

    A 64-year-old man with an *Aspergillus fumigatus* infection disseminated from the lung to the ankle and adjacent bone was successfully treated with posaconazole after failure of itraconazole and amphotericin B lipid complex. There was marked clinical improvement within 6 weeks, and all infection was resolved within 6 months.

43. Pappagianis D, Zimmer BL: Serology of coccidioidomycosis. *Clin Microbiol Rev* 1990;3:247-268.

44. Bayer AS, Guze LB: Fungal arthritis: II. Coccidioidal synovitis: Clinical, diagnostic, therapeutic, and prognostic considerations. *Semin Arthritis Rheum* 1979;8: 200-211.

45. Weinberg JM, Ali R, Badve S, Pelker RR: Musculoskeletal histoplasmosis: A case report and review of the literature. *J Bone Joint Surg Am* 2001;83:1718-1722.

46. Fowler VG Jr, Nacinovich FM, Alspaugh JA, Corey GR: Prosthetic joint infection due to Histoplasma capsulatum: Case report and review. *Clin Infect Dis* 1998;26:1017.

47. Saiz P, Gitelis S, Virkus W, Piasecki P, Bengana C, Templeton A: Blastomycosis of long bones. *Clin Orthop Relat Res* 2004;421:255-259.

    Blastomycosis, like tuberculosis, often is mistaken for a neoplasm. Blastomycosis osteomyelitis can be treated with excellent results. The key is diagnosis and the inclusion of endemic fungal infections in the differential diagnosis of bone tumors. Culturing of specimens obtained at biopsy should be done for every potential neoplasm.

48. Chleboun J, Nade S: Skeletal cryptococcosis. *J Bone Joint Surg Am* 1977;59:509-514.

49. Bayer AS, Choi C, Tillman DB, Guze LB: Fungal arthritis: V. Cryptococcal and histoplasmal arthritis. *Semin Arthritis Rheum* 1980;9:218-227.

50. Lie KW, Yu YL, Cheng IK, Woo E, Wong WT: Cryptococcal infection of the lumbar spine. *J R Soc Med* 1989; 82:172-173.

51. Agrawal A, Brown WS, McKenzie S: Cryptococcal arthritis in an immunocompetent host. *J S C Med Assoc* 2000;96:297-299.

52. Zacharias J, Crosby LA: Sporotrichal arthritis of the knee. *Am J Knee Surg* 1997;10:171-174.

53. DeHart DJ: Use of itraconazole for treatment of sporotrichosis involving a knee prosthesis. *Clin Infect Dis* 1995;21:450.

54. Kauffman CA: Sporotrichosis. *Clin Infect Dis* 1999;29: 231-236.

55. Smith JW, Piercy EA: Infectious arthritis. *Clin Infect Dis* 1995;20:225-230.

56. Kauffman CA, Hajjeh R, Chapman SW: Practice guidelines for the management of patients with sporotrichosis: For the Mycoses Study Group, Infectious Diseases Society of America. *Clin Infect Dis* 2000;30:684-687.

57. Petitjean G, Fluckiger U, Scharen S, Laifer G: Vertebral osteomyelitis caused by non-tuberculous mycobacteria. *Clin Microbiol Infect* 2004;10:951-953.

    Vertebral osteomyelitis caused by nontuberculous mycobacteria is rare. Its clinical features can be indistinguishable from those of pyogenic osteomyelitis, and early diagnosis is challenging because of the microorganisms' slow growth. No consensus guidelines for treatment exist; prolonged antimycobacterial therapy with surgical débridement is recommended.

58. Eid AJ, Berbari EF, Sia IG, Wengenack NL, Osmon DR, Razonable RR: Prosthetic joint infection due to rapidly growing mycobacteria: Report of 8 cases and review of the literature. *Clin Infect Dis* 2007;45:687-694.

    The symptoms and treatment of rare prosthetic joint infections caused by rapidly growing mycobacteria are described, and the current literature is reviewed.

59. Griffith DE, Aksamit T, Brown-Elliott BA: An official ATS/IDSA statement: Diagnosis, treatment, and prevention of nontuberculous mycobacterial diseases. *Am J Respir Crit Care Med* 2007;175:367-416.

    This is the official American Thoracic Society–Infectious Diseases Society of America statement on the diagnosis and treatment of nontuberculous mycobacteria.

60. Clark D, Lambert CM, Palmer K, Strachan R, Nuki G: Monoarthritis caused by Mycobacterium avium complex in a liver transplant recipient. *Br J Rheumatol* 1993;32:1099-1100.

61. Jones AR, Bartlett J, McCormack JG: Mycobacterium avium osteomyelitis and septic arthritis in an immunocompetent host. *J Infect* 1995;30:59-62.

62. Murdoch DM, McDonald JR: Mycobacterium avium-intracellulare cellulitis occurring with septic arthritis after joint injection: A case report. *BMC Infect Dis* 2007;7:9.

    A patient with rheumatoid arthritis developed bilateral shoulder arthritis and cellulitis at corticosteroid injection sites. Culturing and joint aspiration revealed *M avium-intracellulare*. This organism should be considered as the cause of skin and joint infections in all immunocompromised patients, particularly after intra-articular injection. Tissue specimens should always be cultured.

63. Stark RH: Mycobacterium avium complex tenosynovitis of the index finger. *Orthop Rev* 1990;19:345-348.

64. Rotstein AH, Stuckey SL: Mycobacterium avium complex spinal epidural abscess in an HIV patient. *Australas Radiol* 1999;43:554-557.

65. Aberg JA, Chin-Hong PV, McCutchan A, Koletar SL, Currier JS: Localized osteomyelitis due to Mycobacterium avium complex in patients with human immunodeficiency virus receiving highly active antiretroviral therapy. *Clin Infect Dis* 2002;35:E8-E13.

66. McLaughlin JR, Tierney M, Harris WH: Mycobacterium avium intracellulare infection of hip arthroplasties in an AIDS patient. *J Bone Joint Surg Br* 1994;76: 498-499.

67. Frosch M, Roth J, Ullrich K, Harms E: Successful treatment of mycobacterium avium osteomyelitis and arthritis in a non-immunocompromised child. *Scand J Infect Dis* 2000;32:328-329.

68. Pombo D, Woods ML II, Burgert SJ, Shumsky IB, Reimer LG: Disseminated mycobacterium avium complex infection presenting as osteomyelitis in a normal host. *Scand J Infect Dis* 1998;30:622-623.

69. Griffith DE: Therapy of nontuberculous mycobacterial disease. *Curr Opin Infect Dis* 2007;20:198-203.

    Although the introduction of macrolide-containing regimens has improved the treatment of *M avium-intracellulare* complex and other nontuberculous mycobacterial disease, the treatment remains challenging. Protection against the emergence of macrolide-resistant *M avium* complex isolates is critically important.

70. Clinical and Laboratory Standards Institute: *Susceptibility Testing of Mycobacteria, Nocardiae and Other Anaerobic Actinomycetes: Approved Standard M24-A.* Wayne, PA, National Committee for Clinical Laboratory Standards, 2003.

71. Franz A, Webster AD, Furr PM, Taylor-Robinson D: Mycoplasmal arthritis in patients with primary immunoglobulin deficiency: Clinical features and outcome in 18 patients. *Br J Rheumatol* 1997;36:661-668.

72. Ross JJ: Septic arthritis. *Infect Dis Clin North Am* 2005;19:799-817.

The US incidence of septic arthritis is increasing, especially among older patients with chronic illness, who are more susceptible to drug-resistant organisms. Successful treatment requires a high diagnostic suspicion, empiric antibiotic treatment, and joint drainage. Inoculation into blood culture bottles is more successful for a bacteriologic diagnosis than plating on solid media.

73. Waites KB, Rikihisa Y, Taylor-Robinson D: Mycoplasma and ureaplasma, in Murray PR, Baron EJ, Jorgensen JH, Pfaller MA, Yolken RH (eds): *Manual of Clinical Microbiology.* Washington, DC, ASM Press, 2003, pp 972-990.

74. Sneller M, Wellborne F, Barile MF, Plotz P: Prosthetic joint infection with Mycoplasma hominis. *J Infect Dis* 1986;153:174-175.

75. Madoff S, Hooper DC: Nongenitourinary infections caused by Mycoplasma hominis in adults. *Rev Infect Dis* 1988;10:602-613.

76. Fresard A, Guglielminotti C, Berthelot P, et al: Prosthetic joint infection caused by Tropheryma whippelii (Whipple's bacillus). *Clin Infect Dis* 1996;22:575-576.

77. Lange U, Teichmann J: Whipple arthritis: Diagnosis by molecular analysis of synovial fluid. Current status of diagnosis and therapy. *Rheumatology* 2003;42: 473-480.

In a patient with chronic illness consistent with Whipple disease and avascular necrosis of the right hip joint, *T whippelii* was identified without tissue biopsy, using molecular analysis (polymerase chain reaction) in bacterial DNA extracted from the synovial fluid.

78. Fleming JL, Wiesner RH, Shorter RG: Whipple's disease: Clinical, biochemical, and histopathologic features and assessment of treatment in 29 patients. *Mayo Clin Proc* 1988;63:539-551.

79. Perlick L, Sommer T, Zhou H, Diedrich O: Atypical prosthetic loosening in the hip joint. *Radiologe* 2000; 40:577-579.

80. Voutsinas S, Sayakos J, Smyrnis P: Echinococcus infestation complicating total hip replacement: A case report. *J Bone Joint Surg Am* 1987;69:1456-1458.

81. Force L, Torres JM, Carrillo A, Busca J: Evaluation of eight serological tests in the diagnosis of human echinococcosis and follow-up. *Clin Infect Dis* 1992;15: 473-480.

82. Mnaymneh W, Yacoubian V, Bikhazi K: Hydatidosis of the pelvic girdle: Treatment by partial pelvectomy. A case report. *J Bone Joint Surg Am* 1977;59:538-540.

83. Aktan AO, Yalin R: Preoperative albendazole treatment for liver hydatid disease decreases the viability of the cyst. *Eur J Gastroenterol Hepatol* 1996;8:877-879.

4: Specific Situations

Chapter 19
The Treatment of Surgical Site Infections

M.M. Manring, PhD   Jason H. Calhoun, MD, FACS   Camelia E. Marculescu, MD, MSCR

Introduction

Surgical site infection (SSI) occurs after approximately 2.6% of the 30 million surgical procedures performed in the United States each year and accounts for 38% of all nosocomial infections in surgical patients.[1] SSI was found to increase the average length of hospital stay by 1 week and add an average of $3,152 to the cost of a hospital stay.[1-4] Infections involving deep spaces or organs lead to even greater increases in cost and length of stay.[5] Orthopaedic surgeons must be aware of the consequences of SSI and the measures that can be taken to prevent it. Timely treatment is the key to arresting the disease, preserving function, and reducing mortality. The treatment of the most common infections after orthopaedic surgery is outlined in this chapter; prevention is discussed in chapter 4, and diagnosis is discussed in section 2.

Soft-Tissue Management

At the first signs of a surgical wound infection, empiric antibacterial therapy is initiated to prevent the spread of infection. An oral antibiotic (cephalexin or an anti-staphylococcal penicillin such as dicloxacillin) should be directed at the bacteria most commonly responsible for SSI, including staphylococci. The prevalence of community-acquired methicillin-resistant *Staphylococcus aureus* (MRSA) has increased, particularly among athletes, children who attend day care facilities, homeless persons, intravenous drug abusers, men who have sex with men, military recruits, prison inmates, and members of certain minority groups.[6] The β-lactam antibiotics, including methicillin, should not be used for empiric treatment of a patient who is at risk for community-acquired MRSA, has a history of MRSA colonization or infection, has a history of extensive broad-spectrum antibiotic use, or has a possible infection with a coagulase-negative staphylococcus. Instead, antimicrobial agents active against MRSA should be used; these include linezolid, trimethoprim-sulfamethoxazole, and a long-acting tetracycline. Vancomycin, linezolid, daptomycin, and tigecycline can be used in a patient with a complicated infection requiring hospitalization or intravenous therapy, although only limited studies on the treatment of skin and soft-tissue infections with daptomycin or tigecycline are available. Dalbavancin, telavancin, and ceftobiprole are under investigation and may become therapeutic options for infections caused by MRSA.[6,7]

Cultures from wound drainage can help direct therapy but are not as specific as cultures from surgical débridement. Empiric therapy may not eradicate organisms in devitalized tissue or abscesses. If the local or systemic signs of infection are not resolved within 48 to 72 hours, the empiric regimen should be modified by adding agents active against gram-negative organisms or MRSA. If empiric treatment fails and the wound infection becomes deeper, more established, and chronic, usually débridement, irrigation, and drainage are required as well as an extended regimen of antimicrobial therapy. The choice of antibiotics ideally should be based on the results of cultures obtained while the patient is not being treated with antimicrobial agents. The duration of antimicrobial therapy generally is 4 to 6 weeks.

Surgical treatment may carry an unacceptable risk of mortality in a patient who is severely injured or immunocompromised. Long-term management of the infection with oral antimicrobial agents may be acceptable if the patient has no adverse effects and the cause of the infection is a low-virulence microorganism that is highly susceptible to oral antimicrobial agents.[8]

Regardless of the choice of agent or duration of treatment, antibiotic therapy often fails in the absence of aggressive débridement. The skin, fascia, and muscle débridement must be sufficient to remove all devascularized tissue. The remaining tissue bed must be considered contaminated even after all necrotic tissue has been débrided, and thorough lavage using copious sterile saline is required. All abscesses should be drained. The resulting deep dead space can be managed using some combination of antibiotic-impregnated polymethylmethacrylate beads, a spacer, a vacuum-assisted closure system, drains, and, eventually, reconstruction (using muscle flaps, reimplantation of the prosthesis, Ilizarov external fixation, or bone grafts). Serial débridement and staged reconstruction sometimes are

4: Specific Situations

required. The patient typically should be monitored for recurrence of infection once a week during the first month after treatment, twice a week during the second and third months, once a month during the fourth through sixth months, and once every 2 to 3 months for the remainder of the first 2 years; annual follow-up may be sufficient after the first 13 months.

The physician should look for clinical signs of a relapse or recurrence of infection, such as redness, pain, swelling, drainage, and fever. Wound cultures and radiographs may be necessary to confirm or rule out a recurrence of infection. A high index of suspicion for recurrence must be maintained during the first year after treatment.

Procedure-Specific Considerations

Arthroscopy

Arthroscopically assisted repair of a small or medium-size rotator cuff tear (the so-called mini-open procedure) has become increasingly popular. The reported incidence of infection in open rotator cuff repair is 0.27% to 1.7%.[9,10] Limited data are available on rates of infection after mini-open repair. A study of 360 consecutive patients from two institutions found an infection rate of 1.9%; the most common cultured microorganism was *Propionibacterium acnes*, a low-virulence, gram-positive, anaerobic rod.[11] *P acnes* may require 5 to 10 days to grow in culture (often from broth). Although *P acnes* typically is susceptible to penicillin, the tetracyclines, clindamycin, and vancomycin, its resistance to these drugs is increasing because of the widespread use of antimicrobial agents to treat acne vulgaris. Metronidazole has no activity against *P acnes*. Treatment of a deep infection or an infection that persists more than 48 to 72 hours after a mini-open cuff repair requires irrigation and débridement followed by 4 weeks of culture-directed intravenous antimicrobial therapy. Because serial débridement may be necessary, the wound should be loosely closed with sutures. The wound can be definitively closed when all cultures from irrigation and débridement are negative.

The reported incidence of infection after arthroscopic anterior cruciate ligament (ACL) reconstruction is less than 1%. However, the infection can lead to serious consequences, including a loss of hyaline cartilage and arthrofibrosis.[12] Although there is no consensus as to the best course of treatment, recent reports indicate that the infection can be eradicated with combined arthroscopic and open surgical wound irrigation and débridement followed by appropriate antimicrobial therapy. Six patients who developed an infection after ACL arthroscopy were successfully treated with aggressive surgical débridement, hardware removal, and culture-directed antimicrobial therapy; none of the six ACL grafts was removed.[13] Eleven patients with postsurgical septic arthritis after a hamstring autograft were successfully treated with arthroscopic débridement of the joint and local surgical wound irrigation, followed by 4 weeks of intravenous antimicrobial therapy. The graft failed in one patient and was removed; hardware was retained in all patients.[14] Timely intervention is the key to maintaining the graft or hardware. Removal must be seriously considered if the graft or hardware appears to be contaminated.

Fracture Fixation

Infection in the region of a fracture most commonly occurs if the injury is open or the fracture has been treated with internal fixation. The infection is likely to delay or prevent fracture union. A glycocalyx (slime layer) develops on the metal hardware used in fracture fixation and protects bacteria from antibiotic penetration. Thus, it is rarely possible to suppress the infection without implant removal, particularly if the overlying skin breaks down and a sinus develops. However, removal of hardware from an unhealed fracture complicates management of the fracture and prevents union. The traditional approach to this dilemma has been to allow the fracture to heal in the presence of infection (**Figure 1**), provided that the hardware remains stable, while reducing the bacterial load with irrigation and multiple débridements as well as 6 weeks of culture-directed antimicrobial therapy.[15-17] A recent study suggests, however, that this approach may be less successful than is generally believed. For some patients (for example, a patient whose infection does not respond to the traditional approach or an immunocompromised patient with a nonarticular fracture), it may be preferable to remove the hardware and stabilize the fracture until the infection is cleared.[18] Long-term suppression with antibiotic therapy may be preferable if the patient is too ill to undergo surgery or hardware removal is not an option.

External fixation formerly was preferred to internal fixation because of the tendency of medullary rods to become secondarily infected. However, the pin sites necessary for external fixation also can become infected. Depending on wound cultures and sensitivity, pin site infections usually are effectively treated with 7 to 10 days of oral antibiotics, which also reduce the swelling around the pins. Pins that do not go through the zone of injury and have a stable bony construct rarely become infected.[19]

Total Joint Arthroplasty

The number of prosthetic joint infections is increasing in the United States because the population is aging and more adults are undergoing total joint arthroplasty. More than 500,000 primary arthroplasties are done annually in the United States, and more than 1.3 million people are living with a joint prosthesis.[20] It is anticipated that by 2030 more than 4 million primary total hip arthroplasty (THA) and total knee arthroplasty (TKA) procedures will be done each year in the United States.[21] The risk of infection is higher after TKA (1% to 2%) than after THA (0.3% to 1.3%) or shoulder ar-

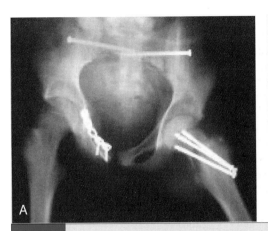
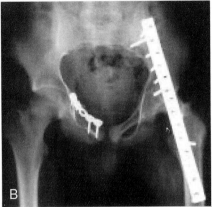
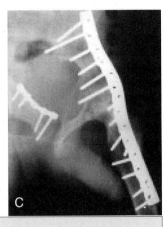

Figure 1 Hardware usually is maintained in an infected fracture. **A,** AP radiograph of a combined pelvic and femoral neck fracture in 16-year-old male patient who developed an intra-articular infection of the left hip 6 months after injury. AP **(B)** and lateral **(C)** radiographs taken 8 months after arthrodesis. The patient was able to bear weight as tolerated. (Reproduced from Beaulé PE, Matta JM, Mast JW: Hip arthrodesis: Current indications and techniques. *J Am Acad Orthop Surg* 2002;10:249-258.)

throplasty (less than 1%).[22-24] SSI can be devastating, leading to pain, surgical revision, and reduced function. Gram-positive cocci cause most prosthetic joint infections. *S aureus* and coagulase-negative staphylococci are the most commonly isolated microorganisms;[25] aerobic gram-negative and anaerobic bacteria are less frequently encountered. Polymicrobial infection is reported in 12% to 19% of patients.[26]

Culture-directed antimicrobial therapy always is required for at least 4 to 6 weeks, regardless of the type of surgical procedure. If the patient is not a candidate for revision surgery, the best option may be long-term suppressive therapy.

The Hip

In a patient with an infection after a THA, treatment with antibiotics alone is used only if the risks of surgery outweigh the benefits. In other patients, revision surgery usually is required, and a two-stage revision procedure is standard. Thorough débridement is required after hardware removal to improve the likelihood of a good outcome. An antibiotic cement spacer is used to deliver a high local concentration of aminoglycoside or vancomycin and maintain the soft-tissue tension. The surgeon must avoid weakening the bone cement by adding no more than 1 to 2 g of antibiotic powder per 40 g of cement for implant fixation.[27,28] The hip is reimplanted if there is no clinical suspicion of infection after 6 weeks of intravenous antimicrobial therapy.

The single-stage revision procedure has had good outcomes in specific circumstances. The patient must be in good general health and have no wound complications after the primary THA, the pathogen must be a methicillin-susceptible staphylococcus or streptococcus, and the microorganism must be susceptible to an antibiotic that can be used in bone cement. Polymicrobial, methicillin-resistant, and gram-negative infections

should be treated with two-stage revision surgery.[25] If revision surgery is not possible because the patient is older than 65 years or very sick, débridement with retention of the infected prosthesis is possible if the prosthesis is stable, the infection is not gram negative, and débridement is performed within 30 days of the onset of clinical symptoms of infection.

In a retrospective study of 91 patients (99 infections) treated with débridement and prosthesis retention, predébridement symptom duration of 8 or more days was associated with an increased risk of treatment failure (hazard ratio, 1.77; 1.02-3.07, 95% CI).[29] The survival rate free of treatment failure was 60% (50%-71%, 95% CI) at 2-year follow-up, the rate after débridement done 8 or more days after the onset of symptoms was 49% (28%-64%, 95% CI).

The Knee

Two-stage revision is the standard treatment for SSI after TKA. The implant is removed, with débridement of all necrotic tissue, and an antibiotic-loaded cement spacer is placed (**Figure 2**). The knee is immobilized for at least 6 weeks using a Jones dressing. The patient avoids weight bearing by using a wheelchair, crutches, or a walker. Culture-specific intravenous antimicrobial therapy is administered during this period, at the end of which inflammatory markers (the erythrocyte sedimentation rate and C-reactive protein level) and wound healing are reevaluated to determine whether the infection has been eradicated; if not, additional surgical débridement and antimicrobial therapy may be required. If there is clinical evidence of an ongoing infection, débridement may be repeated, with an exchange of the antibiotic spacer.[30] The decision to repeat antimicrobial therapy and proceed with revision should be based on the severity of the infection and the patient's overall health. Resection arthroplasty, knee arthrodesis, or amputation may provide a better outcome in a patient

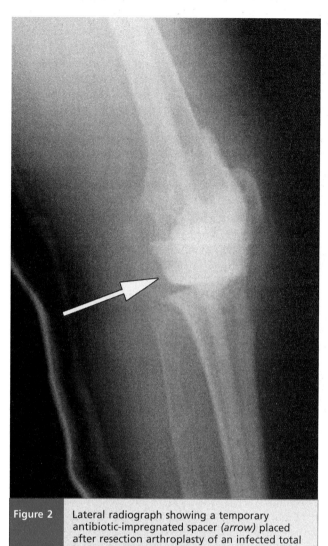

Figure 2 Lateral radiograph showing a temporary antibiotic-impregnated spacer *(arrow)* placed after resection arthroplasty of an infected total knee prosthesis in a 72-year-old man.

with a catastrophic infection. The second procedure may be complicated by osseous deficits in the distal femur and proximal tibia, and a custom-designed prosthesis may be required.[31]

A single-stage revision may be an option if the infection is caused by a low-virulence microorganism, such as a coagulase-negative staphylococcus. Long-term follow-up data on single-stage revisions are limited, although 107 patients were found to have a similar outcome after a two-stage or direct exchange procedure.[32] Arthroscopic débridement and retention of the prosthesis, followed by suppressive antibiotic therapy, may be attempted if the patient has symptoms of less than 7 days' duration and no radiologic signs of prosthesis loosening. This approach may be especially useful in patients who are medically unstable or receiving anticoagulation therapy.[33] If the prosthesis is cemented, an arthroscopic débridement and retention procedure is less likely to be successful because the cement-prosthesis interface probably is protected from both débridement and antibiotic penetration.[34]

The Shoulder

Deep infection is rare after shoulder arthroplasty; the reported incidence is 0.4% to 2.9%, which is similar to the incidence after THA or TKA.[35,36] The treatment options depend on how long after surgery the infection is detected. An acute infection diagnosed within 4 weeks of implant surgery and with no soft-tissue involvement may be successfully treated with arthroscopic synovectomy with lavage and débridement, followed by 4 to 6 weeks of intravenous antimicrobial therapy. Soft tissue usually is involved, however, and open débridement and lavage are required. The implant can be retained after cleansing with jet lavage. Variability in the head-to-taper volume of different implants can complicate the process of cleaning the implant. If the implant is modular, the head-neck taper should be disassembled for cleansing.[37] A two-stage revision usually is required in a patient with a chronic infection or an acute infection diagnosed 4 or more weeks after primary implantation. The implant and all cement are removed, the soft-tissue is débrided, and the wound is rinsed with jet lavage. A temporary spacer made of antibiotic-loaded cement is placed to provide stability and protection of the soft tissues as well as high local concentrations of culture-specific antibiotics. Intravenous antimicrobial therapy is administered for 6 to 8 weeks. At the completion of antimicrobial therapy, inflammatory markers (erythrocyte sedimentation rate and C-reactive protein level) and joint aspirate should be obtained to evaluate the effectiveness of the antimicrobial therapy. A new prosthesis may be implanted if the inflammatory markers are normal and the joint aspirate does not reveal the growth of a microorganism. If the infection has persisted, a second revision procedure using an antibiotic spacer, followed by an additional course of intravenous antimicrobial therapy, may be required before reimplantation.

Spinal Surgery

SSI is among the most common complications of spinal surgery (**Figure 3**). The severity of the infection depends on the complexity of the procedure. The reported risk of infection after lumbar diskectomy with prophylaxis is only 0.7%, but the use of an operating microscope was shown to double the infection rate.[38] The risk of infection after a spinal fusion varies with the instrumentation used. If no instrumentation is used, the risk of infection is 2%; with Harrington rods, the risk increases to 7%.[39] A patient with a traumatic spine injury typically has greater instability and soft-tissue disturbance and spends more time in an intensive care unit than other patients undergoing spinal surgery; the reported rate of SSI is as high as 10%.[40] For some patients with a postdiskectomy infection, antibiotic therapy of 6 weeks' duration is sufficient to resolve the infection;[41] if signs of infection persist, the optimal treatment is débridement of the disk space from an anterior approach. Infection after spinal stenosis decompression rarely responds to antibiotics alone and usu-

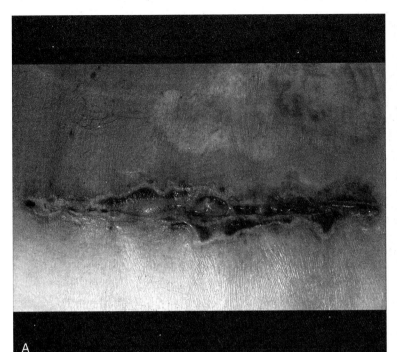
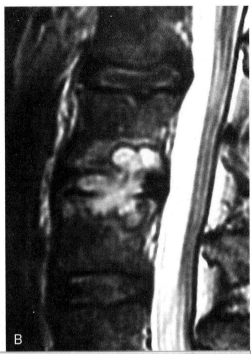

Figure 3 **A,** Intraoperative photograph taken before formal irrigation and débridement of an early, deep postoperative spinal wound infection with aggressive mixed-flora bacteria and extensive myonecrosis in an immunocompromised host. **B,** Sagittal T1-weighted MRI study showing high signal intensity in the disk space. This finding is consistent with diskitis. (Reproduced from Sasso RC, Garrido BJ: Postoperative spinal wound infections. *J Am Acad Orthop Surg* 2008;16:330-337.)

ally requires surgical débridement of necrotic tissue followed by 6 weeks of antimicrobial therapy. An infection after a percutaneous intradiskal procedure, if diagnosed within 4 weeks, often can be successfully treated with antimicrobial therapy and immobilization. Surgical débridement usually is required for patients who do not respond to antibiotic therapy or develop neural deficits.[42] For complex wounds, the use of temporary antibiotic beads and vacuum-assisted closure dressings can significantly aid healing.[43]

The use of antibiotics alone probably will fail to arrest the infection in a patient who has instrumentation, but it can postpone the removal of hardware.[39] After cultures are obtained, broad-spectrum antibiotics should be administered, including vancomycin if MRSA is suspected. Surgical débridement of all layers should be done, with removal of any loose bone graft and revision of any loose fixation. The instrumentation should be removed only as a last resort in a catastrophic infection. If the initial infection is associated with myonecrosis, débridement should be repeated after 48 and 72 hours. The antimicrobial therapy should be adjusted based on the results of culturing and susceptibility testing. Intravenous antimicrobial therapy should be continued for 6 weeks after débridement. Patients should be assessed for pseudoarthrosis after removal of the hardware.

Summary

The treatment of SSI varies slightly depending on the surgical site and procedure, but the same principles apply to all infections. Swift recognition of the clinical signs is essential. Empiric antimicrobial therapy should be initiated at the first signs of an infection and may be sufficient to arrest its spread. Prolonged intravenous antimicrobial therapy should be directed by cultures taken at the time of surgical débridement. In the absence of aggressive débridement, antimicrobial therapy alone usually fails if the infection is well established. The rate of infection is impressively low after many orthopaedic procedures, but the surgeon always must be ready to suspect infection and be prepared to take aggressive action.

Annotated References

1. National Nosocomial Infections Surveillance System: National Nosocomial Infections Surveillance (NNIS) system report: Data summary from January 1992 through June 2004, issued October 2004. *Am J Infect Control* 2004;32:470-485.

   The data collected and reported by hospitals participating in the surveillance of nosocomial infections in the United States are reported and summarized.

2. Martone WJ, Jarvis WR, Culver DH, Haley RW: Incidence and nature of endemic and epidemic nosocomial infections, in Bennett JV, Brachman PS (eds): *Hospital Infections*, ed 3. Boston, MA, Little Brown, 1992, pp 577-596.

3. Boyce JM, Potter-Bynoe G, Dziobek L: Hospital reimbursement patterns among patients with surgical wound infections following open heart surgery. *Infect Control Hosp Epidemiol* 1990;11:89-93.

4. Poulsen KB, Bremmelgaard A, Sorensen AI, Raahave D, Petersen JV: Estimated costs of postoperative wound infections: A case-control study of marginal hospital and social security costs. *Epidemiol Infect* 1994;113: 283-295.

5. Vegas AA, Jodra VM, Garcia ML: Nosocomial infection in surgery wards: A controlled study of increased duration of hospital stays and direct cost of hospitalization. *Eur J Epidemiol* 1993;9:504-510.

6. Marcotte AL, Trzeciak MA: Community-acquired methicillin-resistant Staphylococcus aureus: An emerging pathogen in orthopaedics. *J Am Acad Orthop Surg* 2008;16:98-106.

   Community-acquired MRSA has become increasingly prevalent. The risk factors include antibiotic use within the preceding year, crowded living conditions, compromised skin integrity, contaminated surfaces, frequent skin-to-skin contact, sharing of personal items, and suboptimal cleanliness.

7. Stryjewski ME, Chambers HF: Skin and soft-tissue infections caused by community-acquired methicillin-resistant *Staphylococcus aureus*. *Clin Infect Dis* 2008; 46(suppl 5):S368-S377.

   Skin and soft-tissue infections are the most frequent forms of community-acquired-MRSA. Antibiotic therapy and surgical treatment options are reviewed.

8. Calhoun JH, Manring MM: Adult osteomyelitis. *Infect Dis Clin North Am* 2005;19:765-786.

   The etiology, radiologic signs, diagnosis, antibiotic treatment, and surgical treatment of adult osteomyelitis are reviewed.

9. Post M: Complications of rotator cuff surgery. *Clin Orthop Relat Res* 1990;254:97-104.

10. Settecerri JJ, Pitner MA, Rock MG, Hanssen AD, Cofield RH: Infection after rotator cuff repair. *J Shoulder Elbow Surg* 1999;8:1-5.

11. Herrera MF, Bauer G, Reynolds F, et al: Infection after mini-open rotator cuff repair. *J Shoulder Elbow Surg* 2002;11:605-608.

12. Schollin-Borg M, Michaëlsson K, Rahme H: Presentation, outcome, and cause of septic arthritis after anterior cruciate ligament reconstruction: A case control study. *Arthroscopy* 2003;19:941-947.

    A study of 575 patients who underwent ACL reconstruction found that laboratory studies and aspiration should be performed liberally to avoid a delayed diagnosis of postsurgical septic arthritis.

13. Binnet MS, Başarir K: Risk and outcome of infection after different arthroscopic anterior cruciate ligament reconstruction techniques. *Arthroscopy* 2007;23:862-868.

    Six of 1,231 patients who underwent ACL reconstruction developed an SSI. Aggressive surgical débridement, hardware removal, and appropriate antibiotic therapy were effective in eliminating the infection and allowing retention of the graft.

14. Judd D, Bottoni C, Kim D, Burke M, Hooker S: Infections following arthroscopic anterior cruciate ligament reconstruction. *Arthroscopy* 2006;22:375-384.

    In a retrospective review of 11 infections after 1,615 ACL reconstructions, the key to a good outcome was timely initiation of treatment, including joint lavage, débridement, and antibiotics. Grafts were retained in 10 of the 11 patients. Level of evidence: IV.

15. Court-Brown CM, Keating JF, McQueen MM: Infection after intramedullary nailing of the tibia: Incidence and protocol for management. *J Bone Joint Surg Br* 1992;74:770-774.

16. Fears RL, Gleis GE, Seligson D: Diagnosis and treatment of complications, in Browner BD, Jupiter JB, Levine AM, Trafton PG (eds): *Skeletal Trauma*, ed 2. Philadelphia, PA, WB Saunders, 1998.

17. Meyer S, Weiland AJ, Willenegger H: The treatment of infected non-union of fractures of long bones: Study of sixty-four cases with a five to twenty-one-year follow-up. *J Bone Joint Surg Am* 1975;57:836-842.

18. Rightmire E, Zurakowski D, Vrahas M: Acute infections after fracture repair: Management with hardware in place. *Clin Orthop Relat Res* 2008;466:466-472.

    A study of 69 patients with fracture who developed an infection after open reduction and internal fixation found that 47 (68%) had successful union with hardware in place. Treating infected fractures with hardware in place was found to be less successful than generally believed. Level of evidence: IV.

19. Thompson DM, Calhoun JH: Treatment of foot and ankle deformities with the Ilizarov fixator, in Laughlin RT, Calhoun JH (eds): *Fractures of the Foot and Ankle*. Boca Raton, FL, Taylor & Francis, 2005, pp 439-458.

    Advanced techniques for external fixation and selected internal fixation options for simple and complex foot deformities are reviewed, with the application of Ilizarov fixators and possible complications, including infection.

20. Trampuz A, Osmon DR, Hanssen AD, Steckelberg JM, Patel R: Molecular and antibiofilm approaches to prosthetic joint infection. *Clin Orthop Relat Res* 2003; 414:69-88.

    The pathogenesis of prosthetic joint infection is related to biofilms, which protect bacteria from antimicrobial

4: Specific Situations

agents and host response. Molecular and antibiofilm approaches to prosthetic joint infection are reviewed.

21. Kurtz S, Ong K, Lau E, Mowat F, Halpern M: Projections of primary and revision hip and knee arthroplasty in the United States from 2005 to 2030. *J Bone Joint Surg Am* 2007;89:780-785.

   The Nationwide Inpatient Sample (1990 to 2003) and census data were used to project that by 2030 the demand for primary THA will grow by 174% to 572,000, and the demand for primary TKA will grow by 673% to 3.48 million procedures.

22. Hanssen AD, Rand JA: Evaluation and treatment of infection at the site of a total hip or knee arthroplasty. *Instr Course Lect* 1999;48:111-122.

23. Lidgren L, Knutson K, Stefánsdóttir A: Infection and arthritis: Infection of prosthetic joints. *Best Pract Res Clin Rheumatol* 2003;17:209-218.

   Diagnostics, bacteriologic findings, and treatment options for infection of prosthetic joints are reviewed. Two-stage revision was found to heal the infection in as many as 90% of patients.

24. Sperling JW, Kozak TK, Hanssen AD, Cofield RH: Infection after shoulder arthroplasty. *Clin Orthop Relat Res* 2001;382:206-216.

25. Lentino JR: Prosthetic joint infections: Bane of orthopedists, challenge for infectious disease specialists. *Clin Infect Dis* 2003;36:1157-1161.

   In a review of the costs, risk factors, and treatment of prosthetic joint infections, two-stage revision was found to be superior to either single-stage revision or débridement with prosthesis retention.

26. Sia IG, Berbari EF, Karchmer AW: Prosthetic joint infections. *Infect Dis Clin North Am* 2005;19:885-914.

   The surgical and antimicrobial treatment of prosthetic joint infection should be individualized to the specific infection and patient. The decision-making process is discussed.

27. Ure KJ, Amstutz HC, Nasser S, Schmalzried TP: Direct-exchange arthroplasty for the treatment of infection after total hip replacement: An average ten-year follow-up. *J Bone Joint Surg Am* 1998;80:961-968.

28. Jackson WO, Schmalzried TP: Limited role of direct exchange arthroplasty in the treatment of infected total hip replacements. *Clin Orthop Relat Res* 2000;381:101-105.

29. Marculescu CE, Berbari EF, Hanssen AD, et al: Outcome of prosthetic joint infections treated with debridement and retention of components. *Clin Infect Dis* 2006;42:471-478.

   Retrospective analysis of 99 prosthetic joint infections in 91 patients found that débridement and retention of the prosthesis was a common treatment. The factors associated with treatment failure included the presence of a sinus tract and symptom duration of at least 8 days before débridement.

30. Burnett RS, Kelly MA, Hanssen AD, Barrack RL: Technique and timing of two-stage exchange for infection in TKA. *Clin Orthop Relat Res* 2007;464:164-178.

   A review of 100 studies found the two-stage exchange procedure with antibiotic cement fixation to be effective for treating infection in TKAs, when it is preceded by component removal, irrigation, and débridement as well as 4 to 6 weeks of intravenous antibiotic therapy. Level of evidence: V.

31. Windsor RE, Insall JN, Urs WK, Miller DV, Brause BD: Two-stage reimplantation for the salvage of total knee arthroplasty complicated by infection: Further follow-up and refinement of indications. *J Bone Joint Surg Am* 1990;72:272-278.

32. Bengtson S, Knutson K: The infected knee arthroplasty: A 6-year follow-up of 357 cases. *Acta Orthop Scand* 1991;62:301-311.

33. Waldman BJ, Hostin E, Mont MA, Hungerford DS: Infected total knee arthroplasty treated by arthroscopic irrigation and débridement. *J Arthroplasty* 2000;15:430-436.

34. Dixon P, Parish EN, Cross MJ: Arthroscopic debridement in the treatment of the infected total knee replacement. *J Bone Joint Surg Br* 2004;86:39-42.

   A study of 15 patients found that arthroscopic débridement allowed retention of a stable prosthesis and eradication of the infection if the surgical technique was meticulous and specific antibiotics were taken for a mean of 8 months.

35. Cofield RH, Edgerton BC: Total shoulder arthroplasty: Complications and revision surgery. *Instr Course Lect* 1990;39:449-462.

36. Swanson AB, de Groot Swanson G, Sattel AB, et al: Bipolar implant shoulder arthroplasty: Long-term results. *Clin Orthop Relat Res* 1989;249:227-247.

37. Jerosch J, Schneppenheim M: Management of infected shoulder replacement. *Arch Orthop Trauma Surg* 2003;123:209-214.

   In 12 patients with an infected shoulder replacement, a temporary antibiotic-loaded spacer aided in establishing anatomic stability. Reconstruction of humeral length was possible, even for long implants.

38. Bassewitz HL, Fischgrund JS, Herkowitz HN: Postoperative spine infections. *Semin Spine Surg* 2000;12:203-211.

39. Sasso RC, Garrido BJ: Postoperative spinal wound infections. *J Am Acad Orthop Surg* 2008;16:330-337.

   Surgeons should be aware of the preventive measures and risk factors for SSI after spinal surgery. Postsurgical infections range in severity from a superficial skin incision infection to a deep subfascial infection with myonecrosis. Management is based on etiology, clinical course, and patient risk factors.

40. Rechtine GR, Bono PL, Cahill D, Bolesta MJ, Chrin AM: Postoperative wound infection after instrumentation of thoracic and lumbar fractures. *J Orthop Trauma* 2001;15:566-569.

41. Lindholm TS, Pylkkänen P: Discitis following removal of intervertebral disc. *Spine* 1982;7:618-622.

42. Silber JS, Anderson DG, Vaccaro AR, et al: Management of postprocedural discitis. *Spine J* 2002;2: 279-287.

43. Yuan-Innes MJ, Temple CL, Lacey MS: Vacuum-assisted wound closure: A new approach to spinal wounds with exposed hardware. *Spine* 2001;26: E30-E33.

Chapter 20

Diabetic Foot Infections

Jason H. Calhoun, MD, FACS   *Benjamin A. Lipsky, MD, FIDSA, FACP   M.M. Manring, PhD

4: Specific Situations

Introduction

Diabetes mellitus is a systemic disease that can affect the nervous, vascular, skeletal, immune, and integumentary systems. The treatment of diabetes and its complications requires a multisystem, multidisciplinary approach in which the orthopaedic foot and ankle surgeon plays a critical role. Foot disorders are among the most common and devastating complications of diabetes.[1] The spectrum of diabetic foot disorders includes pain insensitivity, motor deformity, ulcerations, poor wound healing, immunologic perturbations, vascular insufficiency, neuropathic arthropathy, and osteomyelitis.

Several types of infection occur more frequently in patients with diabetes than in the general population. Foot infections are probably the most common. Diabetic foot infections range in severity from relatively mild to limb or life threatening. Most require immediate medical attention, including diagnostic evaluation, treatment, and sometimes hospitalization. Diabetic foot infections are associated with acute morbidity, often requiring surgical resection or amputation.

Almost all diabetic foot infections begin in a wound, which often is a neuropathic ulceration or a traumatic break in the skin envelope. The infection initially may be minor, but if not identified early and properly treated it can rapidly progress to involve deeper soft tissues and ultimately bone and joints.

Infection of the foot in patients with diabetes is predicted to become a progressively greater source of concern in the future. According to the World Health Organization, the worldwide population of people with diabetes will increase 39% by 2030; a single study of health records in Ontario, Canada, revealed a 69% increase between 1995 and 2005.[2] In the general population, greater longevity and a higher incidence of obesity are increasing both the duration and amount of stress on the feet.

*Benjamin A. Lipsky, MD, FIDSA, FACP or the department with which he is affiliated has received research or institutional support from Merck and Pfizer and has received miscellaneous nonincome support, comercially derived honoraria, or other nonresearch-related funding from Merck, Pfizer, Cubist, and Schering Plough/Bayer.

Epidemiology

A diabetic foot infection is commonly defined as any inframalleolar infection in a person with diabetes mellitus. Such infections have a high incidence. In 14 European hospitals, a clinically infected wound was found in 58% of 1,229 patients with a diabetic foot ulcer.[3] A prospective study found that 9% of patients in a diabetes disease management program developed a foot infection during an average 27-month period.[4] Foot ulcers are the most common factor predisposing a patient with diabetes to infection, and a patient's lifetime risk of developing a foot ulcer is as high as 25%[5] (Figure 1). The morbidity associated with chronic or recurring ulceration is one of the greatest obstacles to the patient's quality of life, frequently requiring lengthy hospital stays, repeated surgery, or amputation.[6,7] Two prospective studies found that more than half of diabetic foot ulcers were clinically infected when the patient sought medical care.[3,5]

Foot infection has become the most common diabetes-related cause of hospital admission and the leading cause of lower extremity amputation.[8,9] Retrospective studies found that 25% to 50% of diabetic foot infections result in a minor, foot-sparing amputation, and 10% to 40% require a major amputation.[10] Approximately 10% to 30% of diabetic foot ulcers progress to require an amputation, and nearly two thirds of amputations involving the foot are preceded by an infected foot ulcer.[10] The consequences of lower extremity amputation are dire. The patient's quality of life is dramatically worsened, and in the United States the mortality rate after amputation ranges from 13% to 40% at 1 year to 35% to 65% at 3 years and 39% to 80% at 5 years. This prognosis is worse than that of most malignancies.[11]

Pathophysiology

The foot is an ideal location for a serious infection to develop, as the structure of the compartments, tendons, nerves, and blood vessels of the foot all favor the spread of infection.[12,13] Infection usually is preceded by the complex process of ulceration, which involves peripheral neuropathy, peripheral vascular disease, and failure of wound healing.[14] The factors that predispose patients with diabetes to foot infection primarily

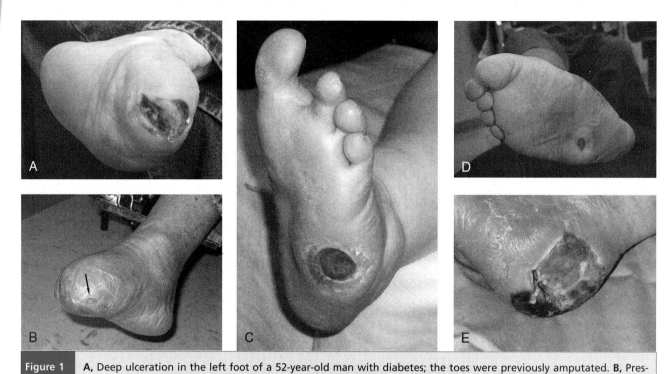

Figure 1 **A,** Deep ulceration in the left foot of a 52-year-old man with diabetes; the toes were previously amputated. **B,** Pressure ulcer *(arrow)* caused by ill-fitting footwear on the right foot of a 69-year-old man. A diabetic foot ulcer on the plantar aspect led to infection necessitating an earlier amputation. **C,** A deep foot ulcer on the lateral plantar aspect of the left foot in a 52-year-old woman with diabetes; the toe was amputated because of infection 1 year earlier. **D,** Charcot foot and a plantar ulcer in the left foot of a 60-year-old man with diabetes. **E,** A heel ulcer in a 69-year-old man with diabetes and peripheral neuropathy, which developed when the patient was confined to bed and the foot became necrotic and infected. Note the extension of the ulceration into deep subcutaneous tissue, the purulent discharge, the small area of necrotic tissue, and the surrounding cellulitis.

involve immune system abnormalities, particularly abnormalities of neutrophil function.[15] However, diabetic foot infection can result from one or more disorders of the nervous, vascular, and immune systems. For example, as many as one third of all diabetic foot ulcers have a mixed neuropathic-ischemic etiology.[16]

Nervous System

Diabetic neuropathy most commonly occurs in patients with poor metabolic control, especially glycemic control. Hyperglycemia probably contributes to abnormalities of the peripheral nerves; it is associated with elevated nerve sorbitol concentrations, myoinositol depletion, increased sodium and potassium stores, and decreased adenosine triphosphatase activity. These metabolic events result in slowed nerve conduction and the development of neural lesions. The loss of myelinated and nonmyelinated nerve fibers is caused by inadequate regulation of microcirculation, oxygen delivery, and extraneural arteriovenous shunting.[17] Sensory neuropathy first appears distally and then progresses proximally in the stocking-glove pattern. Diminution of light touch sensation and proprioception, as a consequence of large-fiber involvement, leads to development of an ataxic gait and muscle weakness in the feet. Small-fiber involvement leads to diminished pain and temperature perception, which leaves the patient vulnerable to burns and repetitive stress injury.

The initial tissue breakdown results from the patient's inability to respond to mechanical stress. Three levels of mechanical stress can lead to tissue ulceration: high stress concentrated in a small area and causing immediate injury such as puncture or tearing; high-tension (shear) stress generated by stepping on a small object that may be inside the shoe; and moderate stress resulting from everyday activities. Moderate stresses are the most common cause of injury in an insensate foot.[18] The consequences of long-term repetition of moderate stress in the insensate foot are underappreciated. The tensile strength of intact plantar skin is approximately 1,200 psi. Average pressure does not exceed 75 psi during normal walking if the person is barefoot or 50 psi if the person is wearing a leather-soled shoe. In a normally sensate foot, pressure of at least 200 psi is necessary to produce pain. However, the combination of pressure as low as 20 psi and 10,000 repetitions per day can cause inflammation by the third day and ulceration by the eighth day.[18] A person with a normally sensate foot feels pain early in the inflammatory stage and seeks relief. In contrast, a person with an insensate foot does not detect pain early enough in the process to avoid tissue damage.[18] Pressure as low as 1 to 2 psi, which is consistent with an overly tight shoe, is sufficient to block capillary flow and cause ischemia. A person with an insensate foot does not notice the cumulative effects of pressure and, because of the absence of sensation, often ignores the effects until tissue damage has occurred.

Several other conditions are associated with diabetic neuropathy, including neuropathic paresthesia, stiff callus, and motor neuropathy. Neuropathic paresthesia can appear as hypersensitivity, superficial burning, or severe deep aching. These sensations may be caused by spontaneous depolarization of nerve fibers as they attempt to heal.

Damage to the autonomic nervous system diminishes its ability to regulate perspiration, skin temperature, and arteriovenous shunting. In response, the plantar skin may form a thick callus in high pressure areas. An absence of normal perspiration causes the callus to become dry, and cracks developing through the dermis serve as a gateway for bacterial infection. As the hard callus thickens, it can cause deep-tissue breakdown, hemorrhage, and necrosis.

Motor neuropathy most commonly is distal. It results in intrinsic muscle dysfunction manifested by the development of claw or hammer toes, depression of the metatarsal heads, and resulting high pressure on the plantar aspect of the forefoot. Less commonly, neuropathy affects a single nerve, such as the common peroneal nerve, and results in drop foot.

Vascular System

Atherosclerotic vascular disease, especially peripheral arterial disease, is common in patients with diabetes and is an independent risk factor for diabetic foot infection.[5] The most common sites of occlusion are the superficial femoral artery at the adductor canal, the aortic bifurcation, the common iliac bifurcation, and the common femoral artery bifurcation. Peripheral vascular disease involves both small and large vessels. Macrovascular disease is the most important cause of ischemia, but microvascular disorders also may contribute. Even in patients with diabetes who do not have critical limb ischemia, impaired foot perfusion secondary to arterial disease is amplified significantly by coexisting microcirculatory disease.[19]

The presence of stiff arteries can cause blood pressure readings to be artificially high. Plain radiographs often provide visual evidence of calcified arteries. The tibial and deep femoral arteries may be occluded in patients with diabetes, and the anterior tibial, posterior tibial, and peroneal arteries are often diffusely involved. In a person who does not have diabetes, collateral circulation often overcomes a single level of occlusion. In a person with diabetes, the involvement of both small and large vessels complicates the treatment of vascular disease. Altered lipoprotein metabolism, hypertension, smoking, and genetic abnormalities have been cited as factors in the accelerated atherogenesis found in patients with diabetes.[20]

Immune System

A person with diabetes may have an abnormal response to a wound infection. Because of the disease's systemic effects on the nervous and vascular systems, the skin of the feet lacks durability. Diabetes inhibits skin elasticity by causing abnormal collagen and keratin formation, and the resulting rigid tissue is vulnerable to fissures, cavities, and ulcers.[21] After pathogens find an opening, they may grow more rapidly because of the altered function of white blood cells. In a person with diabetes, polymorphonuclear leukocytes have altered chemotaxis, migration, phagocytosis, and intracellular bacterial killing activity, and some evidence suggests that cellular immune responses and monocyte function are reduced.[22] This favorable environment for bacteria growth is enhanced by the combination of hyperglycemia and decreased oxygen tension.[23] Insulin deficiency leads to ineffective anaerobic metabolism as well as hypertonicity and edema, creating an even more favorable environment for bacteria growth and a less favorable environment for leukocytes and antibiotics.[24] Wound healing is further compromised by the decreased production and diminished strength of collagen.

Diagnosis

Prompt clinical assessment is crucial for a suspected diabetic foot infection because the infection can spread rapidly. The tools of diagnosis are the patient history and physical examination, selected laboratory tests, and imaging. A patient with a diabetic foot condition should undergo a thorough evaluation of all systems affected by diabetes, beginning with the entire body and progressing to the affected limb and the wound. Because all open wounds are colonized with bacteria, a wound infection must be diagnosed clinically rather than microbiologically. The clinical diagnosis of infection can be difficult, especially in a patient with peripheral neuropathy or ischemia. The patient may not feel ill and may not have a systemic inflammatory response (such as fever or leukocytosis) or typical local signs of infection (such as erythema, induration, warmth, pain, or tenderness).[25] Radiologic findings often are nonspecific; diabetic osteomyelitis may be difficult to distinguish on radiographs from conditions such as neuro-osteoarthropathy.[26]

The average age of a patient with a diabetic foot infection is approximately 60 years. Most patients have had diabetes for 15 to 20 years. Almost two thirds have evidence of peripheral vascular disease, and approximately 80% have lost protective sensation in the feet. Approximately half of these patients already have received antibiotic therapy for the foot lesion, and as many as one third have had the foot lesion for more than 1 month. The infected areas most often are the toes and metatarsal heads, particularly the plantar surface. Because of sensory neuropathy, many patients do not report pain. More than half of the patients, including those with a serious infection, are afebrile, and their white blood cell count and erythrocyte sedimentation rate are not elevated.[27,28] Some patients have

Table 1

Recommended Procedure for Evaluating a Patient With a Suspected Diabetic Foot Infection

1. Describe the lesion (for example, cellulitis, ulcer) and any drainage (for example, serous, purulent).
2. Determine whether signs of inflammation are present and their extent.
3. Determine whether infection is present as well as its extent and probable cause.
4. Examine the soft tissue for evidence of crepitus, abscess, sinus tracts, or foreign bodies.
5. Probe any skin breaks with a sterile metal probe to determine whether bone is exposed or palpable.
6. Measure the wound (length, width, estimated depth); consider photographing the wound.
7. Palpate pedal pulses and record findings, using a Doppler instrument if necessary.
8. Evaluate neurologic status (protective sensation, motor and autonomic function).
9. Cleanse and débride the wound; remove any foreign material, eschar, or callus.
10. Culture the cleansed wound, preferably by curettage, biopsy, or aspiration rather than swab.
11. Order plain radiographs (for most patients), and consider other imaging studies as needed.
12. Determine the consultants who should see the patient as well as the urgency of consultation.

only nonspecific symptoms or unusually poor glycemic control.

Examination

The assessment begins with a careful patient history and a thorough physical examination. Table 1 lists the recommended steps in the examination. The patient's level of sensation can be qualitatively assessed using the light touch and pinprick sensations, two-point discrimination, and proprioception; these are diminished in a patient with sensory neuropathy, usually in a stocking pattern below the knee. Quantitative methods of assessing sensation can offer more objective data. The most common method uses nylon Semmes-Weinstein monofilaments, which are pressed into the skin perpendicularly until they bend and exert force. The patient's sensation threshold is determined by the smallest monofilament that can be felt. Protective sensation is assumed to be present if the patient can feel the 5.07 monofilament, which exerts approximately 10 g of force. However, 10% of patients with diabetes who have this protective level of sensation develop neuropathic joints or ulcerations.[29,30] There is no standard, evidence-based method of applying the monofilaments. Testing at 8 to 10 anatomic sites is generally recommended, although a test of 4 plantar sites on the forefoot (the great toe and the base of the first, second, and third metatarsals) can identify 90% of patients who have an insensate site.[31]

The biothesiometer is an electrical device that delivers measurable stimulatory vibrations. It is not widely used because few studies are available to demonstrate its performance characteristics; it is also more expensive and less widely available than monofilaments. However, a recent prospective study of 103 patients suggested that the biothesiometer is more sensitive in predicting susceptibility to foot ulceration than the 10-g monofilament test or its predecessor, the tuning fork.[32]

The vascular examination findings have the greatest effect on treatment choice. The qualitative assessment focuses on noninvasive measures of pressure, flow, and tissue oxygenation, including pulses, skin temperature, capillary refill, and hair and nail growth. The assessment for vascular disease usually begins with palpating for dorsalis pedis and posterior tibial pulses. The accuracy of Doppler examination depends on the compressibility of the vessels being studied; it yields pressure measurements at multiple levels of the leg, foot, and ankle. The most common measurement used to detect peripheral vascular disease is the ankle-brachial index, which is the ratio of systolic blood pressure in the ankle to that in the brachial artery. An ankle-brachial index of 0.90 or less suggests the presence of peripheral vascular disease; an index higher than 1.1 may represent a false elevation caused by medial arterial calcinosis.[33] Transcutaneous oxygen measurement requires expensive equipment and a trained technician and therefore is less widely used. However, it is the most accurate method of assessing local skin vascularity and wound-healing potential. Transcutaneous oxygen tension greater than 40 mm Hg is correlated with a high likelihood of wound healing.[33]

The metabolic control of diabetes usually is the responsibility of the primary care physician or endocrinologist. To make an informed evaluation of the patient's healing potential, the orthopaedic specialist must be aware of the patient's hemoglobin A1C level, glucose level, and nutritional indices. A total serum protein concentration of 6.2 g/dL, a serum albumin level of 3.5 g/dL, and a total lymphocyte count of 1,500/mm³ are necessary for optimal tissue healing.

Classification of Ulceration

Because ulceration is a precursor of infection, classification of a diabetes-related foot disorder is useful in planning treatment. The Wagner classification (Table 2) was among the first of many suggested classification systems and is among the most widely used. An ulceration is graded on a scale from 0 (no open lesion) to 5 (gangrene of the entire foot). The more recent University of Texas Wound Classification (Table 3) grades the wound on a scale from 0 to 3, based on visual inspection, estimated depth, and the presence of infection or ischemia. The University of Texas system has been validated in prospective studies.[34,35]

Staging of Infection

A diabetic foot infection should be staged to guide treatment decisions such as the need for hospitalization, broad-spectrum parenteral antibiotic therapy, imaging studies, or urgent surgical procedures. In two similar systems developed by committees of the Infectious Diseases Society of America[28] (Table 4) and the International Working Group on the Diabetic Foot,[36] wound severity is characterized as mild (limited in size and involving only the skin and superficial subcutaneous tissues), moderate (larger or deeper, possibly involving the fascia, tendon, joint, or bone), or severe (accompanied by systemic signs or symptoms of infection or severe metabolic derangement).[28]

Table 2

Wagner Classification of Ulceration

Grade	Criterion
0	No open lesion
1	Superficial ulcer
2	Deep ulcer
3	Localized osteomyelitis or abscess
4	Forefoot gangrene
5	Gangrene of entire foot

Table 3

University of Texas Wound Classification

	Grade			
	0	**1**	**2**	**3**
A	Completely epithelialized preulcerative or postulcerative lesion	Superficial wound with no tendon, capsule, or bone involvement	Wound penetrating to tendon or capsule	Wound penetrating to bone or joint
B	Completely epithelialized preulcerative or postulcerative lesion, with infection	Superficial wound with no tendon, capsule, or bone involvement, with infection	Wound penetrating to tendon or capsule, with infection	Wound penetrating to bone or joint, with infection
C	Completely epithelialized preulcerative or postulcerative lesion, with ischemia	Superficial wound with no tendon, capsule, or bone involvement, with ischemia	Wound penetrating to tendon or capsule, with ischemia	Wound penetrating to bone or joint, with ischemia
D	Completely epithelialized preulcerative or postulcerative lesion, with infection and ischemia	Superficial wound with no tendon, capsule, or bone involvement, with infection and ischemia	Wound penetrating to tendon or capsule, with infection and ischemia	Wound penetrating to bone or joint, with infection and ischemia

(Adapted with permission from Lavery LA, Armstrong DG, Harkless LB: Classification of diabetic foot wounds. *J Foot Ankle Surg* 1996;35:528-531.)

Table 4

Infectious Diseases Society of America Simple Clinical Classification of Diabetic Foot Infection Severity

	Criterion			
Severity	**Superficial Ulcer or Cellulitis**	**Deep Soft-Tissue or Bone Involvement**	**Tissue Necrosis or Gangrene**	**Systemic Toxicity or Metabolic Instability**
Mild	Present ($\leq$ 2 cm)	Not present	Not present	Not present
Moderate	Present	May be present (without gas or fasciitis)	May be present (limited)	Not present
Severe	Present	May be present	May be present	Present

(Adapted with permission from Lipsky BA, Berendt AR, Deery HG, et al: Diagnosis and treatment of diabetic foot infections. *Clin Infect Dis* 2004;39:885-910.)

4: Specific Situations

Imaging

Diagnostic imaging is most commonly used to detect evidence of bone pathology, particularly osteomyelitis (**Figures 2** through **4**). Plain radiographs are useful in determining the presence of bony abnormalities, foreign bodies, or gas. Changes characteristic of infection, such as periosteal elevation or cortical destruction, may appear beneath an ulcer on plain radiographs. Peripheral neuropathy can cause osteoarthropathy such as Charcot foot, and therefore identification of bony abnormalities representing infection can be difficult. Radiography is insensitive during the first few weeks of an infection and is most likely to be useful when a bone in-

fection is well established, especially in the forefoot or hindfoot.[37] Soft-tissue pathology such as an abscess or sinus tract is better defined using ultrasonography or CT and best defined using MRI.

The diagnostic role of radionuclide scanning is limited. All types of inflammatory conditions, including arthritis, gout, and tumors, enhance isotope uptake and thus diminish the specificity of the test. Leukocyte scans are more specific than bone scans and have the advantage of showing that an area of infection has subsided; however, they are insufficiently accurate for most evaluations.[38] Many recent comparative studies have found MRI to have the greatest diagnostic accuracy (**Figure 4, B**). An MRI interpreted by an experienced radiologist can reveal bone infection (characterized by

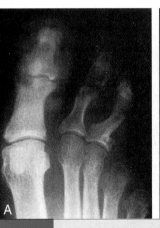
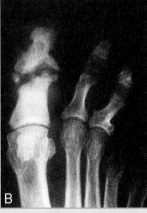

Figure 2   **A,** AP radiograph of the right foot of a 45-year-old man with diabetes and chronic osteomyelitis, showing early bone changes. Note the cortical bone lysis around the medial aspect of the interphalangeal joint of the great toe. **B,** Three months later, an AP radiograph of the foot of the same patient showing progressive erosion of the bone and joint in the great toe.

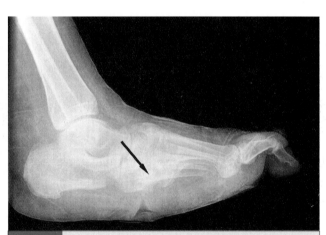

Figure 3   A lateral radiograph of the left foot of a 60-year-old man with diabetes showing severe erosive changes of the midfoot suggestive of Charcot foot. The site of infection is indicated by the arrow.

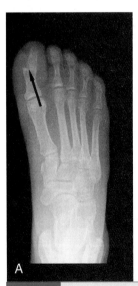
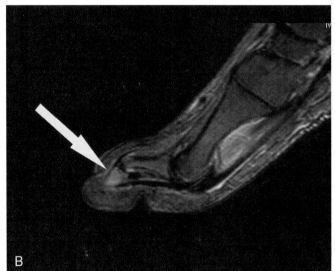
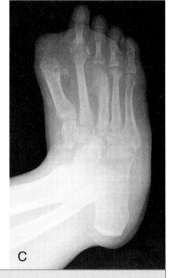

Figure 4   **A,** AP radiograph of a 38-year-old man with diabetes and osteomyelitis in the great toe; the area with infection can be seen as a shadow on the bone *(arrow).* **B,** MRI study showing the infection as a light spot *(arrow).* The toe was later amputated. **C,** Eighteen months later, an AP radiograph of the foot of the same patient showing the development of Charcot foot. Separation can be seen at the metatarsal joint and midfoot bones.

bone marrow edema) with 90% to 100% sensitivity and specificity.[26] However, changes caused by acute Charcot arthropathy, fracture, or postsurgical residue can be overestimated or mistaken for infection on MRI.[39]

Although the findings of clinical evaluation and imaging are useful in deciding whether osteomyelitis is present, bone biopsy is the standard criterion for the diagnosis.[36] A specimen can be obtained percutaneously (usually under fluoroscopic or CT guidance) or during surgery. If possible, the specimen should undergo both microbiologic and histologic processing. The biopsy procedure is relatively easy and safe, and it allows the physician to be certain of the diagnosis as well as the causative organism and its antibiotic susceptibilities before the patient is subjected to prolonged antibiotic therapy.

Surgical Treatment

Minor Débridement

With the exception of a lesion resulting from primary cellulitis, débridement of an infected foot lesion is almost always required to remove full-thickness dead skin, necrotic tissue, foreign material, or surrounding callus.[25] The procedure is designed to allow a full evaluation of the wound, prepare the wound for more accurate cultures and the application of topical antibiotics, and hasten healing by turning a chronic wound into an acute wound.

Débridement is more successful when performed with instruments rather than with enzymatic or chemical agents. Minor foot wounds can usually be débrided in the clinic or at the bedside. Most patients are sufficiently neuropathic that local anesthesia is not required. A scalpel or scissors is used to pare away callus, remove all undermining, and saucerize the wound. Definitive débridement often requires multiple procedures during several visits. Failure to adequately débride the wound is a common cause of persistent infection and failure of healing.

Surgical Débridement and Drainage

A deeper infection often requires surgical débridement and drainage. Early surgical intervention can halt progression of the infection, shorten the duration of antibiotic therapy, decrease the need for major amputation, and hasten the restoration of full ambulation.[39] Fulminant soft-tissue infection, such as gas gangrene or necrotizing fasciitis, requires urgent débridement. In addition, purulent fluid must be drained from enclosed spaces. Ischemic tissue must be débrided to allow endogenous leukocyte formation and absorption of systemic antibiotics. If bone and other dead tissue cannot be resorbed or remodeled, bacteria can establish communities in a biofilm called the glycocalyx, which is a physical barrier to antibiotic therapy. Thus, a thorough

inspection for dead tissue is required; the full extent of tissue destruction, particularly in deep compartments, may not be initially apparent. The surgeon must be knowledgeable about the compartments and spaces of the foot; each of them must be carefully explored because infection can track from one space to another.[40]

Most surgeons attempt to preserve as much tissue as possible. However, adequate débridement and drainage usually cannot be accomplished by performing small stab wounds and inserting drains.[19] In the past, a higher amputation was more often performed.[41] The presurgical and intrasurgical course is determined by evaluating tissue oxygenation using clinical methods (pedal pulses, skin temperature, capillary refill, bleeding from a cut), the ankle-brachial index, and transcutaneous oxygen and carbon dioxide pressure monitoring, as well as the type of infection (for example, cellulitis, ulceration, abscess, or gangrene, usually in the forefoot and plantar areas).[34]

Plantar incisions for drainage or débridement should be made parallel to the blood supply and run from the lesion to the area posterior to the medial malleolus. To explore the plantar space for abscess, the incision may be carried through the plantar aponeurosis to pass through the medial and central spaces. The flexor tendons must be explored by opening the intervening space between the abductor hallucis and flexor digitorum brevis, toward the central space where the plantar nerves and arteries are located. The flexor hallucis longus tendon is separated from the quadratus, and dissection continues distally to the plantar nerves.[34] If the patient has sensation, tissues should be carefully dissected to prevent the development of a sensitive plantar scar. Care must also be taken to avoid injuring the posterior tibial artery, its bifurcations to the lateral and medial arteries, or the digital arteries.

Arresting osteomyelitis is more difficult if limb ischemia is present. Sufficient débridement has been performed when all necrotic bone has been removed and a blood supply adequate for bone healing, antibiotic penetration, and oxygen delivery has been restored. In ischemic bone, in which bleeding may be limited, punctate bleeding of cortical bone (the paprika sign) is the best indicator of sufficient débridement. If possible, the surgery should be performed without a tourniquet so the extent of soft-tissue and bone bleeding can be evaluated and blood vessel damage can be avoided. If a tourniquet is used, it should be released after cultures are taken to ensure that blood flow is adequate, the remaining bone and soft tissues are viable, and irrigation is complete.

Débridement of large bones such as metatarsal heads or tarsal and hindfoot bones is performed using a bone scalpel such as the Midas Rex (Medtronic, Minneapolis, MN) or Anspach (Anspach, Palm Beach Gardens, FL) or a dental-type burr to allow easy visualization of punctate bleeding. Débridement of smaller bones is best performed using a sharp metatarsal rongeur and small curets. Skin and tissue edges are closed using no tension and nonabsorbable sutures. If skin edges cannot be easily closed, additional bone must be resected or the bone most be allowed to granulate closed so as to avoid skin grafting to granulated bone. Additional surgical débridement may be necessary if the wound does not close primarily.[41]

Amputation

Limb salvage or reconstruction is not feasible for some patients, making amputation the best option.[42] Osteomyelitis of the lesser toes sometimes is efficiently treated by enucleation or amputation of the affected phalanx.[43] Total or partial ray resection can be used to treat osteomyelitis of the metatarsals, if there is viable soft tissue. If the infected bone is only partially resected, antibiotic therapy should be administered for approximately 6 weeks, compared with approximately 2 weeks if the infected bone is completely removed. Midfoot osteomyelitis sometimes can be treated with enucleation of the bone, but a midfoot amputation may be needed, especially if the patient has advanced forefoot tissue loss and soft-tissue infection.[44] If calcaneal or talar osteomyelitis cannot be treated with enucleation, a Syme amputation (amputation of the foot with retention of the heel pad) or a below-knee amputation may be needed.[45]

An accurate amputation is essential for producing a residual limb suitable for early fitting of a prosthesis.[46] In general, it is preferable to remove as little of the foot as necessary, while selecting an amputation level that is likely to produce a stable, healing residual limb. The amputation level is determined by vascular status and the potential viability of tissues proximal to the site of infection. Tissue vascularity at the amputation site must be assessed to determine the potential for successful wound healing. Clinical assessment is important, as no test is completely accurate in assessing perfusion status in the lower extremity. However, an ankle-brachial index of 0.5 or a transcutaneous oxygen and carbon dioxide pressure reading above 20 to 30 mm Hg is associated with good healing after amputation in patients with diabetes.[1]

The clinician and the patient must share a clear understanding of the treatment goals and the difficulties that may persist after the initial antibiotic therapy or surgical intervention. Amputation surgery, when required, is not the final treatment step. Instead, it can be thought of as the first step in regaining limb function and developing a strategy that addresses the systemic nature of the disease. The patient must be taught how to prevent future foot complications because approximately half of patients with a diabetic foot wound develop a similar condition in the contralateral foot within 18 months.[47] A delay in recognizing the severity of the disease increases the risk of a major (usually below-knee) amputation.[48]

Offloading

Pressure reduction, called offloading, is a critical element in the treatment of a diabetic foot ulcer. A patient should never be allowed to walk out of the clinic in the footwear that caused the lesion. Excessive pressure in a neuropathic diabetic foot must be alleviated to foster wound healing. The goal of offloading is to reduce pressure at the lesion site while maintaining the patient's ambulation. This goal can be achieved through bed rest or by using crutches or a wheelchair, walker, total-contact cast, leg roller, or orthotic device.

Antibiotic Therapy

Indications

Between 40% and 60% of patients with a diabetic foot ulcer are treated with antibiotics.[25] Although the diagnosis can be difficult to confirm, the available data suggest that more than half of all diabetic foot ulcers are clinically uninfected and that antibiotic therapy does not improve the outcome of an uninfected lesion.[10] Antibiotic therapy is associated with adverse effects, is expensive, and contributes to the development of antibiotic-resistant organisms. It therefore should be used only in conditions for which it has demonstrated effectiveness. Only clinically infected diabetic foot wounds should be treated using antibiotic therapy, unless future data from human trials establish its effectiveness in preventing infection or treating uninfected tissue.

Choice of Antibiotic

Many antibiotic agents are effective in treating diabetic foot infections. The four most important considerations in selecting an antibiotic agent are the intended route of delivery, the antibiotic susceptibility of the likely pathogen, the safety of the agent, and the proof of its effectiveness in similar infections. Other factors also may be important, including patient allergies or comorbidities, the cost and availability of the agent, and the expected duration of therapy.

The initial antibiotic therapy usually is empirically chosen, based on an educated guess as to the causative pathogen. The clinical and laboratory clues listed in Table 5 can help in choosing the most appropriate agent.[49] Often a patient with a mild infection who has not recently received antibiotic therapy can be treated with an agent primarily directed at aerobic grampositive cocci, especially *Staphylococcus aureus*. Most other patients should begin antibiotic therapy with a broad-spectrum regimen to cover the most common pathogens, pending the results of wound cultures[49] (Table 6). In choosing a broad-spectrum regimen, the physician must consider whether the patient has previously received antibiotic therapy or has a known local antibiotic sensitivity pattern. The regimen should almost always include an agent active against staphylococci and

Table 5

Guide to Selecting an Empiric Antibiotic Regimen for Diabetic Foot Infection

Infection Characteristics	Probable Pathogens	Empiric Antibiotic Regimens
Acute Antibiotic naïve Unlikely to be caused by MRSA	Aerobic gram-positive cocci	Penicillin First-generation cephalosporin
Acquired in health care environment Acquired in geographic area with high incidence of MRSA	MRSA	Cotrimoxazole Doxycycline Clindamycin Glycopeptide Linezolid Daptomycin
Chronic Previously treated with antibiotic	Gram-positive cocci ± gram-negative bacilli ± anaerobes	β-lactam β-lactamase inhibitor Second- or third-generation cephalosporin Group-1 carbapenems Fluoroquinolone
Necrotic Gangrenous Ischemic limb with foul odor	Gram-positive cocci ± gram-negative bacilli ± obligate anaerobes	Clindamycin ± fluoroquinolone Metronidazole + fluoroquinolone β-lactam β-lactamase inhibitor Carbapenems
Previous hydrotherapy Green- or blue-colored drainage	Pseudomonas aeruginosa	Antipseudomonal fluoroquinolone Penicillin or cephalosporin

(Adapted with permission from Lipsky BA: Empirical therapy for diabetic foot infections: Are there clinical clues to guide antibiotic selection? *Clin Microbiol Infect* 2007;13:351-353.)

Table 6

Suggested Empiric Antibiotic Regimens for Diabetic Foot Infection

Infection Severity	Method of Administration	Recommended Regimens	Alternative Regimens
Mild or moderate	Oral usually adequate for entire course	Cephalexin (500 mg qid) Amoxicillin-clavulanate (875 mg-125 mg bid) Clindamycin (300 mg tid)	Levofloxacin (500 mg PO qd) ± clindamycin (300 mg PO tid) Trimethoprim-sulfamethoxazole (double strength PO bid)*
Moderate or severe	IV until infection is stable, then oral equivalent	Ampicillin-sulbactam (2.0 g qid) Clindamycin (450 mg PO qid) + ciprofloxacin (750 mg bid)†	Ertapenem (1 gm qd) Linezolid (600 mg bid)* ± aztreonam (2 g tid) Piperacillin-tazobactam (3.375 g qid)†
Life threatening	Prolonged IV often required	Imipenem-cilastatin (500 mg qid)† Clindamycin (900 mg IV tid) + tobramycin (5.1 mg/kg d) + ampicillin (50 mg/kg IV qid)	Vancomycin (15 mg/kg bid)* + ceftazidime (1 g tid) + metronidazole (7.5 mg/kg IV qid) Daptomycin (4 mg/kg qd) + moxifloxacin (400 mg qd)

Bid = twice daily, IV = intravenous, PO = by mouth, qd =daily, qid = four times daily, tid = three times daily
*Consider if MRSA is suspected.
†Consider if *P aeruginosa* is suspected.

streptococci. The rising incidence of methicillin-resistant *S aureus* (MRSA) requires consideration of an agent active against this pathogen. When the results of the wound culture are known, antibiotic therapy should be modified based on the findings as well as the patient's response to the empiric regimen. If the infection is improving and the patient is tolerating the therapy, there may be no reason to change the regimen, even if some or all of the isolated organisms are resistant to the agents being used. If the infection is not

4: Specific Situations

Table 7

Effective Antibiotics for the Treatment of Diabetic Foot Infection

Antibiotic Group	Specific Drug
Penicillin β-lactamase inhibitor congeners	Amoxicillin-clavulanate (oral) Ampicillin-sulbactam (parenteral) Piperacillin-tazobactam (parenteral)* Ticarcillin-clavulanate (parenteral)
Cephalosporins	Cephalexin (oral) Cefoxitin (parenteral) Ceftizoxime (parenteral)
Fluoroquinolones	Ciprofloxacin (oral or parenteral) Ofloxacin (oral or parenteral) Trovafloxacin (oral or parenteral)* Levofloxacin (oral or parenteral) Moxifloxacin (oral or parenteral)
Carbapenems	Imipenem-cilastatin (parenteral) Ertapenem (parenteral)*
Clindamycin (oral or parenteral)	
Vancomycin (parenteral)	
Linezolid* (oral or parenteral)	
Daptomycin (parenteral)	

*US Food and Drug Administration–approved for treatment of diabetic foot infection

responding, the regimen should be changed to cover all isolated organisms. If the infection is becoming worse despite the susceptibility of the isolated bacteria to the regimen, it is possible that a fastidious organism was missed during wound culture. Alternatively, surgical intervention may be needed.

New antibiotic drugs are constantly being developed as some older agents become obsolete or are used for a different purpose. The agents listed in Table 7 were found to be clinically effective in prospective studies of diabetic foot infection. No single agent or combination has emerged as the most effective regimen. Because of hepatotoxicity, trovafloxacin is reserved for the treatment of serious infections in patients who are in a hospital or other health care facility. The clinician needs to have a broad understanding of the principles of antibiotic therapy rather than extensive knowledge of a few agents.

Route of Therapy

Patients who have a systemic illness or severe infection, cannot tolerate oral agents, or are known to harbor a pathogen not susceptible to oral agents should receive intravenous antibiotic therapy. The patient's condition normally stabilizes in 3 to 5 days as the infection responds to therapy, and at that time a change to oral antibiotics is appropriate. More prolonged intravenous therapy may be required for patients with bacteremia, osteomyelitis, or an infection resistant to oral agents. Such a patient often can be treated on an outpatient basis, if a program is available to provide ambulatory parenteral therapy.[50] The presence of peripheral vascular disease may complicate therapy, as the drug concentrations often do not reach a therapeutic level in the foot, even if serum levels are adequate.[51-53] Alternative modes of antibiotic delivery have been used, including retrograde venous perfusion; intra-arterial administration; and intrasurgically implanted antibiotic-loaded beads, flakes, or cement. None of these therapies has been adequately evaluated, and they cannot be recommended for routine use.[54]

Oral antibiotic therapy is less expensive and more convenient than parenteral therapy, and it is sufficient for most patients. The spectrum of organisms that can be treated through oral therapy has been expanded by new oral antibiotics such as the fluoroquinolones[55,56] and linezolid.[57] Although the absorption of oral medications is sometimes poor in patients with diabetes, clindamycin, metronidazole, trimethoprim-sulfamethoxazole, linezolid, and the fluoroquinolones are well absorbed and highly bioavailable after oral administration. In particular, the fluoroquinolones usually achieve a high tissue concentration when administered orally to treat a diabetic foot infection, even in a patient with gastroparesis.

Treatment with a topical antibiotic may be an option for a mildly infected foot ulcer.[58] Topical therapy can achieve a high local concentration of the agent, and it avoids systemic adverse effects. Several agents, including silver sulfadiazine, neomycin, polymyxin B, gentamicin, and mupirocin, have been used to treat soft-tissue infections in other sites, but there are no published data on their efficacy in diabetic foot infections.[59]

Duration of Therapy

For a mild or moderate infection, a 1- to 2-week course of antibiotic therapy has been found to be effective;[27] a more serious infection usually requires a 2- to 4-week course of treatment. Adequate débridement, resection, or amputation of infected tissue may allow a shorter course of therapy. In a patient who develops bacteremia, a 2-week course of antibiotic therapy is prudent.

The duration of antibiotic therapy is determined by the patient's response and the clinician's judgment. Therapy usually can be discontinued when all signs and symptoms of infection are resolved, even if the wound has not completely healed. A patient who refuses or cannot undergo surgical resection may require prolonged suppressive antibiotic therapy.

The number and function of leukocytes in bone are suboptimal for antibiotic therapy, and antibiotics generally are unable to thoroughly penetrate infected bone. As a result, the initial treatment of osteomyelitis is usually parenteral and requires a prolonged course (at least 6 weeks). Treatment of chronic osteomyelitis has been thought to require removal of the infected bone by débridement or resection. Retrospective series have shown, however, that more conservative approaches may be appropriate. Diabetic foot osteomyelitis was arrested for at least 2 years with antibiotic therapy alone in approximately two thirds of patients studied.[37,60] Oral antibiotics with good bioavailability, such as the fluoroquinolones and clindamycin, may be adequate for most or all of the therapy. If all infected bone is removed, a shorter (2-week) course of antibiotic therapy may be sufficient. For some patients, long-term suppressive therapy or intermittent short-term therapy is the most appropriate approach.

Outcome of Therapy

After appropriate antibiotic therapy, a good clinical response can be expected in 80% to 90% of patients with a mild or moderate infection. The response is approximately 50% to 60% in patients with a deeper or more extensive infection. An infection involving deep soft tissue or bone requires thorough débridement, and bone resection or partial amputation is required in approximately two thirds of such patients. The amputation usually is foot sparing, and long-term control of the infection is achieved in approximately 80% of patients.[54,61] However, the infection recurs in 20% to 30% of those patients, many of whom have underlying osteomyelitis. Several factors generally increase the likelihood that treatment of a diabetic foot infection will be successful, including absence of exposed bone and a palpable popliteal pulse, toe pressure of more than 45 mm Hg, ankle pressure of more than 80 mm Hg, and peripheral white blood cell count of less than 12,000/mm^3.[13]

Patients who have had one diabetic foot infection are at substantial risk of a second infection within a few years. Patients must be educated regarding prevention techniques and, if applicable, lifestyle choices, as well as the crucial importance of obtaining prompt medical attention for any foot condition.

Adjunctive Treatments

Treatment of the diabetic foot often involves extensive surgery or amputation, and research has therefore focused on modalities to heal ischemic tissue in a less invasive fashion. Some published data are available on several adjunctive treatments, including revascularization, injections of recombinant granulocyte-colony stimulating factor (G-CSF), and hyperbaric oxygen therapy.

Lower extremity vascular procedures such as angio-plasty, stenting, and bypass grafting have been shown to be safe and effective for patients with a diabetic foot infection. Critically ischemic feet that formerly would have been treated with amputation often can be saved using one of these techniques. A vascular surgeon should be consulted if vessel repair could help to save distal tissue. Early recognition and aggressive surgical drainage of pedal sepsis followed by surgical revascularization were found to be critical to achieving maximal limb salvage.[62]

The addition of subcutaneous injections of G-CSF to customary forms of treatment, including antibiotic therapy, has been studied by several investigators. A meta-analysis of five published randomized controlled studies found that adjunctive G-CSF treatment did not appear to hasten the clinical resolution of diabetic foot infection or the healing of ulceration in a total of 167 patients. However, G-CSF was associated with a significantly reduced rate of amputation and other surgical procedures. This finding suggests that G-CSF should be considered for some patients, especially those with a limb-threatening infection. The drug is expensive, and larger studies are needed to determine whether it can be recommended.[63]

It is reasonable to hope that improving the delivery of oxygen to ischemic tissue can help fight infection and speed recovery in a diabetic foot wound. Although hyperbaric oxygen therapy has been studied for years, most of the published reports are anecdotal or from uncontrolled studies. Hyperbaric oxygen therapy is expensive and has limited availability. The currently prevalent practice is to reserve its use for the treatment of a severe infection that has not responded to other therapies. A 1997 meta-analysis of four prospective randomized studies concluded that hyperbaric oxygen therapy significantly reduced the risk of major amputation and improved the likelihood of healing in a total of 147 patients at 1-year follow-up.[64] These findings must be interpreted cautiously because of the small number of patients and the studies' methodologic shortcomings. A more recent review of the available data concluded that hyperbaric oxygen therapy should not be offered to patients with a diabetic foot wound, pending the availability of large-scale randomized studies with adequate blinding, control, and power. Such studies must clearly demonstrate that hyperbaric oxygen has efficacy and cost effectiveness in healing ulcers and preventing major amputation.[65]

Summary

Diabetic foot disorders present a complex challenge. Orthopaedic surgeons increasingly encounter this common complication of diabetes as the lifespan of patients with the disease continues to increase. Treatment of the diabetic foot requires a team approach to address metabolic disorders in the nervous, vascular, and immune systems and to recognize the interplay among these

4: Specific Situations

systems. Careful clinical evaluation, including microbiologic and imaging studies, can help the clinician devise a course of treatment, usually involving débridement and culture-directed antibiotic therapy. The patient, family members, primary care physician, and orthopaedic surgeon must work together to ensure that the patient is fully informed about the recommended procedures and their likely outcome, as well as the impact of lifestyle factors such as smoking, diet, and weight control on long-term prospects for a healthier life.

Annotated References

1. Philbin TM, Berlet GC, Lee TH: Lower-extremity amputations in association with diabetes mellitus. *Foot Ankle Clin* 2006;11:791-804.

   A multidisciplinary diabetic foot care team can help decrease the rate of major amputations and improve patients' quality of life.

2. Lipscombe LL, Hux JE: Trends in diabetes prevalence, incidence, and mortality in Ontario, Canada 1995-2005: A population-based study. *Lancet* 2007;369:750-756.

   The prevalence of diabetes in Ontario increased substantially over a decade and by 2005 exceeded the global rate predicted for 2030.

3. Prompers L, Huijberts M, Apelqvist J, et al: High prevalence of ischaemia, infection and serious comorbidity in patients with diabetic foot disease in Europe: Baseline results from the Eurodiale study. *Diabetologia* 2007;50:18-25.

   The severity of diabetic foot ulcers in Europe was found to be greater than previously reported. Nonplantar foot ulcers were more common than plantar ulcers, especially in patients with severe disease, and serious comorbidity increased significantly with increasing severity of foot disease.

4. Lavery LA, Armstrong DG, Wunderlich RP, Tredwell J, Boulton AJ: Diabetic foot syndrome: Evaluating the prevalence and incidence of foot pathology in Mexican Americans and non-Hispanic whites from a diabetes disease management cohort. *Diabetes Care* 2003;26:1435-1438.

   The incidence of diabetes-related lower extremity complications is reported for a cohort of patients enrolled in a diabetes disease management program. The incidence of amputation was higher in Mexican-American patients, although their rates of ulceration, infection, vascular disease, and lower extremity bypass were similar to those of non-Hispanic whites.

5. Lavery LA, Armstrong DG, Wunderlich RP, Mohler MJ, Wendel CS, Lipsky BA: Risk factors for foot infections in individuals with diabetes. *Diabetes Care* 2006;29:1288-1293.

   Evaluation of 1,666 consecutive patients in a managed care outpatient setting over 2 years to prospectively determine the risk factors for diabetic foot infection found

   199 foot infections in 151 patients (9%). The authors concluded that efforts to prevent infections should be targeted to people with a traumatic foot wound, especially a wound that is chronic, deep, recurrent, or associated with peripheral vascular disease.

6. Boulton AJ, Vileikyte L, Ragnarson-Tennvall G, Apelqvist J: The global burden of diabetic foot disease. *Lancet* 2005;366:1719-1724.

   The worldwide increase in diabetic foot disease has economic consequences. The authors urge a broader understanding of the resources required to treat the disease and the need for integrated patient treatment.

7. Price P: The diabetic foot: Quality of life. *Clin Infect Dis* 2004;39(suppl 2):S129-S131.

   A literature search to investigate the health-related quality of life of patients with foot complications associated with diabetes found that the health-related quality of life of patients with diabetic foot ulceration may be poorer than of patients who had amputation. Many patients with ulceration live with a fear of recurrence as well as repeated bouts of infection and potential lifelong disability.

8. Lipsky BA: Medical treatment of diabetic foot infections. *Clin Infect Dis* 2004;39(suppl 2):S104-S114.

   Treatment options for diabetic foot infections are reviewed, including nonsurgical and surgical approaches and antibiotic recommendations.

9. Carmona GA, Hoffmeyer P, Herrmann FR, et al: Major lower limb amputations in the elderly observed over ten years: The role of diabetes and peripheral arterial disease. *Diabetes Metab* 2005;31:449-454.

   The incidence, etiology, and prognosis of major lower limb amputations (transtibial or higher) in patients older than 65 years was determined retrospectively.

10. Apelqvist J, Bakker K, Van Houtom WH, Nabuurs-Fransen MH, Schaper NC: *International Consensus on the Diabetic Foot: International Working Group on the Diabetic Foot.* Amsterdam, The Netherlands, International Diabetes Federation, 1999, pp 1-96.

11. Reiber GE: Epidemiology of foot ulcers and amputations in the diabetic foot, in Bowker JH, Pfeifer MA (eds): *The Diabetic Foot.* St. Louis, MO: Mosby, 2001, pp 13-32.

12. Enderle MD, Coerper S, Schweizer HP, et al: Correlation of imaging techniques to histopathology in patients with diabetic foot syndrome and clinical suspicion of chronic osteomyelitis: The role of high-resolution ultrasound. *Diabetes Care* 1999;22:294-299.

13. Eneroth M, Larsson J, Apelqvist J: Deep foot infections in patients with diabetes and foot ulcer: An entity with different characteristics, treatments, and prognosis. *J Diabetes Complications* 1999;13:254-263.

14. Chang BB, Darling RC III, Paty PS, Lloyd WE, Shah DM, Leather RP: Expeditious management of is-

chemic invasive foot infections. *Cardiovasc Surg* 1996; 4:792-795.

15. Boyko EJ, Lipsky BA: Infection and diabetes mellitus, in Harris MI (ed): *Diabetes in America*, ed 2. Bethesda, MD: National Institutes of Health, 1995, pp 485-499.

16. Laing P: The development and complications of diabetic foot ulcers. *Am J Surg* 1998;176:11S-19S.

17. Greene DA: Neuropathy in the diabetic foot: New concepts in etiology and treatment, in Levin ME, O'Neal LW (eds): *The Diabetic Foot*. St. Louis, MO: Mosby, 1988, pp 76-83.

18. Brand PW: The insensitive foot, in Jahss MH (ed): *Disorders of the Foot and Ankle: Medical and Surgical Management*. Philadelphia, PA, WB Saunders, 1991, vol 2, pp 2170-2186.

19. Williams DT, Price P, Harding KG: The influence of diabetes and lower limb arterial disease on cutaneous foot perfusion. *J Vasc Surg* 2006;44:770-775.

Two influences on cutaneous foot perfusion in diabetes were found: global microcirculatory dysfunction, reflected in low-chest and foot transcutaneous oxygen values; and macrovascular disease, as indicated by reduced toe-brachial pressure indices and foot transcutaneous oxygen values.

20. Maggiore P, Echols RM: Infections in the diabetic foot, in Jahss MH (ed): *Disorders of the Foot and Ankle: Medical and Surgical Management*. Philadelphia, PA, WB Saunders, 1991, vol 2, pp 1937-1957.

21. Delbridge L, Ctercteko G, Fowler C, Reeve TS, Le Quesne LP: The aetiology of diabetic neuropathic ulceration of the foot. *Br J Surg* 1985;72:1-6.

22. Sentochnik DE, Eliopoulos GM: Infection and diabetes, in Kahn CR, Weir GC, King GL, Jacobson AM, Moses AC, Smith RJ (eds): *Joslin's Diabetes Mellitus*, ed 14. Philadelphia, PA, Lippincott Williams & Wilkins, 2005, pp 1017-1034.

A general review of issues is provided regarding infection in patients with diabetes.

23. McMahon MM, Bistrian BR: Host defenses and susceptibility to infection in patients with diabetes mellitus. *Infect Dis Clin North Am* 1995;9:1-9.

24. Das Evcimen N, King GL: The role of protein kinase C activation and the vascular complications of diabetes. *Pharmacol Res* 2007;55:498-510.

Protein kinase C activation is probably responsible for some pathologies in diabetic retinopathy, nephropathy, and cardiovascular disease. Protein kinase C isoform-selective inhibitors are a promising therapy to delay the onset or stop the progression of diabetic vascular disease with few adverse effects.

25. Nelson EA, O'Meara S, Craig D, et al: A series of systematic reviews to inform a decision analysis for sampling and treating infected diabetic foot ulcers. *Health Technol Assess* 2006;10:iii-iv, ix-x, 1-221.

An electronic database review of evidence on the diagnostic tests used to identify infection in diabetic foot disorders and interventions to treat them found that the available evidence is too weak to draw reliable implications for practice.

26. Tan PL, Teh J: MRI of the diabetic foot: Differentiation of infection from neuropathic change. *Br J Radiol* 2007;80:939-948.

MRI features can be used to help differentiate osteomyelitis from neuro-osteoarthropathy in the foot.

27. Armstrong DG, Perales TA, Murff RT, Edelson GW, Welchon JG: Value of white blood cell count with differential in the acute diabetic foot infection. *J Am Podiatr Med Assoc* 1996;86:224-227.

28. Lipsky BA, Berendt AR, Deery HG, et al: Diagnosis and treatment of diabetic foot infections. *Clin Infect Dis* 2004;39:885-910.

A consensus framework for treating all patients with a suspected diabetic foot infection is presented by a committee of the Infectious Diseases Society of America. An extensive bibliography is included.

29. Boulton AJ, Malik RA, Arezzo JC, Sosenko JM: Diabetic somatic neuropathies. *Diabetes Care* 2004;27:1458-1486.

The epidemiology, natural history, pathogenesis, clinical features, diagnosis, and treatment of focal and multifocal neuropathies are presented, with screening guidelines for diabetic distal sensory polyneuropathy.

30. Mayfield JA, Sugarman JR: The use of the Semmes-Weinstein monofilament and other threshold tests for preventing foot ulceration and amputation in persons with diabetes. *J Fam Pract* 2000;49:S17-S29.

31. Smieja M, Hunt DL, Edelman D, Etchells E, Cornuz J, Simel DL: Clinical examination for the detection of protective sensation in the feet of diabetic patients: International Cooperative Group for Clinical Examination Research. *J Gen Intern Med* 1999;14:418-424.

32. Miranda-Palma B, Sosenko JM, Bowker JH, Mizel MS, Boulton AJ: A comparison of the monofilament with other testing modalities for foot ulcer susceptibility. *Diabetes Res Clin Pract* 2005;70:8-12.

In this study of the optimal use of 10-g monofilament for the assessment of foot ulcer risk, the threshold number of testing sites and the proportion of insensate sites were determined. The sensitivity and specificity of the 10-g monofilament test are compared with that of other methodologies.

33. American Diabetes Association: Peripheral arterial disease in people with diabetes. *Diabetes Care* 2003;26:3333-3341.

Peripheral arterial disease is characterized by atherosclerotic occlusive disease of the lower extremities and is a major risk factor for lower extremity amputation. Peripheral arterial disease is strongly associated with symptomatic cardiovascular and cerebrovascular disease.

34. Armstrong DG, Lavery LA, Harkless LB: Validation of a diabetic wound classification system: The contribution of depth, infection, and ischemia to risk of amputation. *Diabetes Care* 1998;21:855-859.

35. Oyibo SO, Jude EB, Tarawneh I, Nguyen HC, Harkless LB, Boulton AJ: A comparison of two diabetic foot ulcer classification systems: The Wagner and the University of Texas wound classification systems. *Diabetes Care* 2001;24:84-88.

36. International Working Group on the Diabetic Foot: *Practical Guidelines on the Management and Prevention of the Diabetic Foot* [DVD]. Amsterdam, The Netherlands, International Diabetes Foundation, 2007.

    This interactive DVD includes chapters on footwear and offloading, wound treatment, and osteomyelitis.

37. Jeffcoate WJ, Lipsky BA: Controversies in diagnosing and managing osteomyelitis of the foot in diabetes. *Clin Infect Dis* 2004;39(suppl 2):S115-S122.

    The microbiology of osteomyelitis of the foot in diabetes, the benefits and limitations of various diagnostic procedures, and the evidence for the effectiveness of surgical and nonsurgical treatment are reviewed.

38. Chatha DS, Cunningham PM, Schweitzer ME: MR imaging of the diabetic foot: Diagnostic challenges. *Radiol Clin North Am* 2005;43:747-759.

    This summary of MRI of the diabetic foot focuses on differentiation of diabetic infection from other entities. The optimal pulse sequences are discussed.

39. Ledermann HP, Morrison WB: Differential diagnosis of pedal osteomyelitis and diabetic neuroarthropathy: MR imaging. *Semin Musculoskelet Radiol* 2005;9:272-283.

    MRI can be used to differentiate between osteomyelitis and acute or subacute neuroarthropathy. Careful analysis of the location of bone signal alterations, their distribution, and pattern is required.

40. Armstrong DG, Lipsky BA: Diabetic foot infections: Stepwise medical and surgical management. *Int Wound J* 2004;1:123-132.

    A step-by-step approach to evaluating and treating diabetic foot infections is provided, including empiric and culture-driven antibiotic regimens and surgical intervention.

41. Calhoun JH, Mader JT: Diabetic foot care, in Chapman MW (ed): *Chapman's Orthopaedic Surgery*, ed 3. Philadelphia, PA: Lippincott Williams & Wilkins, 2001, vol 3, pp 3073-3095.

42. Pinzur MS, Sage R, Abraham M, Osterman H: Limb salvage in infected lower extremity gangrene. *Foot Ankle* 1988;8:212-215.

43. Kerstein MD, Welter V, Gahtan V, Roberts AB: Toe amputation in the diabetic patient. *Surgery* 1997;122:546-547.

44. Stone PA, Back MR, Armstrong PA, et al: Midfoot amputations expand limb salvage rates for diabetic foot infections. *Ann Vasc Surg* 2005;19:805-811.

    In an evaluation of transmetatarsal and transtarsal-midfoot amputations performed over 8 years, more than half of the nonhealing transmetatarsal amputations were salvaged using transtarsal amputation, with excellent functional results.

45. Hudson JR, Yu GV, Marzano R, Vincent AL: Syme's amputation: Surgical technique, prosthetic considerations, and case reports. *J Am Podiatr Med Assoc* 2002;92:232-246.

46. Randon C, Deroose J, Vermassen F: How to perform a below-knee amputation. *Acta Chir Belg* 2003;103:238-240.

    In many patients, amputation should be considered the starting point for revalidation and rehabilitation rather than the failure of a revascularization technique. The authors review the steps needed to produce a good-quality stump, allowing early fitting of a prosthesis.

47. Kucan JO, Robson MC: Diabetic foot infections: Fate of the contralateral foot. *Plast Reconstr Surg* 1986;77:439-441.

48. Mills JL, Beckett WC, Taylor SM: The diabetic foot: Consequences of delayed treatment and referral. *South Med J* 1991;84:970-974.

49. Lipsky BA: Empirical therapy for diabetic foot infections: Are there clinical clues to guide antibiotic selection? *Clin Microbiol Infect* 2007;13:351-353.

    Several principles can be applied to avoid selecting an unnecessarily broad or inappropriately narrow antibiotic regimen.

50. Tice AD, Hoaglund PA, Shoultz DA: Outcomes of osteomyelitis among patients treated with outpatient parenteral antimicrobial therapy. *Am J Med* 2003;114:723-728.

    Retrospective chart review of 454 patients treated with intravenous antimicrobial therapy for osteomyelitis revealed that almost all recurrences of osteomyelitis were within 1 year. The recurrence rate of osteomyelitis associated with *S aureus* appeared to be higher after vancomycin was used.

51. Raymakers JT, Houben AJ, van der Heyden JJ, Tordoir JH, Kitslaar PJ, Schaper NC: The effect of diabetes and severe ischaemia on the penetration of ceftazidime into tissues of the limb. *Diabet Med* 2001;18:229-234.

52. Oberdorfer K, Swoboda S, Hamann A, et al: Tissue and serum levofloxacin concentrations in diabetic foot infection patients. *J Antimicrob Chemother* 2004;54:836-839.

The serum and tissue concentrations of levofloxacin were determined after oral administration to patients with an infected diabetic foot ulcer. The results are compared with microbiologic findings.

53. Legat FJ, Maier A, Dittrich P, et al: Penetration of fosfomycin into inflammatory lesions in patients with cellulitis or diabetic foot syndrome. *Antimicrob Agents Chemother* 2003;47:371-374.

The distribution of the broad-spectrum antibiotic fosfomycin in infected soft tissue of patients with uncomplicated cellulitis of the lower extremity or a diabetic foot infection was investigated using in vivo microdialysis. Fosfomycin was found to have good penetration into the fluid of the interstitial space in both inflamed and noninflamed soft tissue.

54. Armstrong DG, Lipsky BA: Advances in the treatment of diabetic foot infections. *Diabetes Technol Ther* 2004; 6:167-177.

Recent improvements in the treatment of diabetic foot infections are reviewed, including newer antibiotics and alternate delivery systems.

55. Greenberg RN, Newman MT, Shariaty S, Pectol RW: Ciprofloxacin, lomefloxacin, or levofloxacin as treatment for chronic osteomyelitis. *Antimicrob Agents Chemother* 2000;44:164-166.

56. Edmiston CE, Krepel CJ, Seabrook GR, et al: In vitro activities of moxifloxacin against 900 aerobic and anaerobic surgical isolates from patients with intra-abdominal and diabetic foot infections. *Antimicrob Agents Chemother* 2004;48:1012-1016.

The in vitro activity of moxifloxacin, ciprofloxacin, levofloxacin, gatifloxacin, imipenem, piperacillin-tazobactam, clindamycin, and metronidazole against 900 surgical isolates was determined using testing methods of the National Committee on Clinical Laboratory Standards.

57. Lipsky BA, Itani K, Norden C: Treating foot infections in diabetic patients: A randomized, multicenter, open-label trial of linezolid versus ampicillin-sulbactam/amoxicillin-clavulanate. *Clin Infect Dis* 2004;38:17-24.

A randomized, open-label, multicenter study compared the efficacy and safety of intravenous and oral formulations of linezolid with those of intravenous ampicillin-sulbactam and intravenous and oral amoxicillin-clavulanate administered for 7 to 28 days.

58. Sibbald RG: Topical antimicrobials. *Ostomy Wound Manage* 2003;49:14-18.

The controversial use of topical antimicrobials is addressed in this description of mechanisms of action, supporting evidence, and perceived limitations.

59. Bergin SM, Wraight P: Silver based wound dressings and topical agents for treating diabetic foot ulcers. *Cochrane Database Syst Rev* 2006;25:CD005082.

A large database review found no randomized or controlled clinical studies evaluating the clinical effectiveness of silver-based wound dressings.

60. Pittet D, Wyssa B, Herter-Clavel C, Kursteiner K, Vaucher J, Lew PD: Outcome of diabetic foot infections treated conservatively: A retrospective cohort study with long-term follow-up. *Arch Intern Med* 1999;159: 851-856.

61. Van Damme H, Rorive M, Martens De Noorthout BM, Quaniers J, Scheen A, Limet R: Amputations in diabetic patients: A plea for footsparing surgery. *Acta Chir Belg* 2001;101:123-129.

62. Sumpio BE, Lee T, Blume PA: Vascular evaluation and arterial reconstruction of the diabetic foot. *Clin Podiatr Med Surg* 2003;20:689-708.

The evaluation of diabetic foot vascularization and principles of drainage, débridement, amputation, and revascularization are reviewed in detail.

63. Cruciani M, Lipsky BA, Mengoli C, de Lalla F: Are granulocyte colony-stimulating factors beneficial in treating diabetic foot infections? A meta-analysis. *Diabetes Care* 2005;28:454-460.

A large database search was performed to assess the value of G-CSF as an adjunctive therapy for diabetic foot infections.

64. Kranke P, Bennett M, Roeckl-Wiedmann I, Debus S: Hyperbaric oxygen therapy for chronic wounds. *Cochrane Database Syst Rev* 2004;2:CD004123.

A large database search was performed to assess adjunctive hyperbaric oxygen therapy for treating chronic ulcers of the lower limb, including those in the diabetic foot.

65. Berendt AR: Counterpoint: Hyperbaric oxygen for diabetic foot wounds is not effective. *Clin Infect Dis* 2006; 43:193-198.

The author argues that hyperbaric oxygen therapy should not be offered for diabetic foot wounds until large-scale randomized studies with adequate blinding, controls, and power have clearly demonstrated its efficacy and cost effectiveness in healing ulcers and preventing major amputation.

4: Specific Situations

Appendix

The American Academy of Orthopaedic Surgeons (AAOS) has developed position and information statements on many topics related to the practice of orthopaedic surgery, including orthopaedic infections. These statements are published on the AAOS website (www.aaos.org) in the "About AAOS" section. This is a dynamic area in which statement updates appear on a continuing basis as new statements are added and old statements are retired. It is highly recommended that readers visit the AAOS website to check for updates. The direct link to the position statements is www.aaos.org/about/papers/position.asp, and the link to the information statements is www.aaos.org/about/papers/advis.asp.

Two AAOS information statements pertinent to the content of *OKU: Musculoskeletal Infection* are printed here for the convenience of readers: "Recommendations for the Use of Intravenous Antibiotic Prophylaxis in Primary Total Joint Arthroplasty" (www.aaos.org/about/papers/advistmt/1027.asp) and "Antibiotic Prophylaxis for Bacteremia in Patients With Joint Replacements" (www.aaos.org/about/papers/advistmt/1033.asp).

American Academy of Orthopaedic Surgeons Information Statement

Recommendations for the Use of Intravenous Antibiotic Prophylaxis in Primary Total Joint Arthroplasty

This Information Statement was developed as an educational tool based on the opinion of the authors. It is not a product of a systematic review. Readers are encouraged to consider the information presented and reach their own conclusions.

Background

Surgical site infections (SSIs) are a major source of postoperative illness, accounting for nearly 25% of all nosocomial infections in the United States each year.[1] The Centers for Disease Control and Prevention (CDC) estimate that approximately 500,000 SSIs occur annually in the United States.[2] The risks for patients who develop SSIs include:

- 60% more likely to spend time in an intensive care unit
- Five times more likely to be readmitted to the hospital
- Twice the mortality rate as patients without wound infections.[3]

Studies have demonstrated that prophylactic antibiotics reduce the incidence of infection after orthopaedic surgery in patients without known infection, and their use is considered routine for primary total joint arthroplasty.[4-7]

The National Surgical Infection Prevention Project (SIPP) was initiated in August of 2002 as a joint venture between the Centers for Medicare and Medicaid Services (CMS) and the CDC. By promoting the appropriate selection, timing, and duration of administration of prophylactic antibiotics, the project seeks to reduce the morbidity and mortality related to postoperative infections in the Medicare population. Experts in surgical infection prevention, hospital infection control, and epidemiology developed three performance measures for national surveillance and quality improvement.[8] The American Academy of Orthopaedic Surgeons was instrumental in developing the following three measures: 1) the proportion of patients who receive prophylactic antibiotics consistent with current recommendations; 2) the proportion of patients who receive antibiotic prophylaxis within 1 hour before the surgical incision; and 3) the proportion of patients whose prophylactic antibiotics were discontinued within 24 hours of the end of surgery.[8] Preliminary data from this surveillance indicates that antibiotic prophylaxis is not always administered in a manner that is supported by scientific evidence. Inappropriate use of antibiotics does not prevent postoperative infections, but contributes to antibiotic resistance, increases the risk of adverse reactions, predisposes the patient to infections, and increases health care costs.

The American Academy of Orthopaedic Surgeons recommends the following evidence-based practices for the appropriate use of intravenous antibiotic prophylaxis in primary total joint arthroplasty to reduce the risk of infection.

Recommendation 1

The antibiotic used for prophylaxis should be carefully selected, consistent with current recommendations in the literature, taking into account the issues of resistance and patient allergies.

Currently, cefazolin or cefuroxime are the preferred antibiotics for patients undergoing orthopaedic procedures.[9-12] Clindamycin or vancomycin may be used for patients with a confirmed ß-lactam allergy. Vancomycin may be used in patients with colonization with methicillin resistant *Staphylococcus aureus* (MRSA) or in facilities with recent MRSA outbreaks.[13] In multiple studies, exposure to vancomycin is reported as a risk factor in the development of vancomycin-resistant enterococcus (VRE) colonization and infection.

Therefore, vancomycin should be reserved for the treatment of serious infection with ß-lactam-resistant organisms or for treatment of infection in patients with life-threatening allergy to ß-lactam antimicrobials.[14]

Recommendation 2

Timing and dosage of antibiotic administration should optimize the efficacy of the therapy.

Prophylactic antibiotics should be administered within one hour prior to skin incision.[15-19] Due to an extended infusion time, vancomycin should be started within 2 hours prior to incision. If a proximal tourniquet is used, the antibiotic must be completely infused prior to the inflation of the tourniquet. Dose amount should be proportional to patient weight; for patients > 80 kg the doses of cefazolin should be doubled.[20] Additional intraoperative doses of antibiotic are advised if:

1. The duration of the procedure exceeds one to two times the antibiotic's half-life.
2. There is significant blood loss during the procedure.[10,21,22]

The general guidelines for frequency of intraoperative administration are as follows (Table 1).[13]

Table 1

Antibiotic	Frequency of Administration
Cefazolin	Every 2-5 hours
Cefuroxime	Every 3-4 hours
Clindamycin	Every 3-6 hours
Vancomycin	Every 6-12 hours

Recommendation 3

Duration of prophylactic antibiotic administration should not exceed the 24-hour postoperative period.

Prophylactic antibiotics should be discontinued within 24 hours of the end of surgery.[9-12,23-29] Medical literature does not support the continuation of antibiotics until all drains or catheters are removed and provides no evidence of benefit when they are continued past 24 hours.[30-47]

References

1. Haley RW, Culver DH, White JW, Morgan WM, Emori TG: The nationwide nosocomial infection rate: A new need for vital statistics. *Am J Epidemiol* 1985;121:159-167.

2. Wong ES: Surgical site infection, in Mayhall DG (ed): *Hospital Epidemiology and Infection Control*, ed 2. Philadelphia, PA, Lippincott, 1999, pp 189-210.

3. Kirkland KB, Briggs JP, Trivette SL, Wilkinson WE, Sexton DJ: The impact of surgical site infections in the 1990s: Attributable mortality, excess length of hospitalization, and extra costs. *Infect Control Hosp Epidemiol* 1999;20:725-730.

4. Fogelberg EV, Zitzmann EK, Stinchfield FE: Prophylactic penicillin in orthopaedic surgery. *J Bone Joint Surg Am* 1970;52:95-98.

5. Pavel A, Smith RL, Ballard A, Larsen AJ: Prophylactic antibiotics in clean orthopaedic surgery. *J Bone Joint Surg Am* 1974;56:777-782.

6. Boxma H, Broekhuizen T, Patka P, Oosting H: Randomized control trial of a single dose antibiotic prophylaxis in surgical treatment of closed fractures: The Dutch trauma trial. *Lancet* 1996;347:1133-1137.

7. Gillespie WJ, Walenkamp G: Antibiotic prophylaxis for proximal femoral and other closed long bone fractures. *Cochrane Database Syst Rev* 2001;1:CD000244.

8. Bratzler DW, Houck PM, Surgical Infection Prevention Guidelines Writers Workgroup, et al: Antimicrobial prophylaxis for surgery: An advisory statement from the National Surgical Infection Prevention Project. *Clin Infect Dis* 2004;38:1706-1715.

9. Page CP, Bohnen JM, Fletcher JR, et al: Antimicrobial prophylaxis for surgical wounds: Guidelines for clinical care. *Arch Surg* 1993;128:79-88.

10. Dellinger EP, Gross PA, Barrett TL, et al: Quality standard for antimicrobial prophylaxis in surgical procedures: Infectious Diseases Society of America. *Clin Infect Dis* 1994;18:422-427.

Appendix

11. Antimicrobial prophylaxis in surgery. *Med Lett Drugs Ther* 2001;43:92-97.

12. Gilbert DN, Moellering RC, Sande MA.

13. American Society of Health-System Pharmacists: ASHP Therapeutic Guidelines on Antimicrobial Prophylaxis in Surgery. *Am J Health Syst Pharm* 1999;56:1839-1888.

14. American Academy of Orthopaedic Surgeons: The use of prophylactic antibiotics in orthopaedic medicine and the emergence of vancomycin-resistant bacteria. 2002. http://www.aaos.org/about/papers/position/1116.asp.

15. Burke JF: The effective period of preventative antibiotic action in experimental incisions and dermal lesions. *Surgery* 1961;50:161-168.

16. DiPiro JT, Vallner JJ, Bowden TA, Clark BA, Sisley JF: Intraoperative serum and tissue activity of cefazolin and cefoxitin. *Arch Surg* 1985;120:829-832.

17. Classen DC, Evans RS, Pestotnik SL, et al: The timing of prophylactic administration of antibiotics and the risk of surgical wound infection. *N Engl J Med* 1992;326:281-286.

18. Fukatsu K, Saito H, Matsuda T, et al: Influences of type and duration of antimicrobial prophylaxis on an outbreak of methicillin-resistant Staphylococcus aureus and on the incidence of wound infection. *Arch Surg* 1997;132:1320-1325.

19. Burke JP: Maximizing appropriate antibiotic prophylaxis for surgical patients: An update from LDS hospital, Salt Lake City. *Clin Infect Dis* 2001;33(suppl 2):S78-S83.

20. Hanssen AD, Osmon DR: The use of prophylactic antimicrobial agents during and after hip arthroplasty. *Clin Orthop Relat Res* 1999;369:124-138.

21. Bratzler DW, Houck PM, Surgical Infection Prevention Guidelines Writers Workgroup, et al: Antimicrobial prophylaxis for surgery: An Advisory Statement from the National Surgical Infection Prevention Project. *Clin Infect Dis* 2004;38:1706-1715.

22. Gross PA, Barrett TL, Dellinger EP, et al: Purpose of quality standards for infectious diseases: Infectious Diseases Society of America. *Clin Infect Dis* 1994;18:428-430.

23. Auerbach AD: Prevention of Surgical site infections. http://www.ahrq.gov/clinic/ptsafety/pdf/ptsafety.pdf.

24. Pollard JP, Hughes SP, Scott JE, Evans MJ, Benson MK: Antibiotic prophylaxis in total hip replacement. *Br Med J* 1979;1:707-709.

25. Williams DN, Gustilo RB, Beverly R, Kind AC: Bone and serum concentrations of five cephalosporin drugs: Relevance to prophylaxis and treatment in orthopedic surgery. *Clin Orthop Relat Res* 1983;179:253-265.

26. Nelson CL, Green TG, Porter RA, Warren RD: One day versus seven days of preventative antibiotic therapy in orthopaedic surgery. *Clin Orthop Relat Res* 1983;176:258-263.

27. Heydemann JS, Nelson CL: Short-term preventative antibiotics. *Clin Orthop Relat Res* 1986;205:184-187.

28. Oishi CS, Carrion WV, Hoaglund FT: Use of parenteral prophylactic antibiotics in clean orthopaedic surgery: A review of the literature. *Clin Orthop Relat Res* 1993;296:249-255.

29. Mauerhan DR, Nelson CL, Smith DL, et al: Prophylaxis against infection in total joint arthroplasty: One day cefuroxime compared with three days of cefazolin. *J Bone Joint Surg* 1994;76:39-45.

30. Chandratreya A, Giannikas K, Livesley P: To drain or not drain: Literature versus practice. *J R Coll Surg Edinb* 1998;43:404-406.

31. Ovadia D, Luger E, Bickels J, Menachem A, Dekel S: Efficacy of closed wound drainage after total joint arthroplasty: A prospective randomized study. *J Arthroplasty* 1997;12:317-321.

32. Jackson JP, Waugh W: Tibial osteotomy for osteoarthritis of the knee. *J Bone Joint Surg Br* 1961;43-B:746-751.

33. Varley GW, Milner SA: Wound drains in proximal femoral fracture surgery: A randomized prospective trial of 177 patients. *J R Coll Surg Edinb* 1995;40:416-418.

34. Cobb JP: Why use drains? *J Bone Joint Surg Br* 1990;72:993-995.

35. Hadden WA, McFarlane AG: A comparative study of closed-wound suction drainage vs. no drainage in total hip arthroplasty. *J Arthroplasty* 1990;5(suppl):S21-S24.

36. Ritter MA, Keating EM, Faris PM: Closed wound drainage in total hip or total knee replacement: A prospective, randomized study. *J Bone Joint Surg Am* 1994;76: 35-38.

37. Reilly TJ, Gradisar IA Jr, Pakan W, Reilly M: The use of postoperative suction drainage in total knee arthroplasty. *Clin Orthop Relat Res* 1986;208:238-242.

38. Beer KJ, Lombardi AV Jr, Mallory TH, Vaughn BK: The efficacy of suction drains after routine total joint arthroplasty. *J Bone Joint Surg Am* 1991;73:584-587.

39. Esler CN, Blakeway C, Fiddian NJ: The use of a closed-suction drain in total knee arthroplasty: A prospective, randomized study. *J Bone Joint Surg Br* 2003;85: 215-217.

40. Adalberth G, Bystrom S, Kolstad K, Mallmin H, Milbrink J: Postoperative drainage of knee arthroplasty is not necessary: A randomized study of 90 patients. *Acta Orthop Scand* 1998;69: 475-478.

41. Niskanen RO, Korkala OL, Haapala J, Kuokkanen HO, Kaukonen JP, Salo SA: Drainage is of no use in primary uncomplicated cemented hip and knee arthroplasty for osteoarthritis: A prospective randomized study. *J Arthroplasty* 2000;15:567-569.

42. Drinkwater CJ, Neil MJ: Optimal timing of wound drain removal following total joint arthroplasty. *J Arthroplasty* 1995;10:185-189.

43. Browett JP, Gibbs AN, Copeland SA, Deliss LJ: The use of suction drainage in the operation of meniscectomy. *J Bone Joint Surg Br* 1978;60-B:516-519.

44. Willett KM, Simmons CD, Bentley G: The effect of suction drains after total hip replacement. *J Bone Joint Surg Br* 1988;70:607-610.

45. Sorensen AI, Sorensen TS: Bacterial growth on suction drain tips: Prospective study of 489 clean orthopedic operations. *Acta Orthop Scand* 1991;62:451-454.

46. Overgaard S, Thomsen NO, Kulinski B, Mossing NB: Closed suction drainage after hip arthroplasty: Prospective study of bacterial contamination in 81 cases. *Acta Orthop Scand* 1993;64:417-420.

47. Manian FA, Meyer PL, Setzer J, Senkel D: Surgical site infections associated with methicillin-resistant Staphylococcus aureus: Do postoperative factors play a role? *Clin Infect Dis* 2003;36:863-868.

48. Cruse PJ, Foord R: A five-year prospective study of 23,649 surgical wounds. *Arch Surg* 1973;107:206-210.

Appendix

Antibiotic Prophylaxis for Bacteremia in Patients With Joint Replacements

This Information Statement was developed as an educational tool based on the opinion of the authors. Readers are encouraged to consider the information presented and reach their own conclusions.

More than 1,000,000 total joint arthroplasties are performed annually in the United States, of which approximately 7% are revision procedures.[1] Deep infections of total joint replacements usually result in failure of the initial operation and the need for extensive revision, treatment, and cost. Due to the use of perioperative antibiotic prophylaxis and other technical advances, deep infection occurring in the immediate postoperative period resulting from intraoperative contamination has been markedly reduced in the past 20 years.

Bacteremia from a variety of sources can cause hematogenous seeding of bacteria onto joint implants, both in the early postoperative period and for many years following implantation.[2] In addition, bacteremia may occur in the course of normal daily life[3-5] and concurrently with dental,

urologic, and other surgical and medical procedures.[5] The analogy of late prosthetic joint infections with infective endocarditis is invalid as the anatomy, blood supply, microorganisms, and mechanisms of infection are all different.[6]

It is likely that bacteremia associated with acute infection in the oral cavity,[7,8] skin, respiratory, gastrointestinal, and urogenital systems and/or other sites can and do cause late implant infection.[8] Practitioners should maintain a high index of suspicion for any change or unusual signs and symptoms (eg, pain, swelling, fever, joint warm to touch) in patients with total joint prostheses. Any patient with an acute prosthetic joint infection should be vigorously treated with elimination of the source of the infection and appropriate therapeutic antibiotics.[8,9]

Patients with joint replacements who are having invasive procedures or who have other infections are at increased risk of hematogenous seeding of their prosthesis. Antibiotic prophylaxis may be considered, for those patients who have had previous prosthetic joint infections, and for those with other conditions that may predispose the patient to infection[8,10-16] (Table 1). There is evidence that some immunocompromised patients with total joint replacements may be at higher risk for hematogenous infections.[10-18] However, patients with pins, plates, and screws, or other orthopaedic hardware that is not within a synovial joint are not at increased risk for hematogenous seeding by microorganisms.

Given the potential adverse outcomes and cost of treating an infected joint replacement, the AAOS recommends that clinicians consider antibiotic prophylaxis for all total joint replacement patients prior to any invasive procedure that may cause bacteremia. This is particularly important for those patients with one or more of the risk factors listed in Table 1.

Table 1

Patients at Potential Increased Risk of Hematogenous Total Joint Infection[8,10-16,18]

- All patients with prosthetic joint replacement
- Immunocompromised/immunosuppressed patients
- Inflammatory arthropathies (eg, rheumatoid arthritis, systemic lupus erythematosus)
- Drug-induced immunosuppression
- Radiation-induced immunosuppression
- Patients with comorbidities (eg, diabetes, obesity, HIV, smoking)
- Previous prosthetic joint infections
- Malnourishment
- Hemophilia
- HIV infection
- Insulin-dependent (type 1) diabetes
- Malignancy
- Megaprostheses

Prophylactic antibiotics prior to any procedure that may cause bacteremia are chosen on the basis of its activity against endogenous flora that would likely to be encountered from any secondary other source of bacteremia, its toxicity, and its cost. In order to prevent bacteremia, an appropriate dose of a prophylactic antibiotic should be given prior to the procedure so that an effective tissue concentration is present at the time of instrumentation or incision in order to protect the patient's prosthetic joint from a bacteremia-induced periprosthetic sepsis. Current prophylactic antibiotic recommendations for these different procedures are listed in Table 2.[19]

Occasionally, a patient with a joint prosthesis may present to a given clinician with a recommendation from his/her orthopaedic surgeon that is not consistent with these recommendations. This could be due to lack of familiarity with the recommendations or to special considerations about the patient's medical condition which are not known to either the clinician or orthopaedic surgeon. In this situation, the clinician is encouraged to consult with the orthopaedic surgeon to determine if there are any special considerations that might affect the clinician's decision on whether or not to premedicate, and may wish to share a copy of these

Table 2

Procedure	Antimicrobial Agent	Dose	Timing	Duration
Dental	Cephalexin, cephradine, amoxicillin	2 g PO	1 hour prior to procedure	Discontinued within 24 hours of the procedure. For most outpatient/office-based procedures a single preprocedure dose is sufficient.
Ophthalmic	Gentamicin, tobramycin, ciprofloxacin, gatifloxacin, levofloxacin, moxifloxacin, ofloxacin, or neomycin-gramicdin-polymyxin B cefazolin	Multiple drops topically over 2 to 24 hours or 100 mg subconjunctivally	Consult ophthalmologist or pharmacist for dosing regimen	
Orthopaedic†	Cefazolin Cefuroxime OR Vancomycin	1-2 g IV 1.5 g IV 1 g IV	Begin dose 60 minutes prior to procedure	
Vascular	Cefazolin OR Vancomycin	1-2 g IV 1 g IV	Begin dose 60 minutes prior to procedure	
Gastrointestinal				
Esophageal, gastroduodenal	Cefazolin	1-2 g IV	Begin dose 60 minutes prior to procedure	
Biliary tract	Cefazolin	1-2 g IV		
Colorectal	Neomycin + erythromycin base (oral) OR metronidazole (oral)	1 g 1 g	Dependent on time of procedure, consult with GI physician and/or pharmacist	
Head and neck	Clindamycin + gentamicin OR cefazolin	600-900 mg IV 1.5 mg/kg IV 1-2 g IV	Begin dose 60 minutes prior to procedure	
Obstetric and gynecologic	Cefoxitin, cefazolin Ampicillin/sulbactam	1-2 g IV 3 g IV	Begin dose 60 minutes prior to procedure	
Genitourinary	Ciprofloxacin	500 mg PO or 400 mg IV	1 hour prior to procedure Begin dose 60 minutes prior to procedure	

† If a tourniquet is used the entire dose of antibiotic must be infused prior to its inflation.

recommendations with the physician, if appropriate. After this consultation, the clinician may decide to follow the orthopaedic surgeon's recommendation, or, if in the clinician's professional judgment, antibiotic prophylaxis is not indicated, may decide to proceed without antibiotic prophylaxis.

This statement provides recommendations to supplement practitioners in their clinical judgment regarding antibiotic prophylaxis for patients with a joint prosthesis. It is not intended as the standard of care nor as a substitute for clinical judgment as it is impossible to make recommendations for all conceivable clinical situations in which bacteremias may occur. The treating clinician is ultimately responsible for making treatment recommendations for his/her patients based on the clinician's professional judgment.

Any perceived potential benefit of antibiotic prophylaxis must be weighed against the known risks of antibiotic toxicity, allergy, and development, selection and transmission of microbial resistance. Practitioners must exercise their own clinical judgment in determining whether or not antibiotic prophylaxis is appropriate.

References

1. Number of Patients, Number of Procedures, Average Patient Age, Average Length of Stay: National Hospital Discharge Survey, 1998-2005. Data obtained from US Department of Health and Human Services Centers for Disease Control and Prevention National Center for Health Statistics.
2. Rubin R, Salvati EA, Lewis R: Infected total hip replacement after dental procedures. *Oral Surg Oral Med Oral Pathol* 1976;41:18-23.
3. Bender IB, Naidorf IJ, Garvey GJ: Bacterial endocarditis: A consideration for physicians and dentists. *J Am Dent Assoc* 1984;109:415-420.
4. Everett ED, Hirschmann JV: Transient bacteremia and endocarditis prophylaxis: A review. *Medicine (Baltimore)* 1977;56:61-77.
5. Guntheroth WG: How important are dental procedures as a cause of infective endocarditis? *Am J Cardiol* 1984;54:797-801.
6. McGowan DA: Dentistry and endocarditis. *Br Dent J* 1990;169:69.
7. Bartzokas CA, Johnson R, Jane M, Martin MV, Pearce PK, Saw Y: Relation between mouth and haematogenous infections in total joint replacement. *BMJ* 1994;309:506-508.
8. Ching DW, Gould IM, Rennie JA, Gibson PH: Prevention of late haematogenous infection in major prosthetic joints. *J Antimicrob Chemother* 1989;23:676-680.
9. Pallasch TJ, Slots J: Antibiotic prophylaxis and the medically compromised patient. *Periodontol 2000* 1996;10:107-138.
10. Rubin R, Salvati EA, Lewis R: Infected total hip replacement after dental procedures. *Oral Surg Oral Med Oral Pathol* 1976;41:18-23.
11. Brause BD: Infections associated with prosthetic joints. *Clin Rheum Dis* 1986;12:523-536.
12. Jacobson JJ, Millard HD, Plezia R, Blankenship JR: Dental treatment and late prosthetic joint infections. *Oral Surg Oral Med Oral Pathol* 1986;61:413-417.
13. Johnson DP, Bannister GG: The outcome of infected arthroplasty of the knee. *J Bone Joint Surg Br* 1986;68:289-291.
14. Jacobson JJ, Patel B, Asher G, Wooliscroft JO, Schaberg D: Oral Staphylococcus in elderly subjects with rheumatoid arthritis. *J Am Geriatr Soc* 1997;45:1-5.
15. Murray RP, Bourne WH, Fitzgerald RH: Metachronous infection in patients who have had more than one total joint arthroplasty. *J Bone Joint Surg Am* 1991;73:1469-1474.
16. Poss R, Thornhill TS, Ewald FC, Thomas WH, Batte NJ, Sledge CB: Factors influencing the incidence and outcome of infection following total joint arthroplasty. *Clin Orthop Relat Res* 1984;182:117-126.
17. Council on Dental Therapeutics: Management of dental patients with prosthetic joints. *J Am Dent Assoc* 1990;121:537-538.
18. Berbari EF, Hanssen AD, Duffy MC, et al: Risk factors for prosthetic joint infection: Case-control study. *Clin Infect Dis* 1998;27:1247-1254.
19. Antibiotic prophylaxis for surgery. *The Medical Letter* 2006;4:83-88.

Index

Index

Index